EMERGING TRENDS IN MEDICAL PLASTIC ENGINEERING AND MANUFACTURING

Plastics Design Library

PLASTICS DESIGN LIBRARY (PDL)
PDL HANDBOOK SERIES
Series Editor: Sina Ebnesajjad, PhD (sina@FluoroConsultants.com)
President, FluoroConsultants Group, LLC
Chadds Ford, PA, USA
www.FluoroConsultants.com

The **PDL Handbook Series** is aimed at a wide range of engineers and other professionals working in the plastics industry, and related sectors using plastics and adhesives.

PDL is a series of data books, reference works and practical guides covering plastics engineering, applications, processing, and manufacturing, and applied aspects of polymer science, elastomers and adhesives.

Recent titles in the series

Biopolymers: Processing and Products, Michael Niaounakis (ISBN: 9780323266987)
Biopolymers: Reuse, Recycling, and Disposal, Michael Niaounakis (ISBN: 9781455731459)
Carbon Nanotube Reinforced Composites, Marcio Loos (ISBN: 9781455731954)
Extrusion, 2e, John Wagner & Eldridge Mount (ISBN: 9781437734812)
Fluoroplastics, Volume 1, 2e, Sina Ebnesajjad (ISBN: 9781455731992)
Handbook of Biopolymers and Biodegradable Plastics, Sina Ebnesajjad (ISBN: 9781455728343)
Handbook of Molded Part Shrinkage and Warpage, Jerry Fischer (ISBN: 9781455725977)
Handbook of Polymer Applications in Medicine and Medical Devices, Kayvon Modjarrad & Sina Ebnesajjad (ISBN: 9780323228053)
Handbook of Thermoplastic Elastomers, Jiri G Drobny (ISBN: 9780323221368)
Handbook of Thermoset Plastics, 2e, Hanna Dodiuk & Sidney Goodman (ISBN: 9781455731077)
High Performance Polymers, 2e, Johannes Karl Fink (ISBN: 9780323312226)
Introduction to Fluoropolymers, Sina Ebnesajjad (ISBN: 9781455774425)
Ionizing Radiation and Polymers, Jiri G Drobny (ISBN: 9781455778812)
Manufacturing Flexible Packaging, Thomas Dunn (ISBN: 9780323264365)
Plastic Films in Food Packaging, Sina Ebnesajjad (ISBN: 9781455731121)
Plastics in Medical Devices, 2e, Vinny Sastri (ISBN: 9781455732012)
Polylactic Acid, Rahmat et al. (ISBN: 9781437744590)
Polyvinyl Fluoride, Sina Ebnesajjad (ISBN: 9781455778850)
Reactive Polymers, 2e, Johannes Karl Fink (ISBN: 9781455731497)
The Effect of Creep and Other Time Related Factors on Plastics and Elastomers, 3e, Laurence McKeen (ISBN: 9780323353137)
The Effect of Long Term Thermal Exposure on Plastics and Elastomers, Laurence McKeen (ISBN: 9780323221085)
The Effect of Sterilization on Plastics and Elastomers, 3e, Laurence McKeen (ISBN: 9781455725984)
The Effect of Temperature and Other Factors on Plastics and Elastomers, 3e, Laurence McKeen (ISBN: 9780323310161)
The Effect of UV Light and Weather on Plastics and Elastomers, 3e, Laurence McKeen (ISBN: 9781455728510)
Thermoforming of Single and Multilayer Laminates, Ali Ashter (ISBN: 9781455731725)
Thermoplastics and Thermoplastic Composites, 2e, Michel Biron (ISBN: 9781455778980)
Thermosets and Composites, 2e, Michel Biron (ISBN: 9781455731244)

To submit a new book proposal for the series, or place an order, please contact David Jackson, Acquisitions Editor at david.jackson@elsevier.com

EMERGING TRENDS IN MEDICAL PLASTIC ENGINEERING AND MANUFACTURING

Markus Schönberger
Frank Plastic AG, Waldachtal, Germany

Marc Hoffstetter
MAVIG GmbH, Munich, Germany

ELSEVIER

Amsterdam • Boston • Heidelberg • London
New York • Oxford • Paris • San Diego
San Francisco • Singapore • Sydney • Tokyo

William Andrew is an imprint of Elsevier

William Andrew is an imprint of Elsevier
The Boulevard, Langford Lane, Kidlington, Oxford, OX5 1GB, UK
225 Wyman Street, Waltham, MA 02451, USA

ISBN: 978-0-323-37023-3

British Library Cataloguing-in-Publication Data
A catalogue record for this book is available from the British Library

Library of Congress Cataloging-in-Publication Data
A catalogue record for this book is available from the Library of Congress

Publisher: Matthew Deans
Acquisition Editor: David Jackson
Production Project Manager: Susan Li
Designer: Mark Rogers

Contents

About the Authors

Dr Markus Schönberger holds a diploma (MSc equivalent) and a PhD (Dr.-Ing.) in Mechanical Engineering. He developed profound knowledge in medical device engineering, plastic manufacturing, and 3D-printing technologies during his previous research at the Institute of Medical and Polymer Engineering of the Technische Universität München. Dr Markus Schönberger is employed currently as Head of R & D at Frank plastic AG (Waldachtal, Germany).

Dr Marc Hoffstetter holds a diploma in Mechanical Engineering (MSc equivalent) and a PhD (Dr.-Ing.) in Biomedical Engineering. He developed profound knowledge in medical device development, injection molding and biomaterials during his previous research at the Institute of Medical and Polymer Engineering of the Technische Universität München and as Manager Medical Devices at Scholz-HTIK GmbH (Kronach, Germany). Currently, Dr Hoffstetter is employed as Head of R&D at MAVIG GmbH (Munich, Germany).

Preface

Plastics are gaining more and more importance within the medical device world as we speak. Historically, most medical devices were made of metals, ceramics, or glasses. Along with enormous research and development efforts within plastic materials and their manufacturing, the medical device industry discovered the advantages of plastic materials for countless applications and substituted metallic, ceramic, or glass materials consequently. Additionally, many new forms of applications would not be possible without the design freedom, material behavior, and manufacturing opportunities of plastic materials.

Medical device engineering cannot be classified simply within a standard engineering discipline. There are more electronic- or physics-based technologies (e.g., X-rays), or more biomechanical engineering-based implants. However, most technologies have in common that they are not thinkable anymore without some sort of plastic application. You might wonder now what a titanium trauma nail has to do with plastic materials. Think about how the trauma nail may be transported to a hospital in a sterile and protective manner: you're right; trauma nails are transported and stored in plastic packaging systems. Plastics have many advantages, but also cause some issues to concern about like biocompatibility, sterilization, or hygienic manufacturing. Not every plastic material, not every manufacturing approach, not every design can be just thrown into the medical device world without the number one burden: regulatory affairs. It is not enough to expect having good biocompatibility or sterile conditions; they have to be approved in a recognized way.

The medical device world offers so many opportunities for plastic engineering and manufacturing, if the general understanding of this branch is present. Then, it is highly interesting looking into emerging trends for plastic engineering and manufacturing for medical devices. Our branch is not the simplest one for introducing new approaches, technologies, or ideas. Introducing a new biocompatible material causes enormous efforts in verification, validation, additional testing, and—don't forget about—convincing. Due to the high complexity of introducing new devices and manufacturing (or even changes in manufacturing), there is always a steady "let's have a look how it works out" thinking within the medical device world. Sometimes, it is easier to keep a system running, even if you already know there is x-times better alternative, just to the fact of the cost and time-consuming introduction processes, which have to take place. But, is this really worth not to think about what is or might be coming next?

During our study and research at the Technical University of Munich, Germany, we have discovered our personal ambition and passion about improving the medical device world with new approaches for plastic manufacturing, design, and treatment integration. Surely, we might be blindfolded on the nonplastic-related eyes for medical devices, but there is still such an enormous potential available, which has not been exploited at all. It is our aim to bring this passion within this book to show future and residing engineers, what will be or at least might be next in the great world of plastic medical device design, engineering, and manufacturing.

For this book, we have activated our network in countless times, which we could develop during our research and industrial employments. In about a year, this book has been developed by the great team of Elsevier (special thanks to David Jackson and Peter Gane) and us. We, Marc, and Markus have discussed hours about the existing situation and what is coming next in our opinion. Several times we have recognized that we have learned so much during that time for ourselves. Each of us has its own focus and view, which made this book even more delicate in our opinion.

We wrote this book in our perspective of the plastics and medical devices and how the future might look alike. Our approach was to present quickly the current situation of regulatory affairs, device design, and manufacturing, before getting into emerging trends, we have discovered. The emerging trends are like a weather forecast: the more information and approaches available, the more concrete the picture is, we were able to paint. But, we want also to look a little bit further by adapting more general trends into the medical device world and carving out impacts on plastic medical devices.

Finally, it is just to say: Enjoy reading; hopefully you may discover new ideas, thoughts, or approaches, which might lead to new plastic medical devices. We are looking forward to get feedback from you, the readership. The future will show how many of our emerging trends will be implemented and how. It will be exciting to see. And in case you make the first contact to the world of medical devices, don't get scared by its complexity or the fear that your engagement somehow could harm anybody someday. Medical engineering may be a complex and highly interdisciplinary field; however, you always should be aware…

> Beside its complexity and multidisciplinarity, (bio)-medical engineering first and foremost is a subset of engineering.

Munich, wonderful state of Bavaria, July 2015.

Dr Marc Hoffstetter Dr Markus Schönberger

Acknowledgments

Definitely one of the top moments writing a book is to think about the acknowledgments, because it can be translated into being almost finished with quite a lot of work. Both of us, Marc and Markus, have their scientific roots traced back to Professor Wintermantel's Institute of Medical and Polymer Engineering at the Technische Universität München. He taught us the ability of not simply accepting everything but keeping future opportunities in mind within our engineering field of plastic and medical engineering. During our research periods, he also reminded us about one fact about writing: in average one page a day. Apparently the unwritten rule appears to be correct, at least with our style of collecting information, discussing the facts, and the actual writing procedure. Beginning in summer 2014, it took us about a year creating this book in its first edition. This year was filled with tremendous support for our project. Many unnamed friends, colleagues, coworkers, and professionals provided us with details, general understanding, or meaningful figures. Especially, Mona supported our efforts marvelously by helping us with medical knowledge plus psychological backing during challenging moments. We both had to manage a work life balance plus writing a scientific book. It wouldn't be possible without the hidden family and friends who supported us regularly. Writing a book without the backing of our editors wouldn't be possible as well. Therefore, we are choosing this acknowledgment page to express our gratitude to Dave Jackson and Peter Gane of Elsevier, Oxford. It has been and hopefully will be a great pleasure working with them. Thanks a lot!

Markus Schönberger and Marc Hoffstetter
December 2015

1 Introduction

OUTLINE

1.1 Introduction

Compared to other elaborate disciplines like medical or pharmaceutical sciences, medical engineering is a rather young discipline, however, well established for some decades already. Although professional medicals in fact use tools and devices to back up their efforts in healing injuries and diseases from their very first beginnings; technical professionals were involved as executing contractors only for very long time. It appears to be obvious that who else than a practicing surgeon knows the best what his instruments should be designed and manufactured like. Therefore, for centuries, medical doctors

Emerging Trends in Medical Plastic Engineering and Manufacturing
http://dx.doi.org/10.1016/B978-0-323-37023-3.00001-4

asked blacksmiths and precision mechanics to manufacture devices following their specifications. Still, developing and manufacturing medical devices is a complex and interdisciplinary field to what the input of the final operator is crucial. However, as a relatively young discipline that came into existence roughly at the beginning of the twentieth century, medial engineering mainly adapted existing knowledge and technologies for its specific needs, making it a **unique blend of sciences** like medicine, biology, (bio) chemistry, pharmacy, classical mechanical engineering, and many more. Moreover, no one is capable of covering all this in the profoundness required. Even today, many people imagine that developing medical devices is still a job for medical professionals, just alike the art of healing. This effect does include frequently professional medics, patients, and even engineers. But if you compare it to the world of aviation: do you want to board a jet plane designed and manufactured by the specifications of the pilot only, or would you prefer one that had professional engineers involved? You see, developing and manufacturing medical devices is a discipline that requires professionals from many disciplines, however, at least medical professionals and engineers.

1.1.1 Plastics and Medical Device Manufacturing or Engineering

Plastic materials and modern medical devices make a perfect fit. Many designs would not be feasible without this extensive collaboration of both engineering entities. In a view of a medical device engineer, it is easy to enthuse about the advantages of plastic utilization. Simply spoken, plastic materials meet the established requirements like process ability, resistance, mechanical properties, biocompatibility, and sterilization capability for the majority of engineered medical devices. As you would expect, plastic materials play a major role for most medical device fields and are processed regularly. At the beginning of the introduction of plastics in the medical device world, standard materials, often addressed as technical type, had been used due to the lack of specific **medical grade**[1] plastic materials.

1. It is worth mentioning some facts about the term **medical grade** within introductory chapter already, because it describes quite well the often established mantra about the complexity within the medical device engineering and manufacturing world. The term medical grade is used for plastic materials, which have been developed and produced by the chemical industry especially for medical device applications. However, it does not exist in a worldwide-approved definition, which standards have to be met. Some medical grade labeling refer to successful biocompatibility tests, while others just mean a clean production environment. Outsiders may imply the tough requirements within the term medical grade, which is nothing specific actually.

In accordance with the general awakening need for specific regulatory boundaries, intended to increase consumer protection and device quality, specialized plastic materials and hygienic manufacturing plus packaging techniques have been introduced for plastic medical devices for decades and since improved constantly. It is an interesting circulation system: new technical opportunities lead to new regulatory measures and vice versa. The technical development regarding plastics, medical device design and its manufacturing, is changing constantly and offers uncountable possibilities for current and future medical device engineers to participate with this world. However, the aspect of **emerging technologies for plastic medical** devices must always be seen in combination with changing or evolving regulatory boundaries. A highly interesting arising manufacturing technology like industrial 3D printing can be considered worthless as manufacturing approach for the medical device industry, if regulatory aspects are not identified adequately and correspondingly addressed.

1.1.2 Regulatory Affairs—Just like Sports

When getting engaged in medical devices as professional engineer, it is crucial for you to have some understanding for facts and correlations that clearly are not covered by technology in its classical understanding. Some of them may appear interesting but still eerie to you, like surgical techniques or the medical basics of some diseases. Others, like aspects of **rules and regulations** (often referred as regulatory affairs), seem to be useless or you are aware of their crucial importance, but still could not develop a passion, yet. Put simply, you tend to think about some aspects, especially regulatory affairs, as boring. Like most young and probably many old engineers, we sensed about regulatory frameworks the same way at the beginning of our career as medical engineering professionals. After getting in touch more deeply, we have developed a different impression and recognize these to be not a necessary evil. Now, we rather see these as useful and valuable tools backing up our engineering work (and hopefully yours as well) and help us to work within the rocky world of liability issues or simply spoken the biological system, often referred as the human body. We understand the difficulty to see the actual importance of regulatory for young and elaborating engineers. You may compare it with baseball, a sport that is not really appreciated in most of the world, but has an enormous background in some countries, where the rules and general understanding of the sport is widely known. As young and skilled batter you clearly focus on hitting the ball as hard as you can. Aspects like techniques for training, advices from the trainer or tactics basing on the games of the rule are anything but interesting for you. You (should) know about their importance, but you probably deal with them only half-assed. However, when becoming a more experienced and elaborate player, you will see, hitting the ball is only the last act in a sequence of actions that is embedded in a complex field of knowledge and experience, many of them from beyond the world of sports. Moreover, **knowing the rules** of a sport sometimes is more important for winning the match than personal skills or fitness. Therefore, our intention is to give you a comprehensive set of facts and correlations that are essential and useful for you as an (young) engineer, who is or will be involved in the world of engineering or manufacturing plastic medical devices. We strongly encourage you to mess around with the sometimes ill-reputed aspect of rules and regulations. It is impossible to cover all imaginable aspects and situations you might encounter, but considering our set of tools, you will develop a way of thinking that is useful to deal with them. One of the most important one is clearly you are and should **remain engineer**. Your comprehensive knowledge upon technology, design and manufacturing is your asset, and the object of desire within the process of medical device development and manufacturing. Today's medical professionals usually are aware that beyond your classical skills you could acquire a broad understanding of their work and needs, making you an intermediator between both worlds. As this is the very understanding of our own engagement in medical devices, we both take always clearly the view of an engineer in this book. May it become a companion for your first step into, or a personal trainer for your daily work within the wonderful and amazing world of medical device engineering.

1.2 The Books Target Group

By reading this introduction, you obviously show increased interest in the world of medical devices or maybe you are already more or less deeply involved in it. This is the first match between you, as valued reader, and us, as the authors, who are seeking to provide you a comprehensive set of knowledge and tools for this world. While developing this book, we both did reflect designated target groups whom to dedicate it to, and thus did define three major groups:

1. Engineering students ogling with medical device world
2. Non-Engineer professionals engaged in medical devices
3. Experienced engineers interested in emerging technologies

This does require to briefly introduce the basics, that you either never heard before, or you simply want to repeat or engross. For professionals involved in medical devices as non-Engineers, we provide basic understanding for technologies and processes utilized, giving them a clue about what technicians are currently and might be in the future thinking and working. Finally, professional medical engineers will find interesting aspects and emerging trends, ranging from the latest state of the art to future developments in medical devices. However, what in precise is the object of interest?

1.2.1 What Is a Medical Device?

As object of a rather young scientific discipline, the term medical device is used in many aspects and in consequence is subject to many definitions. For layperson, it does include any apparatus or device intended for application by a medical professional within his work, ranging from a surgical blade, rather simple in design, to elaborate machines for modern medical imaging like X-ray or computer tomography. A recurring **characteristic** of medical devices is that they are intended in some way to detect, prevent, monitor, treat or alleviate diseases, injuries, or disabilities. They are intended mainly for application by trained and experienced medical professionals and their primary mode of action is physical in nature, contrary to drugs, that exhibit a chemical mode of action. This understanding of medical devices is used by close to all competent authorities that regulated their markets, and thus will be subject to this book. Further, today an increasing number of medical devices are partly or entirely based on polymer materials, and in consequence within this book we focus on these types. This does include frequently mentioned buzzwords like caps and closures, single-use devices, instruments, orthopedic or dental implants, prostheses, in vitro diagnostics, lab-on-chip devices, and many more. Anyhow, the facts presented remain valid for all medical devices, regardless if based on different types of materials, electronic devices, or medical software.

You now are aware if this book does cope your interests in medical devices and does comply with your understanding and approach to them. In case by that you are encouraged to proceed, we will provide you some information about **how to use the book** for your purposes the most convenient way. Moreover, to give you a teaser we will show you a picture from a typical medical treatment that does demonstrate the overwhelming number of plastic medical devices that make an integral part of modern medicine (Figure 1.1).

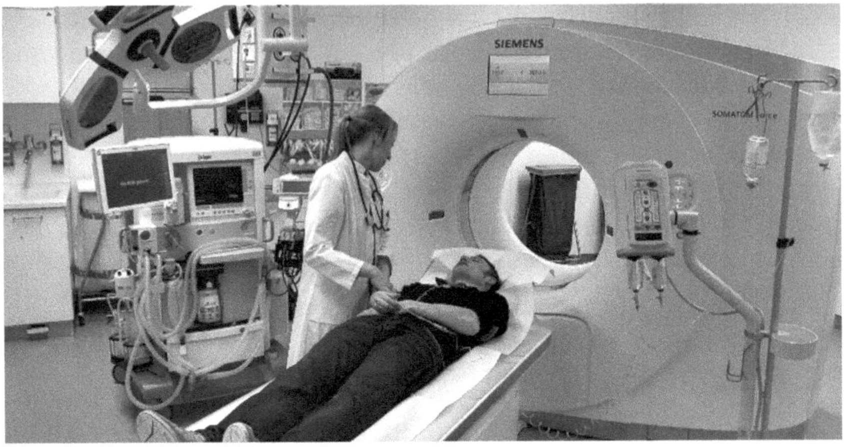

Figure 1.1 Image of a state-of-the-art trauma room in a hospital. You easily will discover the overwhelming presence of polymer-based medical devices. This may give you an impression about the superior role that polymers take within medical device engineering. *Image courtesy of the Institute of Clinical Radiology, University of Munich–Grosshadern Campus.*

1.3 User's Manual

Within each chapter and paragraph, you will find basic facts that are essential for working within the medical device world. They should become your fundamental set of tools necessary to collaborate with colleagues and third parties, such as customer, clients, medical professionals, and representatives of competent authorities. As experienced professional, regardless if engineer or not, you might find it useful to get a **quick refresh** or engross your knowledge in these basics: as there could be some stuff, you might have missed. A following central section is intended to give an insight into the **current state-of-the-art** or as it is about to be implemented. It is designed to give lateral entrants a thorough understanding upon the process of current and evolving medical device engineering. Last but not least as professional and experienced engineer you presumably will focus on the rear section that depicts **evolving trends** and technologies. Anyhow, we encourage you to deal with the initial parts too, as these might provide facts that aim to look beyond the end of one's nose.

1.3.1 Useful Landmarks in This Book

Probably alike most people, we seldom happen to read a book entirely from first to last page. As matter of fact, most readers show a tendency to **pick out chapters of interest** and will start reading somewhere right in the book. We strongly encourage to do so, as anything like the ideal approach to medical device engineering does not exist. This is why we made strong efforts to implement each chapter as suitable for stand-alone. In consequence, when reading the entire book, you might get the impression we repeat identical topics. But in fact, we rather aim to show a different view on the very same topic, and so always provide additional facts and correlations relevant for the particular aspect.

For the cases you will use this book to repeat knowledge you already have learned, or as a quick reference, we did implement additional markers. These are **bold-marked** phrases or keywords that provide landmarks within the running text or that subdivide it. This will be useful to find sections of interest more easily, regardless whether searching a topic of interest or seeking a quick reference. In cases where this approach is not suitable, we decided to use **bullet points** as appropriate way to:

- highlight a set of multiple aspects
- explain facts, too bulky and long for a running text
- provide additional landmarks within the book

The referencing of *Organizations* or *rules and regulations* done in italics and abbreviations (abr.) will be introduced repeatedly with respect to readers taking direct access. Tables and figures are intended self-explaining, once more encouraging you to directly jump into any chapter. Definitions and catch phrases of superior importance that should become your mantras are enclosed in an individual frame.

> Definitions and catch phrases of superior importance!

Sometimes, additional information is helpful for a better understanding. Footnotes are used to include further details, which are not absolutely necessary to work with the chapter, but will lead to an increased understanding of the actual topic or will give some interesting facts and background information.

When using an e-book, you will find a couple of links implemented in the running text, marked by an underline. These refer to resources with additional information, like product data sheets and brands mentioned or full text of rules and regulations cited. Wherever possible, we tried to avoid naming companies and brands. If unavoidable, we tried to reference competitors too, as we do not intend to prefer or advertise any product commercially available.

1.4 Medical Device Engineering—Advantages of Polymers

A well-known scientist at the Technical University of Munich expressed "somebody, who knows polymers, will take steel" regularly during his basic subject lectures. You have probably heard similar statements, which show a general lack of information or knowledge about current possibilities with state-of-the-art polymers. Usually, the medical device industry can be considered more conservative in adopting general technological trends, but in regards of utilization of polymers it has adopted the major advantages of polymers in most applications for decades. For a better understanding of the often existing advantages of polymers, it is worth having a lock into times, when metals and ceramics had been the primal materials for medical devices.

1.4.1 Metals and Ceramics as Primal Materials to Plastic Application

For decades, all disciplines of engineering were and still are heavily influenced by the application of metals (in contrast to most new medical device applications). Knowledge about smelting ores and processing metals triggered leaps in technology and had significant impact on the development from the Bronze Age to Modern Eras such as the time of space travel and the Digital Age. A comparable influence can be seen in the evolving use of ceramics, as these are fundamental for technologies as electronics and semiconductors. As these both were the first man-made materials, the very first medical devices manufactured by mankind were based on these too and the first devices basing on these materials can be traced back to the ancient Egyptians and Etruscans. Anyhow, many well-established medical devices are redesigned with plastic materials and most new devices are unthinkable with at least some plastic parts, as this comes along with some decisive advantages from a technical as well as a biomedical point of view.

The phrase polymer is a summarizing expression for many different types, which can be subdivided in the major classes' thermoplastics, elastomers, and thermoset plastics. Some types of polymers cannot be easily classified in one of the major classes, like UV-curing photopolymers that are some kind of thermoset plastic, but will not cure under heat application like typical representatives. On the other hand, thermoplastic elastomers, that combine properties of rubber (thermoset) and thermoplastics, are state of the art. The wide range of available polymers and the ongoing developments for new approaches have led to uncountable amounts of applicable plastics for medical devices. Additionally, inserting additives like reinforcement fibers, color pigments, drugs, and many more, can alter many polymers easily. It is essential having a good overview about existing and available plastic materials. Therefore, an extra chapter for material selection is added (Chapter 3.1.2), which should give some more details about the plastic materials themselves. Especially for the less-experienced readers, a general understanding about polymers is helpful to derive possibilities of emerging technologies for plastic medical devices.

But coming back to the fact, why most modern medical devices are unthinkable or at least less likely without the possibilities of modern polymers and the derived manufacturing opportunities.

1.4.2 Technical Advantages of Polymers

Plastic materials have technical advantages regarding manufacturing procedures as well as characteristic material properties in comparison to metal or ceramic materials. Generally spoken, raising research and development efforts has led to an enormous range of available plastic materials with nearly uncountable variations regarding mechanical properties, density, processing, optics, haptics, biocompatibility, resistance, altogether with relatively easy adaptions with additives like softeners, antimicrobial substances, or fiber reinforcements. Hand in hand with material efforts, manufacturing technologies have been established and further developed manifoldly to achieve highly geometric complex, relatively cheap and automated manufactured plastic devices, which can be considered unthinkable often with other types of materials including their manufacturing approaches.

Summarizing the utilization of plastic materials for technical devices may offer following technical advantages:

- suitability of fully automated mass production lanes,
- countless variation of available materials (from optical clear, over biodegradable to high-tensile plastic plus carbon composites),
- adaptation by additives inline possible,

- countless combination possibilities for manufacturing steps, materials, and additives (like surface treatment, inserts, more component, foam structures),
- normally less energy-consuming than metal or ceramic manufacturing,
- mostly recycling processes are suitable or at least energetic recycling,
- cheaper production with comparable or optimized device characteristics.

This list should be considered as general overview of many opportunities regarding plastic materials, device design, and manufacturing. Surely, there exist many more aspects for the individual technical situation.

1.4.3 Technical Advantages for Medical Devices

This book is based on the use and manufacturing of plastic materials for medical devices. Regardless the actual application, plastic materials offer many advantages as material for medical devices. Most of them were mentioned in the section before. These general technical advantages play a major role for plastic medical device design and manufacturing, of course, especially, if you bring the fact into your mind that many medical devices are single use with relatively low mechanical requirements in comparison to other engineering fields.

However, some specific characteristics about plastic materials make their application for medical devices even more interesting in many cases. Surely, not every plastic material meets the following criteria, but for each of the mentioned aspects suitable, and more than one, plastic alternative is available and already widely in use within in the medical device world.

Additional advantages of plastics within medical devices in a biomedical point of view:

- many plastic materials can be altered toward an increased biocompatibility level,
- antimicrobial properties can be inserted by additives or compounds,
- surface structures can be adapted (partially) toward a better tissue interaction (in the desired way),
- many plastic materials offer a good resistance against bio fluids,
- many plastic materials are disinfectable or serializable with state-of-the-art approaches,

- differing from metals and ceramics, plastic materials are mostly compliant to modern technologies of medical imaging,
- most raw plastic materials are not known for causing chronic allergies,
- and uncountable more situation-specific advantages in a biomedical point of view.

The consideration of emerging plastic technologies for medical devices comes with a profound knowledge about plastic materials, manufacturing and design in general. This book does not focus on existing technologies and should not be considered a regular textbook about plastics, but we try to give some further introduction at the given points within the upcoming sections. However, it is not our aim to bring your knowledge about plastics up to speed, beginning with all basics. Therefore, it might be helpful to have a certain understanding of the plastic and medical engineering world or at least having interest in gaining additional information with further reading.

1.5 Medical Devices—a Conservative World?

In general, the world of medical device is considered as rather conservative by engineers in comparison to other engineering disciplines like consumer electronics or automotive. Established methods and practices are evolved and refined usually rather than rashly replaced by novel approaches. This may sound narrow-minded but is due to several reasons.

1.5.1 Complexity

The interaction of a medical device with the patient during application is very complex. Design and manufacturing modifications that appear to be negligible may suddenly show severe adverse effect during device application. Further, the effect of some interactions may be undiscovered for very long time and thus be hard to detect. In consequence, novel medical devices and manufacturing approaches are subject to thorough testing in order to evaluate their performance and safety. This process is regularly very time and money consuming. Engineers from fast-moving industries like consumer electronics and software may get the impression; this is rather done to thwart innovations than to assure the patient's safety. Anyhow, history has shown that jumping the gun may show catastrophic effects. In the 1960s, thousands of children were born with severe birth defects, caused by the painkiller Contergan (http://www.ncbi.nlm.nih.gov/pubmed/23138926), which was tested and found suitable for pregnant women, but then turned out to show horrible undiscovered side effects. You consider this rather a topic of the pharmaceutical industry? The history of medical devices has seen a highly comparable disaster, which leads us to the issue of legal and ethical liability.

1.5.2 Legal and Ethical Liability

The development of innovative medical devices does induce risks that may be reduced only but not eliminated fully. In case of occurring complications, the way you might have handled these risks will be thoroughly investigated and evaluated by many parties. Investigative authorities may consider prosecution that might result in company or even personal liability. In parallel, a public discussion will debate about an ethical liability. Even if acquitted from any legal charges, a company, brand, or person associated with a scandal in public health care may encounter consequences as if condemned. A prominent example for this is a contraceptive intrauterine device called Dalkon Shield (http://www.britannica.com/EBchecked/topic/1951988/Dalkon-Shield), developed and marketed in the 1970s. The design of the device promoted infections of the uterus in an unforeseen way, inducing severe injury to its users and causing manifold fatalities. Despite ample indications for this problem, marketing of the device continued for years before removed from market. The resulting litigations lasted for decades. You see, beyond the patient's health, great values may be at stake when developing medical devices. The combination of complexity and legal and ethical liability has caused major hurdles for implementing new medical devices or even manufacturing approaches by the introduction of countless regulatory issues by legislations or approved organizations worldwide. Innovation and development has to encounter these aspects consequently, which may differ from economic area to another additionally.

1.5.3 Medical Work Environment

Often forgotten, but a so-called end-consumer exists within the medical device world as well: medical professionals or patients themselves. Especially, medical professionals are often rather conservative in adopting new technologies than ultramodern. Do not think about high-tech medical facilities like university hospitals, like these frequently are depicted in television series, and which are focused on adopting the latest trends. The regular medical facilities, which account for most medical device applications worldwide, are the major market for the medical device industry.

The daily routine of medical professionals features a considerate responsibility and frequently comes along with a heavy workload. Therefore, it makes sense that medical professionals will preferably follow established therapies that base on medical devices he is familiar with. The medical industry addresses this situation by introducing device changes or brand new applications usually in small steps and a well-prepared way, accompanied by much kind of marketing efforts.

1.5.4 Profit Margin versus Medical Device Innovations

The existing and probably tightening regulatory boundaries must primarily be seen as efforts for consumer protection. In fact, the very first regulations for medical devices were enforced in response to health system–related scandals. Regulatory boundaries represent tough market entrance barriers for possible new players or competitors within the medical device world. In contrast to the IT world, where anywhere and anybody with a certain idea and skill set is able to develop apps and sell it on app-stores easily, just having enthusiastic ideas and a start-up environment will not lead to successful medical device developments. An interesting sidekick: so-called medical apps are gaining more and more attention by regulatory bodies. These apps have been developed to give advice for healthier lifestyle based on measured information like heart rates, temperature, or to provide simply a digital counterpart of a medical professional (see Chapter 6.7). The actual same situation is evolving comparable with conventional medical devices decades ago: unprofessional or not well-setup apps offer poor or even wrong advice for private consumers, which may lead to severe damages.

Simply spoken, regulatory boundaries ensure a certain market protection versus new competitors. This effect may lead to less pressure for innovation to gain market share, revenue growth, and profit margin. To a certain extent, it is practicable to participate on the medical device market as old-established competitor without severe efforts regarding development and innovation. Surely, market forces to bring the costs down exists as well, but the relatively constant growth of the medical device market over many years, mainly decoupled from the general economic developments, along with a certain level of market protection supports the more conservative few about new developments additionally to the discussed points before.

Simply summarized: If established as a player within the medical device world using its (maybe self-developed) technology: why should the company or most medical professionals, like long-trained surgeon, be interested in highly innovative new approaches?

1.6 Forces behind Future Design and Manufacturing Trends

We discussed reasons why the medical device world may be considered as a conservative world. The mentioned issues support definitely this theory, but even the most conservative engineering field is subject to emerging design and manufacturing trends, and it is not our intention to leave the general impression that the plastic medical device world has to be described as unduly conservative and noninnovative. Our chosen field should be described mainly as a highly complex and innovative but meantime carefully working entity. The interesting question is now, which forces are major driving forces behind future design and manufacturing trends for plastic medical devices? For medical devices, it is important to see social and political issues. In contrast to less emotional fields, medical devices deal usually with some sort of health-related problems. Health is definitely a key factor for all human individuals, especially for elderly people. The older someone is, the more medical care is required in general. The majority of health-related costs occur during the last-living years due to rapidly increasing illnesses. A second driving force behind raising health-care costs is the demographic trend within industrialized countries: the share of elderly persons is raising consequently. So, on the one hand more patients want to be treated adequately with at least state-of-the-art equipment, and on the other hand the general costs for health care should raise at the lowest pace possible to keep health insurance or payment systems intact or at least working.

1.6.1 Demographic Trend and Cost Reduction

Transferred to the medical device world, this fact leads to increased efforts to develop medical devices, which help to bring the cost of health care down (e.g., by reducing treatment periods, less invasive operation techniques, or self-treatment opportunities), or are cheaper than existing alternatives. A good example of a medical device, which has helped to decrease treatment costs enormously, is the vascular stent of clotted heart arteries, which allows reopening these arteries in a minimal invasive procedure without a long-lasting surgery. The development of stents and corresponding application systems decreased costs, lead to intensified efforts of optimization, and finally stents are definitely cheaper to manufacture and sold than at the beginning. This can be described as a typical cycle of medical device development driven by cost reduction. Surely, the stent application offers definitely good medical reasons, why the application has become so popular, but the cost reduction effort made it possible to establish this technology to the current level. The cost topic brings us to the major payment factor in health-related questions: health insurance systems.

1.6.2 Health Insurance Systems

Health insurance or payment systems have an enormous effect as a force behind future design and manufacturing. More lucrative health systems lead to more medical device developments specific for such an entity with the restriction that it must have a certain market volume. The US market is highly interesting for medical device companies regarding reimbursement issues (let us put liability and regulatory affairs aside at this moment). The reimbursement field is less restrictive regarding costs in comparison to single payment system countries (e.g., UK or Sweden) or highly regulated countries (e.g., Germany, Austria, France). The adaptation of state-of-the-art devices, which are not classified as extremely risky, the US market is definitely more interesting than others. New devices may be developed faster for such markets than in other parts of the world. An example is sewing templates for surgical procedures, which are manufactured individually for each patient to increase the outcome of standard procedures like knee implant surgery (see Chapter 4.2.1). These sewing templates have been introduced within the US market first due to its ability to reimburse the additional cost of treatment easier than in other health-care markets. But, as you should have recognized already, every already mentioned or upcoming aspect of driving forces is embedded into a complex correlation between mutually dependent influences. The effect of the health insurance systems is accompanied by the actual size or volume of health-care system, political measures, and of course regulatory efforts.

1.6.3 Regulatory Efforts and Legislative Measures

Regulatory efforts cannot be considered without political influences. Each major health-care market (European Union, USA, China, among others) has its own medical device legislation passed to ensure end-consumer protection as good as possible. As expectable, each region has some unique characteristics with its regulatory systems. A change within the approved regulatory systems can trigger enormous development efforts. However, the aspect of development must be understood in a way of product and its manufacturing compliance improvement with regulatory regulations.

A fictional example may help to understand the correlation of new regulatory measures as a driving force for design and manufacturing. Think about a well-established manufacturing technology, which cannot be transferred into a hygienic design version. State of the art is to produce with such a technology under regular conditions, followed by some sort of cleaning process to meet the requirements regarding hygienic medical devices. A new regulatory measure may demand that every technology has to comply with the rules of hygienic manufacturing. The effect is foreseeable: the used technology must be fitted toward hygienic issues in some way, or a new technology has to be developed. Surely, regulatory attempts can be triggered by political considerations as well. Reasons may be a political agenda to push certain technological attempts or sort of devices, to protect the own market or to comply simply with a negative atmosphere within the electorate toward a certain issue like some sort of additives within a material, which is under scrutiny to have some impact on the human body, but which cannot be approved finally. The example behind is the Bisphenol-A topic, among others mainly found in polycarbonate polymers. Polycarbonate is a widely processed plastic material within the medical device world, but Bisphenol-A is suspected of causing negative interferences with the human body. Though no significant evidences have been presented so far, a European country decreased enormously the allowed Bisphenol-A share in processed polycarbonate devices without focusing on possible effects for medical device companies and their manufacturers (e.g., necessary validation efforts may lead to long-lasting delivery problems of many medical devices). Political topics must not be only negatively driven, but can be also caused by the idea of enhanced new technologies. A good example is the 3D-printing technology, which is pushed heavily by US politicians to raise the US manufacturing share again. Of course, the availability of research grants lead to interesting efforts within the medical device world as well. Due to its highly interesting opportunities, the topic of 3D printing is discussed in a separate chapter.

1.6.4 Engineering Developments and Consumer Markets

The 3D-printing topic is a good start for our last topic about forces behind future trends, which we want to address: generally engineering developments and consumer markets. The engineering world is currently full of many highly interesting developments, especially for the private consumer market, which offers also interesting new opportunities for the medical device world. Getting back to the 3D printing: generative manufacturing technologies are getting more and more attention by the media due to their opportunities plus by engineers as well. The different approaches have become so sophisticated that the medical device industry has to consider evolving possibilities to profit from arising advantages in many fields. Surely, 3D printing will not become the state-of-the-art manufacturing technology for many medical devices, but the technology may offer cost-saving potentials or opportunities of whole new treatment approaches, which are unthinkable without such a technology. Easily spoken, major trends within the engineering world have usually an impact on future design and manufacturing trends of medical devices. Even highly specific trends like automated flying systems like drones, that see first utilizations for automated parcel delivery, may lead to new approaches for medical devices. The following picture shows an automated flying drone, which is activated by emergency units to support first responders in rural areas with a defibrillator to treat cardiac defibrillation before professional units may arrive on scene. This idea will not be probably a high-volume market success, but it is a perfect example for what ideas can be developed if general engineering trends are broken down into the medical device world (Figure 1.2).

The introduced forces behind future medical device trends help us to understand better the complex medical device world. Based on these facts in combination with our experience, we have collected and summarized the major emerging aspects for future medical device design and manufacturing within the upcoming chapters. The wished objective with this

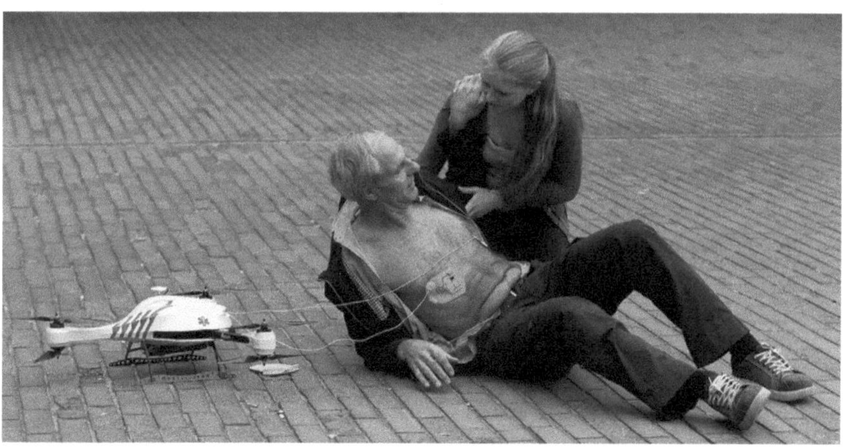

Figure 1.2 Automated flying drone with included defibrillator to support first responders of heart-related emergencies in rural areas. *Image courtesy of TUDelft & Alec Momont.*

introduction is to show you, as the honorable reader of our book, a first impression how the medical device world is connected. The upcoming chapters may help to deepen the knowledge, do bring up interesting and maybe unknown trends and decrease possible reservations to the medical device world.

2 Regulations for Medical Devices

OUTLINE

Emerging Trends in Medical Plastic Engineering and Manufacturing
http://dx.doi.org/10.1016/B978-0-323-37023-3.00002-6

If you get in touch with the world of medical devices for the first time, you might be scared or frightened about appearing complexity, even as experienced engineer. Potentially, you feel overwhelmed by requirements that are pushing in from elaborated scientific disciplines like chemistry, biology, and of course human medicine. Maybe you commence to reflect the impressive complexity of human anatomy and physiology, or maybe you start calling into mind individual experiences or stories you have heard from friends and relatives concerning medical treatments. It is well conceivable that you might think, even a tiny mistake occurring during medical device design or manufacturing might result in severe harm to a patient—or even death! However, by making first contacts to the world of medical technology, you always must remember that it is a subset of **general engineering**. Basic requirement for any medical device must be its ability to perform the intended functionality and in consequence, all principles of good engineering practice remain valid. A medical device may be subject to more requirements that will be handled like any other, even if derived from most elaborate biochemical correlations. Development and manufacturing of medical devices is an interdisciplinary collaboration between biologists, medical professionals, and engineers (and many more) and every party will bring in its own unique expertise. Understanding for the involved sciences will always give you an advantage, but as an engineer involved in medical device development you should clearly **focus on your own discipline**—and that is developing technology.

Within the last decades, a wide range of regulations for medical devices (development plus manufacturing) have been enacted by legislation across the world. These regulations proclaim the intention to protect end-consumer (that is the patient or operator), but also give engineers procedures to follow and help to stay within demanded standards for medical devices. It is our aim to show the reader the benefit of these regulations.

2.1 Special Requirements within the Biomedical Field—Fundamentals

During application, most medical devices will directly or indirectly make contact to or penetrate the surface of the human body for varying durations during utilization. The device material(s) will get in contact with body liquids and consequently interact with living tissue, and thus most likely will influence metabolic processes in a physical and/or chemical (thus commonly labeled as physicochemical) way. This does induce manifold aspects of concern that in classical technical fields like consumables, electronics, or automotive are not relevant and thus commonly not known by conventional engineers. However, the industrial sectors of cosmetics, food, and pharma share most of these aspects with the medical device industry, which is why all four of them are commonly summed up as the field of **Life Sciences**. Actually, many more scientific disciplines such as biology, genomics, and biotechnology are regarded as Life Sciences as well, but will be considered as a subset of the four initially listed. Many aspects regarding medical devices that are dealt with in this book consequently are relevant and handled in comparable ways in any field of the Life Sciences. However, before transferring rules or methods from any field to another, you must consider its respective landscape of established methods, regulations, and laws. These may differ significantly, albeit dealing with the very same scientific correlations.

Cosmetics, Food, Pharma & Medical Devices are **Life Sciences!**

Close to all **Life Science products** make **contact** to, or penetrate the **human body** and thus most likely will influence metabolic processes!

Identical scientific **correlations** may be handled with **significantly differing regulations** and **laws** in each Life Science!

2.1.1 Leachables and Extractables

Polymers are a blend of manifold inorganic and organic chemical compounds, whereas the constituents beyond the synthesized plastic itself may be divided in two groups. Some are **intended** to modify the plastic properties. This may include, among others, pigments for dyeing, softeners to adjust hardness or flexibility, stabilizers that improve environmental resistance, processing aids or any additives. Others are **unintended,** but not preventable. Synthesizing of the polymer itself can cause impurifications, whereas these may consist of unprocessed raw material(s), remaining processing aids (e.g., catalysts, plasticizers, scavengers), or unwanted by-products of the chemical reaction. Further converting of the plastic will amplify this pollution, as any contact to secondary material(s) such as processing machinery, manufacturing equipment, or packaging materials possibly may add contaminations or induce further reactions. Especially, the issue of thermal-induced degradation must be highlighted, why heating up plastic must be seen critically. The influence of elevated temperature, combined with remaining moisture and present impurifications (desired or undesired) will induce physicochemical reactions that, fueled by the presence of heat energy, modify and/or dismantle the polymer and thus generate generally unwanted by-products. Albeit at much slower rate, these processes will continue at room temperature and thus influence the plastic product over its entire life cycle. Moreover, during application, many medical devices will be exposed to aggressive body fluids like sweat, urine, or blood that are likely to enhance polymer degradation. Further, any contact between the (inevitably contaminated) polymer and a pharmaceutical may induce reactions between both of them. Besides further polymer degradation, this may damp, alter, or inhibit the drug's desired effect.

Polymers are a blend of manifold chemical compounds, inevitable **containing** unwanted **impurities**!

Any **further processing** or contact to **body fluids** is very likely to **trigger** polymer **degradation** and **pollution**!

Thereby, the risks to health arise from the fact that any constituent of the polymer will find its way to the devices surface by diffusion. These diffusing compounds generally are divided in two groups. **Extractables** are substances that migrate when the device is exposed to more challenging surrounding conditions, such as aggressive aquatic systems, elevated temperatures, or prolonged contact to the human body. Simply, extractables describe "what can come out" of the device. Compounds that will migrate at normal surrounding conditions are labeled **leachables,** embracing anything that "will come out." In consequence, leachables make a subset of extractables.

2.1.2 Cause of Foreign Body Reactions

A chemical compound present on the surface of a human body will migrate into deeper layers of the skin (or mucosa) and thus finally get in contact with living cells. This is the mechanism of action for any body lotion, beauty cream, or ointment, regardless if applied as cosmetic or pharmaceutical. The gastrointestinal tract does represent an internal surface of the body, and absorbing of nutritive substances or drugs when digesting does represent the identical correlation. Same thing in the lungs, where respiratory gases or aerosol pharmaceuticals will diffuse through the surface of the alveoli into the blood stream. Beyond the migration through an outer or inner body surface, drug may be administered via a direct injection, bypassing the body's ways to absorb any substance, thus labeled as parenteral administration (Greek for "bypassing the digestive system"). Depending on the location of a medical device during application, its leachables and extractables will find their way into the human body. By circulating body fluids, these will be dispersed inside the human body and may induce body-wide or systemic effects. Table 2.1 does illustrate the path of access for a Life Science product (or compounds of it) into the human body.

Almost any exogenous (not body's own) substance or object getting in contact with living tissue will cause a foreign body reaction. Beyond the physical and chemical nature of the unfamiliar substance, the reaction's nature and intensity will be determined by the quantity involved, the path of access, location within the human body, and duration of exposure. Usually, observed immediate effects comprise weak to intense immune reactions and/or inflammatory processes, necrosis of affected tissue, systemic toxicity, or (sudden) death. Due to their late occurrence, long-term effects are more difficult to detect and, moreover, sometimes not linked appropriately to their real cause. These effects may encompass hemolysis, chronic

Table 2.1 Illustration of the Path of Access of Life Science Products (or Their Compounds) to Living Tissue, Influencing Its Metabolism and Causing Biological Reactions. From a Physiological Point of View, the Digestive Systems Does Represent Body Surface as Well, Still It Is Useful to List Is Separately

Life Sciences		**Path of Access**					**Human Body**
Cosmetics	**Leachables/extractables**	X	X			**Contact to living tissue**	**Influencing metabolism** and **Causing biological reactions**
Food				X			
Medical devices		X	X	X	X		
Pharma		X	X	X	X		
		Skin	Mucosa	Digestive tract	Parenteral		

inflammations, benign or malignant tissue degeneration, development of cancer, and death resulting from chronic intoxication.

> Almost every exogenous compound (not body's own) will provoke a foreign body reaction!

Anyhow, the body's first reaction to most (but not every) foreign compounds usually is fever as immediate immune response, which is why these materials are labeled as exogenous **pyrogens** (from Greek *pyros* = fire and *genesis* = origin, creation). Thereby, it makes no difference if these compounds are, for example, pathogenic germs, polymer particles, viruses, or leachables, whereas especially particles from elastomer or rubber abrasion are known to show a big potential to provoke fever. Same thing is with bacteria, as pretty much everyone knows from his/her very own experience. However, even devitalized bacteria may cause fever. This is due to large molecules called lipopolysaccharides or **endotoxins** and that are found in the cell wall of a specific type of bacteria (Gram-negative) and consequently make a subset of pyrogens. So even bacteria killed by any process of sterilization, still sticking to a medical device, may provoke an intense immune response.

> Compounds inducing **fever** as immune response are labeled **pyrogens**, whereas those originating from **killed bacteria** are called **endotoxins**.

In order to handle these risks, it is inevitable to consider many aspects from biology and human medicine with their manifold scientific subdisciplines such as microbiology, biochemistry, physiology, human biology, and genetics. Nevertheless, before you start feeling deterred: although it might be undoubtedly from great benefit to study some or even all of them, it is anything but necessary to do so when dealing with medical devices as engineer. In interdisciplinary collaboration, all the sciences mentioned developed a manageable set of biological aspects and demands that found expression in relevant legal demands. The most relevant ones will be covered by the next sections. This will give you the necessary basic set to work in the medical device field. In addition, as time will go by, you automatically will learn many more of them, expanding your set of tools for the fascinating science of medical technology.

2.2 Biological Demands

The application of most medical devices involves inevitable undesired biological reactions, mainly by the tissue being in direct contact. Therefore, a key demand when designing medical devices must be to reduce these reactions to a minimum. The keyword in this case is **biocompatibility**, indicating that the selected combination of material(s), design, manufacturing, and application appears suitable for the intended use as medical device. Unfortunately, sometimes there is still some confusion about the meaning of this term. It may suggest to engineers, not familiar with the dynamics of interaction in-between device and organism, that a group of material does exist that may be used without any further concern. Additionally to technical polymers, there are many available that are marketed as medical grade, advertised as being tested for biocompatibility and hence suitable for medical devices, thus encouraging this misunderstanding. However, such thing as materials that are automatically suitable for application in a medical device does not exist. Furthermore, a material known to be biocompatible for an intended application may lose this property by processing or exposition to inappropriate surrounding conditions. Any polymer interacts in a certain way with a living biological system and it can be only evaluated in each specific case if the occurring reactions are acceptable in order to reach a higher aim. A suitable definition of **biocompatibility** must consider these correlations and therefore should read:

> Biocompatibility refers to the ability of a material to perform with an appropriate biologic response in its intended use.

In the context of medical devices and (bio) materials two other terms are often used that frequently are interpreted in different ways. These are toxicity and biological safety. **Toxicity** in general does describe the degree to which a substance may cause harm to living cells and subsequent to the entire organism. It is generally accepted[1] that every substance may do so,

1. The idea that any substance is toxic, depending on the dose applied, is credited to the medieval scientist Paracelsus who stated: "Dosis facit venenum" (translated does say "Dose makes the poison").

depending on quantity and location of application. Accordingly, its meaning is closely linked to biocompatibility. A meaningful definition in the context of medical devices should read:

> Toxicity is the inherent property of a substance to cause an adverse effect in a biological system

The term **biological safety** is used in a wide range but generally does refer to either any kind of potential harm to a biological system (e.g., human body) or, turned around and used more frequently, any health risk arising from a biological system (e.g., pathogen bacteria). Anyhow, the difference between most definitions is subtle. If dealing with medical devices, it is from great importance to deal with biological hazards that menace the health of patients and professionals involved in device manufacturing and application. The risks induced by the biological response to a device or bioactive substance (e.g., carcinogenic or mutagenic compounds) rather should be seen as a topic of biocompatibility, although logically an issue of biological safety. Many hazards may arise from bacteria, viruses, or biomaterials and thus are related to the field of microbiology. These must be encountered by approaches such as clean production environments, appropriate hygienic standards, or validated processes of sterilization, always enclosed by a comprehensive risk management (see Section 2.3.7). If all relevant risks are reduced to a level acceptable, the device may be considered as biologically safe. Further, biological hazards in the field of Life Sciences may arise from carcinogenic or mutagenic chemicals, bioactive molecules, or highly toxic compounds. These are handled by regulations and guidelines for biosafety and biosecurity, issued by regulatory authorities such as the Food and Drug Administration (FDA). Nevertheless, as these are usually from minor importance for medical devices, it is a justifiable simplification to neglect them within the context of this book. Hence, it is an appropriate definition and frequently encountered understanding that:

> Biological safety is the **absence** of unacceptable **risks** arising from **(micro)biology**

However, not the materials of a medical device alone influence the properties such as biocompatibility, biological safety, and toxicity. In fact, the very same polymer may provoke significantly different biological reactions, among others, depending on the **shape and surface** being in contact with the tissue. The micro- and nanomorphology exhibits a significant impact on mutual reactions on cellular level, as well as the **surface-area-to-volume ratio** of the foreign body. The precise correlations are not fully understood yet and still subject to current research. Anyhow, even if you are not involved in basic research on biomaterials, you should remember: the very same amount of material processed by identical technologies and parameters may exhibit excellent biocompatibility as monolithic sphere, but may induce massive inflammatory processes, if presented as a multitude of micro- or nanospheres. Moreover, even the general **shape of the device**, for example, may influence the biological safety. It is well known that tubular structures like urinary catheters, feeding tubes, or intravenous needles may serve as guide rail for bacteria and germs. Placed too long or inappropriately, a biofilm will grow on the device and expand along its surface and so eventually find access to the body and cause an infection. A material that is known to be biocompatible for the intended application may lose this property by **processing** or further treatment or even may become toxic. These issues can and thus should be considered in medical device designs.

Now, you see clearly that the properties of biocompatibility, biological safety, and toxicity (or its absence) have relevance in pretty much every Life Science, however, sometimes they are understood and thus defined in different ways. It should be clear that all form **three key properties** that are **mandatory** for any medical device, regardless its intended application. Thereby, biological safety is from superior importance to evaluate a medical device, even if the others seem to be violated. For example, a toxicity that is limited to a defined duration or spatial extension may be desired, assuming it still does not break the demand for biological safety by means of inducing intolerable biological responses. This may sound noncredible to you, but is found in intrauterine devices for contraception or antimicrobiological compounds (Section 5.3) that are added to biomaterials (e.g., antimicrobial-modified catheters). All three key properties show mutual influence and are individually or in sum affected by many aspects resulting from design, manufacturing, postprocessing, application, and waste management of the medical device. The meshwork of interdependencies and most common engineering-related influences are illustrated in Figure 2.1.

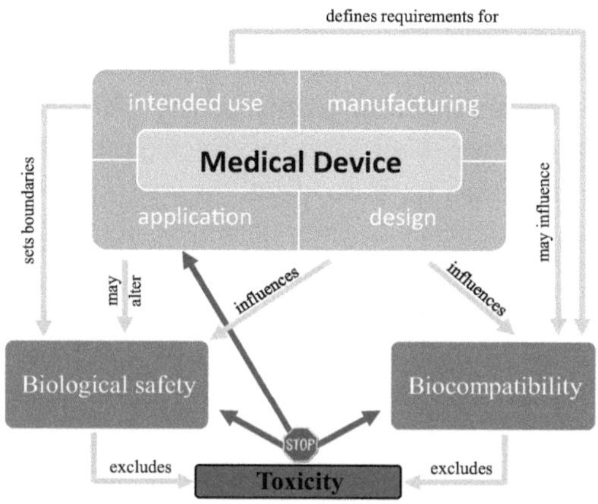

Figure 2.1 Any medical device is characterized by its design, manufacturing, and intended application and must comply with three key features: biological safety, biocompatibility, and absence of toxicity. All of them show mutual influences as displayed.

2.3 Legal Demands

The only appropriate and ethically justifiable approach to assure that the previously introduced key properties are implemented at satisfying extent can only be a comprehensive set of biological and biomedical tests. Over the past decades, many techniques and guidelines for **testing of medical devices** were developed or adapted from other Life Sciences, mainly the pharmaceutical industry, as it is very familiar with the concepts of toxicity and biological safety. Other requirements cover topics such as **quality management systems** (QMS) or tools to **manage risks** involved. Nowadays, almost any regulatory landscape either directly demands or makes references to those that are relevant for the specific device. The following section will give you an overview upon the most important ones.

2.3.1 Pharmacopeia of the United States Class Plastics

A pharmacopoeia is a reference book, issued by a medical or pharmaceutical society in recognition of (or directly by) a governmental authority, providing the general accepted rules for quality, testing, denomination, and storage of pharmaceuticals. Additionally, it does list all compounds, materials, and methods allowed to utilize for drug making, hence defining the regulatory boundary conditions when dealing with pharmaceuticals. All materials getting in direct or indirect contact with drugs during their manufacturing, processing, and packaging must comply with the relevant specifications. As plastic materials found wide applications as packaging materials, nowadays every pharmacopoeia defines types allowed for applications and does describe in precise how these materials must be tested for compliance. At the time when polymers found applications as implant materials, no appropriate methods for testing were developed and established at that time. Facing the lack of appropriate guidelines, one decided to test the materials following the specifications of the **Pharmacopeia of the United States** (USP), as these comprise animal experiment based in vivo testing. This does include subcutaneous (under the skin) implantation of polymer specimens and subsequent evaluation of the biological response. As this testing does correspond highly to the intended use, it is a meaningful method to assess the materials biocompatibility. Within its general chapter <88>, the USP defines a set of three tests for in vivo screening of plastic materials, designed to evaluate the biological response to them. The tests comprise injection (subcutaneous and intravenous) of extracts, prepared from the plastic material, and the implantation of test stripes subcutaneous and/or intramuscular. The tissue and body reactions are evaluated in order to determine the potential to cause irritations or an acute systematic toxicity. Basing on these investigations, the material is **assigned to one of six classes** that are named in Latin numerals, whereas only the strictest Class VI is considered to be appropriate as implant material. Therefore, many plastic materials are advertised as USP class VI tested, suggesting their suitability for medical devices. It is worth mentioning that preparation of the extracts has to be performed at 50, 70, or 121 °C, respectively, and the temperature utilized must be added to the classification. Accordingly, a material labeled as USP class VI tested formally should provide information upon the temperature (e.g., for class VI-121° extracts were prepared at 121 °C), although this is very rarely found in material data sheets or promotional literature. It is important for you to remember that USP material testing never was intended to be used to evaluate biocompatibility of materials for or even entire medical devices. This rather should be done following a comprehensive set of ISO standards that utilize comparable techniques and that will be introduced in the following chapter. Nevertheless, you still frequently will encounter USP classification in product requirements and material specifications, and it still may be mandatory for medical devices that deal with pharmaceutical products.

USP plastic material testing is for **Pharma** applications.
State of the art for **medical devices** is **ISO 10993**.

2.3.2 Limulus Amebocyte Lysate Test

Endotoxins that are found in their cell wall of some bacteria (Gram-negative) may provoke fever as immune response even if devitalized by sterilization. Therefore, it is from great importance to check pharmaceuticals and medical devices that make contact with blood on the presence of these endotoxins. Fist approaches to do so were based on animal testing, comparable to USP material classification, but these are comparatively slow, cost-intensive and the results may be superimposed by other effects. In 1956, it was discovered that the blood of the Atlantic horseshoe crab (*Limulus polyphemus*) will turn into a semisolid state when in contact with endotoxins. This is due to a substance called **limulus amebocyte lysate** (LAL) that is expressed by the immune cells of the horseshoe crab, and the clogging of the blood is supposed to contain intruding bacteria. Basing on these findings, the LAL test for endotoxins was developed in the 1970s and was incorporated into the USP (<85>) as well as regulations issued by the FDA. For the test, blood is harvested from the crabs that are returned to the water afterward. The relevant blood cells (amebocytes) are separated by centrifugation and placed into distilled water, where these start to swell and burst (lyse). This does release the chemicals of interest (called "lysate") that will be purified and freeze-dried until utilization. Currently, the LAL test basing on the blood of horseshoe crabs is still state-of-the-art to check surfaces of medical devices regarding the existence of endotoxins.

Due to the heavy use of horseshoe crabs, all three of its species are on the red list of threatened species and practically no method for farming could be established yet, which is why the sustainability of this approach is subject questioned. Moreover, welfare for animal used for scientific purposes plays a bigger role in emerging regulations (see Section 2.4.2). Modern techniques of bioengineering enable to utilize other sources than the blood of the horseshoe crab to harvest the lysate of interest, or follow different approaches. A very promising one does mimic the human fever reaction. It does base on monocytes that are a subtype of white blood cells and play a central role in the innate immune response. These may be harvested easily from human blood and used for the test that is called **monocyte activation test** (MAT). Since 2009, it is part of the European Pharmacopoeia as monograph 2.6.30 and recommended as replacement for the rabbit implantation test. Thereby, MAT just alike all other approaches are ideally suited to be implemented as lab-on-chip applications, as presented in (Section 6.3), that feature improved sustainability due to less impact on the environment.

2.3.3 Colony Forming Units

The problems arising from endotoxins require to keep the amount of bacteria sticking to a medical device as low as possible, even if it will be sterilized prior use. This is the reason for strong attempts to keep devices as clean as possible during manufacturing with clean room manufacturing as prominent example. Therefore, a meaningful definition of sterility should read.

> Sterility is the **absence of living or devitalized** microorganisms.

Consequently, a technique is required that enables to roughly determine the quantity of living germs present in a given sample. State of the art is a technique for microbiological examination called plate count. Basic tool is a sterile agar plate, a **petri dish usually filled with agar** (a sticky and jelly-like substance gained from algae) and nutrients. The plate is contacted with the sample, whereupon most bacteria (but not all) present on the surface will be transferred to the agar. Subsequently, the plate is covered and incubated for several days at conditions ideal for the growth of bacteria (37 °C, high humidity). Finding ideal conditions, every single bacterium will perform rapid reproduction and create a colony that is visible as dot on the agar plate with the naked eye. Probably, you happened to see this miracle of biology on the surface of meat or marmalade that is no longer fit for consumption. By counting the colonies on the plate, the number of bacteria that were present on the sample easily can be determined. As the nucleus of each colony may be a single bacterium, a group of them sticking together or any other viable microorganism, the term **colony forming unit (CFU)** is utilized. Consequently, the result of plate counting is the number of CFUs per plate and allows deriving the number of bacteria per unit square that were present on the initial specimen.

Samples inappropriate for direct sampling with plates require additional techniques for indirect contacting. In order to determine the number of CFUs present on a complex surface or on an entire medical device, the sample thoroughly is **rinsed** with purified and sterile **water**. The resulting solution is **filtered** and subsequently, the entire filter is placed on the agar plate. For sampling the surrounding air, an agar plate is placed uncovered for several hours or days. Any CFU present in the air will follow gravity and so eventually make contact with the plate, an approach known as settling plate.

Interestingly, wherever required, contact plates are the standard technique to determine CFUs within every Life Science like food, pharma, and cosmetics. So these are utilized in vast numbers and two types evolved as quasi standard. **Settle plates** usually are **90 mm** in inner diameter (resulting surface ~64 cm^2) and base on the petri dish, the standard tool in microbiology since the late nineteenth century. The typical height is 15 mm whereas only a few millimeters is filled with growth medium, so direct contacting of flat surfaces is unfeasible. They are typically utilized for samples gained by indirect contacting or for testing air. **Contact plates** usually are **55 mm** in inner diameter (resulting surface ~24 cm^2), and the growth medium does exhibit a convex meniscus poking out of the plate to facilitate sampling. A broad rim gives good grip during sampling and the bottom exhibits a 1 cm^2 square grid, which facilitates the counting of grown microbes. They are used to sample smooth and dry surfaces, typically within the manufacturing environment, and for personnel hygiene monitoring, by contacting clothing, hands, or gloves. When engaged with CFU determination, you may encounter the abbreviation **RODAC-plates**, the short version for **R**eplicate **O**rganism **D**etection **a**nd **C**ounting.

If sampling surfaces are frequently treated with disinfectant, some disinfection agent might migrate into the growth medium during contacting. This would inhibit the growth of the bacteria and thus falsify the result. So contact plates usually are prepared with a **neutralizing agar**, a compound that inhibits the influence of remaining disinfectant. Beyond simply counting the number of CFUs present after incubation, a task not requiring much training, the different types of bacteria and spores can be derived from the shape and morphology of the respective colony, whereas this action requires comprehensive knowledge in microbiology. In consequence, while sheer counting frequently is performed in-house, further evaluation is assigned to third-party laboratories. Further, there is a vast number of differing growth media available on the market that allows to test on more complex aspects of microbiology. The considerable gap between sampling and receiving results (several days) generates the demand for considerable faster detection of CFUs. Currently, there are some in-line measurement systems in development, but none of them has received approval by any competent authority.

2.3.4 ISO 10993

The former lack of appropriate standards for the evaluation of biocompatibility for entire medical devices, or materials as components of them, was addressed for the first time by the regulatory authorities of Canada (Health and Welfare Canada), the UK (Health and Social Services UK), and the US (FDA) by issuing the *Tripartite Biocompatibility Guidance* (GPM#87-1) as draft in 1987. Although this guideline never emerged the status of a draft, it was utilized by device manufacturers until 1993, when the *International Organization for Standardization* (ISO) as nongovernmental body issued its standard ISO 10993, named "Biological Evaluation of Medical Devices Part 1: Evaluation and Testing." It gained significant regulatory relevance in 1995 when the FDA issued its blue book memorandum #G95-1 that is closely related to a modified version of ISO 10993-1 and explains how to deal with it, replacing the tripartite standard previously recommended. Since then, the ISO 10993 was evolved consistently by adding more parts that directly address topics that are relevant to evaluate toxicity, biocompatibility, and biological safety, making it a comprehensive set of currently 20 standards (as of 2015) that address guidelines for testing medical devices. It was adapted by many more organizations like the European Committee for Standardization (CEN) or the Chinese FDA, clearly making it the gold standard for biological device testing.

Part 1 of ISO 10993 is designed as header does embrace a general procedure applicable for the biological evaluation of any medical device regardless its intended use (see Figure 2.2). All definitions, terms, and

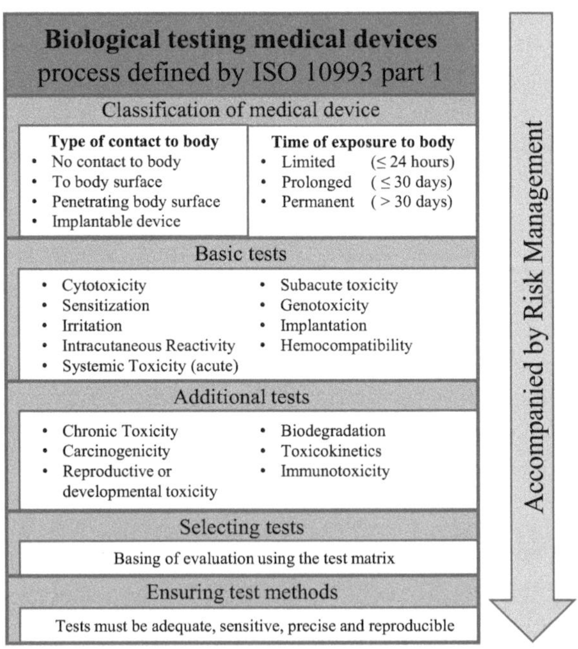

Figure 2.2 Flowchart displaying the process of Biological Evaluation of Medical Devices as described in ISO 10993 part 1. It is not to be confused with the flowchart provided within the standard itself. The actual testing conditions are described in subsequent parts of ISO 10993.

correlations used in the standard are congruent to those presented in this book (refer Sections 2.1 and 2.2). First recommended step is to classify the device according to the type of body contact and time of exposure. This classification is not to be confused with the general risk classification (Classes I–III) you will encounter in many regulations, and that is intended to index categories of medical devices. Subsequently, a set of basic biologic tests is presented and explained, complemented by another set dealing with more elaborate aspects, whereas all of them are linked to the respective parts of ISO 10993. You will find all of them listed in Table 2.2. Basing on the characteristic of the medical device and its unique risk profile, methods for adequate testing now will be selected. To do so, you will find added to the standard a matrix, reflecting device classification and thus guiding your assessments. A medical device must not be automatically tested for all biological aspects, but rather for those found to be relevant for its intended use. Although ISO 10993 does embrace most aspects of biological testing to the greatest possible extent, those not covered must not be neglected but rather handled using test methods with congruent design. Thereby these, just alike those covered by the standard, must be adequate, sensitive, precise, and reproducible. For additional support ISO 10993-1 is completed by a flowchart that does support your line of action when biologically evaluating a medical device. This chart is not to be confused with the one presented in Figure 2.2 as this displays the general proceeding according to the standard. Like any process related to medical devices, any action must be accompanied by a comprehensive Risk Management (see Section 2.3.7).

Like any other standard, ISO 10993 was adapted in some aspects during transfer into the respective national version. Hence, you must consider the one relevant for the country of approval. The understanding of the FDA toward biological testing is explained more detailed in Section 2.4.1 as these differ in some aspects.

2.3.4.1 ISO 10993—Tested Materials

Nowadays many polymer materials are marketed as medical grade and frequently advertised with catchphrases like "tested with 10993" or "biocompatible according to ISO 10993." These promises must be handled with care. First of all, it is very unlikely that a polymer material was tested by all biological aspects as presented within the standard—a task inducing considerable time, effort, and costs. Most frequently these materials were tested according to **ISO 10993-5** only. This test is designed to evaluate the reaction of living cells to the polymer material (or extracts prepared from it) within a laboratory environment cell

Table 2.2 Overview Upon ISO 10993 With All Its Respective Parts. While Part 1 Is Designed as Head of the Standard, Providing a General Introduction, the Others Directly Refer to Specific Tests (Please Note That Part 8 Was Withdrawn). A Medical Device Must Be Tested for Those Aspects Found to Be Relevant for Its Intended Use

Content of ISO 10993	
#	**Title of Respective Part**
1	Evaluation and testing in the risk management process
2	Animal welfare requirements
3	Tests for genotoxicity, carcinogenicity and reproductive toxicity
4	Selection of tests for interactions with blood
5	Tests for in vitro cytotoxicity
6	Tests for local effects after implantation
7	Ethylene oxide sterilization residuals
8	Selection of reference materials (withdrawn)
9	Framework for identification and quantification of potential degradation products
10	Tests for irritation and delayed-type hypersensitivity
11	Tests for systemic toxicity
12	Sample preparation and reference materials
13	Identification and quantification of degradation products from polymeric medical devices
14	Identification and quantification of degradation products from ceramics
15	Identification and quantification of degradation products from metals and alloys
16	Toxicokinetic study design for degradation products and leachables
17	Establishment of allowable limits for leachable substances
18	Chemical characterization of materials
19	Physicochemical, morphological, and topographical characterization of materials
20	Principles and methods for immunotoxicology testing of medical devices

culture and will give a first indication concerning biocompatibility. Cells that are severely harmed or even killed in contact with the polymer indicate a toxic reaction which concludes an inadequate biocompatibility and vice versa. In fact, testing a material according to part 5 is considered to be equivalent to biocompatibility—an undue simplification, as you know when reflecting the correlations presented in Section 2.2. Additionally, some materials are tested for **ISO 10993-10** to prove their suitability for contact to the skin. Anyhow, it is important to remember that any testing performed by the polymer manufacturer is valid for the raw material only. Any properties found for the plastic during biological testing may be altered significantly by processing. This is why the standard strongly does recommend always to test the final device. Further aspects of pretested materials are covered in Section 3.1.2.

> Many medical grade polymers are **advertised** as **ISO 10993** tested.
> To do so, additional information upon the respective parts considered must be given, unless it was tested for **all parts**.

2.3.5 Standards and Regulations for Specific Devices

The tests presented so far are designed to test any medical device on its biological safety or its biocompatibility. Anyhow, up to date many more national and international standards and regulations were developed that are specific for the respective type of medical device, reflecting its unique requirements during application. While many of these cover mechanical testing to avoid harm to the patient's health due to device failure, and thus reflect the common knowledge upon how these medical devices should be designed, some provide specific guidelines how to evaluate their biocompatibility. As these are to manifold to be presented fully, you will be given a few examples to give you an insight into the complexity. The sets of standards ISO 7206, ISO 14243, or ASTM F2033-12 deal with biological and mechanical testing for bone and joint replacements. As for most load-bearing implants, beyond testing on stress during life cycle it is from great importance to evaluate the influence of abrasion on the human body. Thereby, the guidelines provided by ISO 10993 are not sufficient and thus are supplemented by additional standards. And as explained in Section 2.1, microscopic particles of elastomer or rubber materials show a big influence to provoke fever. As these materials frequently are utilized in systems delivering fluids to a patient, such as drips, parenteral nutrition, or blood transfusions, several sets of standards that deal with those devices, like ISO 1135 or ISO 8536.

Additionally to those covering mechanical and biological testing of medical devices, many more standards and regulations do exist. These deal with aspects such as labeling requirements, layout of user instructions, or instructions for user safety. So it is strongly recommended to thoroughly review the regulatory landscape for those regulations and standards that are relevant for the respective medical device.

2.3.6 Quality Management System

Design, manufacturing, and application of medical devices come along with a hazard potential that must be addressed by appropriate QMS, which are mandatory for any company marketing medical devices and for those contractors whose services might affect the patient's health. The most common way in the European Union (EU) (including EU-based companies seeking market approval in China) is to establish a quality system according to ISO 13485 and subsequent certification by a notified body. In fact, this standard is based on the worldwide utilized standard ISO 9001 "Quality management systems—Requirements," adapted to the field of medical devices. Legal boundary conditions allow to utilize any kind of QMS (contrary to automotive suppliers, where certification to ISO/TS 16949 in mandatory), as long as all relevant means are covered sufficiently, but this is useful only for very few special cases. Certification is not mandatory for contractors, but the legal risks involved will be transferred to the company placing the order. In consequence, certification de facto is a barrier to enter the medical device market.

Companies that market medical devices in the **United States** (and US-based companies seeking market approval for China) are required to establish a QMS that is compliant to 21 CFR 820 and will be audited by the FDA followed by a listing in its database. Subcontractors are required to comply with the sections of the law relevant for the respective services provided and may (but not automatically will) be inspected by the FDA. Alternatively, a company may participate in the **Medical Device Single Audit Program** (MDSAP) launched in 2014. Thereby, a party accredited by the MDSAP will perform an audit on compliance to ISO 13485 that may replace FDA inspection. This is an interesting approach for established EU-based companies seeking access to the US market as manufacturer. Anyhow, product approval for the US market still requires participation of the relevant competent authorities.

2.3.7 Risk Management

The process of designing, manufacturing, and distributing a medical device must be accompanied by an adequate process that deals with the risks involved, just like any task in engineering. As a matter of fact, **risk management** is seen as a crucial aspect within any relevant standard or regulation for medical device-related QMS. This does include hazards arising from both, device failure as well as incorrect application, thus not automatically exempting the medical device company from responsibility for any harm resulting from user error. ISO 13485 does use the term risk management in several of its sections and even directly does cite the standard **ISO 14971** "Medical devices—Application of risk management to medical devices" that consequently is the de facto approach to this topic within the EU and is relevant for European Companies seeking market approval in China. Interestingly, the codification of **21 CFR 820**, relevant as law for the US market, does use this term only once within its body, namely in subchapter 820.40(g) that deals with the topic of design validation. The FDA's position toward risk management rather may be understood when looking at the law's preamble, where ISO 9001, ISO 13485, and the Global Harmonization Task Force (GHTF) (now *International Medical Device Regulators Forum* (IMDRF)) are named directly. Further sources are a set of FDA guidance documents as listed in Table 2.3.

Table 2.3 Overview Upon All Documents Issued by the FDA Covering the Aspect of Risk Management for Medical Devices. Interestingly the Word "Risk" Is Only Used Once within the Body of 21 CFR 820, but within the Preface, ISO 9001, ISO 13485, and the GHTF (Now IMDRF) Are Named Directly

Title	Issued
Do it by Design	December, 1996
Design Control Guidance for Medical Device Manufacturers	March, 1997
A Guide to Inspections of Quality Systems	August, 1999
Medical Device Use–Safety: Incorporating Human Factors Engineering into Risk Management	July, 2000
Quality System Information for Certain Premarket Application Reviews; Guidance for Industry and FDA Staff	February, 2003

When taking the challenge to read all documents mentioned, you easily will get the impression that the FDA's fundamental understanding of risk management is very closely related to the basic means of ISO 14971. But if so, you must consider that some important aspects differ in detail. And you should not be confused that the FDA issued some documents dealing with risk management (such as Guidance for Industry—Q9 Quality Risk Management) that are intended for application in other regulated industries like pharma or food. However, the ISO 14971 will give you a good understanding of how risks in the medical device industry should be dealt with.

Basic understanding of ISO 149714 is that any risk is defined by combination of probability and severity of harm. Using both aspects, you may generate easily a graph that usually draws the severity as X-axis, quantified numerically or by an adjective, and its probability in comparable way as Y-axis. The result is an array that does display any characteristic of risk as individual field, as displayed image 2.3. Any risk with high probability that will lead to severe harm is not acceptable and thus labeled red. Those exhibiting a moderate combination are colored yellow, indicating that the risk basically is acceptable but should be reduced ***a**s **l**ow **a**s **r**easonably **p**racticable,* abbreviated as **ALARP**[2]. Prior to 2012, the standard additionally comprised fields colored in green, indicating a risk with low probability and/or negligible harm that consequently were considered acceptable. Now, every risk is considered as reducible, which is why green fields no longer exist. Anyhow, you probably still will encounter them from time to time. The precise layout of the two areas (red and yellow), as well as scaling of the axes, may be adapted to the individual needs, but must be reasonable and reflecting the definitions of ISO 14971 (Figure 2.3).

To get closer to the process of risk management, it is important to know that the standard explains that it is impossible to eliminate an existing risk fully, but reducing it as much as reasonably practical is mandatory. Embracing the entire life cycle of a medical device, periodically repeating, all imaginable risks are identified, evaluated, and charted in the graph. Each entry of a risk in red or yellow fields will require action, either to reduce probability or severity of harm, ideally both. If the action defined is found to be effective, the risk will be

2. The term ALARP was first used in the UK as part of the "Health and Safety at Work etc. Act" of 1974.

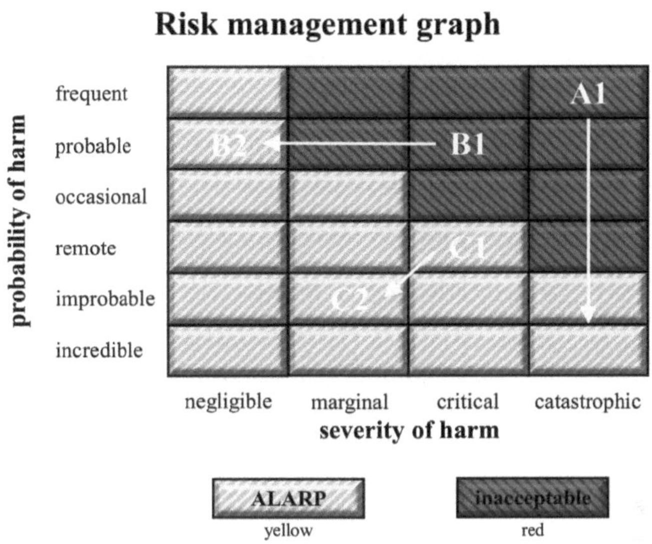

Figure 2.3 Graph as it may be applied during the process of risk management. Any risk is defined by the severity of harm involved (X-axis) and its probability of occurrence (Y-axis). Those combining high probability and severe harm are not acceptable (red (black in print version) area). A moderate combination (yellow (white in print version) area) should be reduced as low as reasonably practicable (ALARP). Prior to the revision of 2012, the standard did comprise risks to be considered as acceptable that were colored green. This no longer does exist, but probably you still will encounter these from time to time. The combinations of letter and number serve as an example. The entries within the respective fields correspond with the risk analysis of a fictional medical device, as displayed in Table 2.4.

reevaluated and its new position charted in the graph. You will be given an example dealing with a fictional medical device (Table 2.4).

Beyond ISO 14971, there are more standards that find application for risk management in medical engineering, such as IEC 62304, IEC 62366, or IEC 60601-1. Combining them sometimes is not very easy, a problem that was addressed by the technical report ISO TR 24971:2013 "Medical devices—Guidance on the application of ISO 14971." It definitely is a useful tool to get closer to the process of risk management.

2.3.8 Validation

Although considered to be of major importance, there often is confusion about the term validation. In fact, you will find different definitions and understanding in almost every single industry, just compare software

Table 2.4 Example for the Risk Management for a Fictional Medical Device. Every Single Risk Identified Will Be Documented and Evaluated by Its Probability and Severity of Harm. Those Found to Be Not Acceptable Must Be Addressed By an Appropriate Action, Whereas Its Effectiveness Must Be Verified. Now the Risk May Be Reevaluated. The Risks Presented (A–C) Are Charted in Figure 2.3

Fictional Medical Device				
Risk Identified and Evaluated		**Action Defined and Evaluated as Effective**	**Risk Reevaluated Considering Defined Action**	
A1	Device is toxic (p: frequent) (s: critical)	Negative in vitro test for toxicity	A2	Final test for no toxicity (p: incredible) (s: critical)
	New materials frequently show severe toxic influence on living tissue, harm defined as catastrophic, but in vivo testing could prove contrary. Consequently, severity remains the same, but probability could be reduced by defined action.			
B1	Design supports biofilm (p: probable) (s: critical)	Redesign considering microbiology	B2	New design hampers formation of biofilm (p: probable) (s: negligible)
	It was found, generation of a biofilm can't be avoided, but may be hampered by appropriate device design. Thus, probability of occurrence remains the same, but severity may be reduced.			
C1	Processing occasionally impairs materials biocompatibility (p: remote) (s: critical)	Adapted processing, known to less likely and less severe influencing material	C2	New processing reduces severity and possibility of negative influence (p: improbable) (s: marginal)
	The intended processing is known to occasionally show critical influence on the materials biocompatibility. By adapting the process, the influence on biocompatibility may be reduced as well as its possibility of occurrence. Hence, both properties could be lowered.			

Table 2.4 Example for the Risk Management for a Fictional Medical Device. Every Single Risk Identified Will Be Documented and Evaluated by Its Probability and Severity of Harm. Those Found to Be Not Acceptable Must Be Addressed By an Appropriate Action, Whereas Its Effectiveness Must Be Verified. Now the Risk May Be Reevaluated. The Risks Presented (A–C) Are Charted in Figure 2.3—cont'd

Fictional Medical Device				
Risk Identified and Evaluated		**Action Defined and Evaluated as Effective**	**Risk Reevaluated Considering Defined Action**	
D1	...	...	D2	...

programming to civil engineering. In addition, even within the medical device industry, you will encounter slightly differing definitions or you may experience vivid discussion upon this topic. To get closer to a well-suited understanding for the term validation, it is useful to look at the term verification that is related closely. A definition issued by the GHTF (now IMDRF) does state that:

> **Verification** is the confirmation by **examination** and provision of objective evidence that the specified requirements have been fulfilled.

You should remember that **verification** always does require hands on every single product. It is obvious that this is close to or even absolutely **unfeasible** for products that may be examined destructive only or are manufactured in mass production. This aspect is found in many industrial fields and commonly addressed by statistical analyses intended to evaluate the process capability. To put it briefly, as result you obtain evidence about the probability that a product manufactured does not meet its requirements. If the probability is evaluated as acceptable, the process of manufacturing may be regarded as stable and will be utilized, monitored by established tools for quality control. Within the world of medical devices, the analysis on process capability does follow the same principles, but compared to traditional manufacturing industries probably does consider more aspects. Additionally, risk management and comprehensive documentation must accompany process analysis. Therefore, a meaningful definition should read:

> **Process validation** means to establish by objective evidence that a process consistently produces a result or product meeting its predetermined requirements.

Of course, validation is not mandatory for the process of manufacturing only but for all aspects of medical devices that may have impact on the patient's health. In consequence, a process of validation must also accompany the process of device development. That is named commonly **design controls**. To put it briefly, you must analyze and find evidence that the design you created is suitable to assure the functionality you desire. Therefore, a meaningful definition should read:

> **Validation** means to confirm through provision of objective evidence that the requirements for a specific intended use or application have been fulfilled.

Of course, this only can be a brief introduction to the complex aspects of process and design validation for medical devices. Further, any preprocessing or postprocessing of a product like cleaning or sterilization must be a subject of validation. If you want to get more into details, please refer to further literature, e.g., the documents issued by the FDA or IMDRF.

2.3.9 21 CFR Part 11

The development, manufacturing, and distribution of medical devices require statutory comprehensive documentation. The legal requirements affect primarily data and documents that are essential to prove safety of the device, such as the design history files, test certificates, work procedures, or tracking and tracing of manufactured materials and products. Nowadays, this takes place close to exclusively with tools for electronic processing of data. External and internal communication happens with e-mail, product development bases on CAD-systems, data from quality inspection are acquired and stored by computers, work instructions are distributed electronically, and the flow of goods is controlled with enterprise recourse planning (ERP) software. Thereby, any action in an FDA-regulated industry is subject to part 11 of the Title 21 of the Code of Federal Regulation that is labeled "electronic records and electronic signatures." This law defines the criteria that make electronic records and signatures—a trustworthy and reliable equivalent to paper-based documentation. And many actions of daily business generate data that are handled ideally electronically. These may include the following:

- The history of device design is documented in CAD-systems
- Risk Management is supported with specialized software
- Data from in-process quality control are stored in databases
- Work instructions are provided as electronic documents
- The flow of goods is managed with ERP software
- Batch numbers and labels are generated automatically

All these actions are subject to the regulations of 21 CFR part 11, if performed electronically. Thereby, the legal requirements are rather challenging and induce many **pitfalls**. To give some examples: It is a common practice to record data from quality inspection in **spreadsheets** or minutes of meeting as **text files**. Both may be manipulated ex post, and thus basically are not compliant to part 11. Usually, **login** to a computer is controlled by username and password. This enables tracking of any action performed within the system, and consequently this approach is utilized as system for electronic identification, and thus considered as electronic signature. Anyhow, this frequently is not compliant to the FDA regulation that requires any user to be provided a unique ID number and personal PIN number, to avoid feigning a foreign identity. Although implementing electronic records and signatures within the entire company offers great benefits in terms of efficiency and costs, the hurdles induced by part 11 are considerably high. Therefore, it is recommendable to thoroughly examine the advantages and disadvantages.

2.4 Regulatory Affairs—Upcoming Restrictions

The global regulatory landscape for medical devices is subject to consistent evolution. Driving forces are new scientific evidences, higher demands on safety of devices, incidents that reveal loopholes and deficiencies in existing regulations, and the increasing globalization of trade. There are a number of rules and regulations issued recently, hence becoming valid after a short period of transition, or that currently are prepared for publication. All of them will have considerable impact on the entire world of medical devices, which is why knowledge upon them is from great importance for anyone working in this field. Thereby the overarching theme is a strong effort for a **global harmonization** of rules and regulations. Not least due to this fact, any new country-specific regulation for medical devices should be considered, regardless of affecting a market of interest or not.

2.4.1 New FDA Guideline to Use ISO 10993

In 2013, the FDA issued the draft of a guideline for its staff and the industry, which will supersede the existing *Blue Book Memorandum #95* when finalized. Although not part of the original ISO standard and no relevant FDA guideline yet, it gives an insight into the agency's understanding upon biological testing, and thus should be considered by medical device manufacturers. The main aspects of this may be listed as below:

2.4.1.1 General Considerations for Biocompatibility Testing

- Although intentionally excluded from the ISO standard, the FDA believes that biological hazards should be considered for biocompatibility testing
- Subject to any test should be the final device or representative coupon devices, considering the volume to surface ration when preparing extractions
- Following the good laboratory practice (GLP) is mandatory
- Manufacturers are encouraged to discuss planned testing with the FDA, as using an appropriate animal model may justify omissions in some basic biocompatibility tests
- Some specific considerations on tests for cytotoxicity, sensitization, pyrogenicity, implantation, genotoxicity, carcinogenicity, and reproductive toxicity (all these subjects of ISO 10993 subsets) are discussed in more detail
- Beyond nature, degree, frequency, and duration of body exposure, considering the chemical characteristics of device materials (including color additives), eventual target population, and target organs is recommended

2.4.1.2 Considerations to Specific Issues

- Instead of labeling a product as free from a defined substance (e.g., **Latex-free**, DEHP-free, pyrogen-free) a manufacturer rather should use the term "not made with..." and give additional information, such as "The product is not made with natural rubber latex"
- FDA believes that there can be unique properties associated with submicron or **nanotechnology** components such as, aggregation, agglomeration, immunogenicity, or toxicity. These must be considered when designing a test, as classical approach may prove to be insufficient
- Comprehensive definition of applicable **color additives**, as these are listed by the FDA

Just alike ISO 10993, the FDA guidance does provide a matrix for test selection and a flowchart for the general line of actions, whereas both are comparable yet not identical. Generally spoken, the recommendations of the FDA are more comprehensive and may give a good indication for the future developments of the standard.

2.4.2 Revisions of ISO 10993

The technical committee (TC) ISO/TC 194, responsible for the standard ISO 10993, does revise currently many existing parts of the standard and is about to develop some genuine as well. These developments are complex and voluminous, and many of them only are from concerns for laboratories performing biological evaluation of medical devices. Hence, you only will be given an outline covering those that are likely to influence the daily business of medical device companies.

2.4.2.1 Animal Welfare

Some aspects of biological evaluation of medical devices necessarily require animal testing. Anyhow, animal welfare is a relevant issue within the medical device industry and consequently is addressed by **ISO 10993-2**. In order to reduce the number of animal tests performed, it is discussed how these may be replaced by tests basing on bioassays. It is very likely that these developments will result in a set of assays, designed to evaluate irritation, sensitization and genotoxicity, and that are considered appropriate to **replace animal tests** currently established as standard procedures. Beside an improvement in animal welfare, this has the potential to significantly reduce costs and time required to biologically evaluate medical devices.

2.4.2.2 Respiratory Devices

Major aspect for this revision is respiratory medical devices, such as ventilators, masks, and inhalers, that make indirect contact to the human body via gas pathway. The current layout of ISO 10993 allows broad room of interpretation on how to apply the standard. To play safe, many companies in consequence follow approaches that include implantation tests for manifold of components, a challenging approach when considering the time and costs involved. This aspect will be addressed by the TC via a **new set of standards** that currently is developed and the name ISO/CD 18562 *Biocompatibility evaluation of respiratory gas pathways in healthcare applications*. It will have major influence on companies dealing with these devices and is expected to assure patient's health more appropriate while reducing the effort required for device development.

2.4.2.3 Nanomaterials

The application of nanomaterials in medical devices gives room for manifold innovations but involves the potential unforeseeable risks. From major concern are long-term effects on biological systems that are difficult to evaluate and consequently thorough investigations on them are a current topic within research and development. To give a regulatory framework, their application in medical devices was addressed by a technical guideline, published by the FDA in 2013 (see Section 2.4.1). Anyhow, the TC of ISO 10993 is pretty aware about the urgent need for guidelines that address the application of nanomaterials. To do so, a new technical report labeled "Guidance on nanomaterials" currently is under development, intended to become part 22 of ISO 10993. It was approved as new project by the ISO committee in mid-2014 and thus still is in its early phase of creation. Anyhow, medical device companies dealing with nanomaterials should keep a close look on these developments as these are very likely to have major impact on the utilization of nanomaterials.

2.4.3 Revision of ISO 13485

With its latest revision in 2012, the responsible TC ISO/TC 210 did reflect significant changes in the worldwide regulatory landscape. Among other things, these were triggered by emerging markets (BRIC-states) and strong attempts for global harmonization (consider IMDRF).

Major scope was to reflect besides FDA requirements those derived from the EU medical device directive (MDD), thus linking the directive to the standard. A revised version of the standard was published as Draft International Standard (DIS) ISO DIS 13485:201X in early 2014 and is expected (as of 2015) to be released as final version 1 year later. With a transition of 3 years, it is intended to become effective. Major aspects of revision are given below:

- Convergence of the ISO 13485 body with the respective regulatory systems of Brazil, Japan, and the United States
- Better alignment with the EU MDD
- Supporting the goals of the MDSAP as currently is launched in Australia, Brazil, Canada and the United States
- More flexible for integration of other frequently applied standards (e.g., ISO 14001 *environmental management systems* or ISO 27001 *information security management*)
- Making the standard more applicable to the entire supply chain in the medical device industry
- Greater emphasis on risk management
- Expanded focus on safety of patient and user
- Mandatory validation of all computer softwares that are used as part of the quality system
- Stronger emphasis on corrective and protective actions

Anyhow, the changes are likely to be from moderate concern for medical device companies but probably will help to further evolve ISO 13485 as global standard for medical devices.

2.4.4 EU Medical Device Regulations

Last revision on the EU MDD took place in 2007, and was published as 2007/47/EC. Embedded in this regulation, the French company *Poly Implant Prothèse* (PIP), producing and globally selling breast implants, commenced illicitly to use industrial instead of medical grade silicones for filling. When surgeons reported more and more concerns about inappropriate high rates of implant failures, the responsible French health authorities issued a general recall, which released a flood of law suits that eventually resulted in the company's bankruptcy and liquidation in

2010. Anyhow, the production process was audited by the French subsidiary of a German notified body and PIP did possess market approval (valid *Conformité Européenne* (CE) mark) for Europe at that time. However, the relevant quality certificates did not apply to the silicone material used. This unprecedented scandal did induce a lively (and still ongoing) debate upon weaknesses and room for improvement in Europe's medical device regulatory frameworks. Frequently expressed objections concern the legal liability, authority, and supervision of notified bodies. In response to this debate, the European Commission (EC) issued a proposal for improved regulations in late 2012 as 2012/0266(COD) *Medical Devices* and 2012/0267(COD) *In vitro diagnostic medical devices*. The final regulation is expected for release in 2015 and will merge the two preexisting directives 90/385/EEC *Active implantable medical devices* and 93/42/EEC *Medical devices* in a new European Medical Device Regulation (EMDR). The amendment to the preexisting regulations for in vitro diagnostics (IVDs) clearly underlines the EC's understanding that these are considered as medical devices too. Contrary to a directive, which must be transferred to national law by every single member state individually, a regulation becomes enforceable law across all EU countries simultaneously. This shall prevent nation specific variations as these may result from using directives. Anyhow, considering the empiric time frame for legislations and assuming a usual transferal period, the regulation is expected to become effective for medical device companies 3 years after final release (2018). The most relevant revisions proposed are related to the work of the notified bodies and their respective governmental surveillance, thus only indirectly affecting medical device companies. Anyhow, many of them certainly will have direct impact on manufacturers as the general scope and requirements of the medical device regulation (MDR) will be significantly expanded. The proposed revisions comprise the following:

2.4.4.1 Impact on Notified Bodies Mainly

- Only, newly to create, special notified bodies will be permitted to issue CE marks for class III devices
- Installation of a Medical Device Coordination Group that will be involved in a newly to-establish scrutiny process for Class III devices, comparable to the premarket approval in the United States
- Notified bodies will be audited jointly for compliance by the http://ec.europa.eu/health/medical-devices/files/bse_tse_en.pdf of all member states, rather than by the respective national only

2.4.4.2 Impact on Medical Device Companies Mainly

- Unannounced audits by the notified body will become mandatory
- The EC authority to create common technical specifications will be expanded to medical devices
- Some devices, e.g., those controlling or monitoring active implants, nanomaterials and any products combined with substances will be classified as Class III
- Invasive products or devices, not intended for medical use but exhibiting a comparable risk profile (e.g., aesthetic implants, cosmetic contact lenses), will be considered as medical devices
- Most devices for IVDs will require involvement of a notified body (you should consider the additional IVD regulation)
- Labeling must include a unique device identification (UDI) number
- Reprocessing used devices, that was identified for single use only by its original manufacturer, will be considered as manufacturing
- Patients provided with an implant must be issued a card providing details, such as expected lifetime and relevant precautions and warnings
- Installation of a qualified person, responsible for regulatory compliance, will become mandatory
- Alterations that significantly alter the characteristic of the device will require anew full process of CE marking
- Manufacturers of Class III devices will be obliged to make publicly accessible information upon safety, clinical performance, and supporting clinical data

It is worth mentioning that the proposed regulations currently are discussed vividly, and some aspects presented are likely to be withdrawn. Anyhow, as the formally still are part of the proposals, we decided to present these without further details.

2.4.5 Unique Device Identifier

As part of the *Food and Drug Administration Amendments Act* of 2007, the request for a *Unique Device Identifier* (UDI) System was signed into law. Motivation to do so was to increase patient's safety by establishing a unique identifier for any medical device that is intended for **sales in the United States**. The system will allow to better analyze reports about adverse events or failures that occur during medical device application. The final rule for the UDI system was released by the FDA in late 2013 and will be phased in over several years, having started 1 year later with Class III (high risk) devices and ending with unclassified or Class I (low risk) devices in 2018. It does require a UDI to be included on every device label and package in *Human Readable Interpretation*, put simply in plain text, as well as in compliance to *automatic identification and data capture* systems of international standards or practice (readable by machines). Thereby, the UDI is a worldwide unique (alpha) numeric code consisting of two components: a device identifier (DI) as fixed portion, providing information about the labeler and details specific for the device type or model, and a product identifier as variable information, encoding information upon lot or batch number, serial number, date of manufacturing, and use-by date. Further, any device labeler is required to provide DI information to the FDA-administered *Global Unique Device Identification Database* (GUDID). That way anyone gets via the Internet publicly access to basic information about any medical device. Figure 2.4 does illustrate the UDI and GUDID system design.

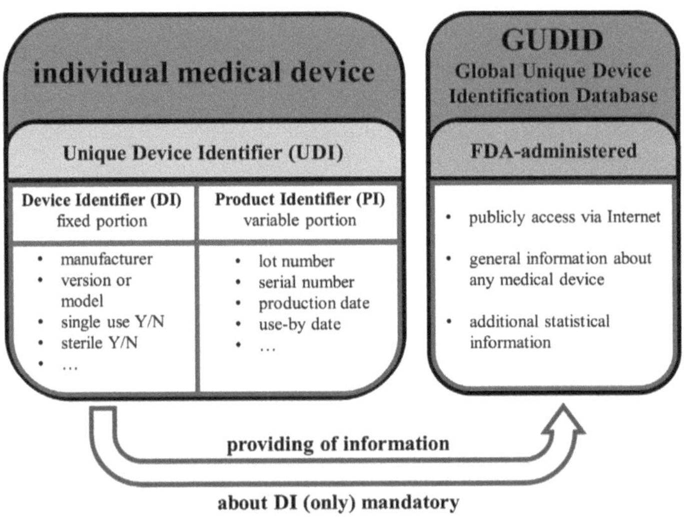

Figure 2.4 The Unique Device Identifier (UDI) is composed of two parts, the device identifier (DI) containing data that are identical for the product line (static portion), and the product identifier (PI) providing information that do vary during serial production, giving every single medical device a worldwide unique number. The PI is listed in the *Global Unique Device Identification Database* (FDA administered) and is accessible to public via the Internet.

While developing the UDI system, the FDA clearly focused on its suitability for global application, as clearly is expressed by the database name. This was done in close coordination with the IMDRF, which issued its highly comparable international guideline *UDI Guidance—Unique Device Identification (UDI) of Medical Devices* shortly after the FDA released its rules. This guidance was developed flexible enough so it may be adapted to national needs by respective competent authorities without losing its compliance to the principle of three pillars. The majority of national competent authorities for medical devices (including all IMDRF members and the EU) announced to, or currently do implement a UDI system compliant to the guideline. Anyhow, the precise approach may vary as three approaches to do so may be used simultaneously, namely labeling according to the standards *Global Standards One* (GS1), *Health Industry Business Communications Council* (HIBCC), and the *International Council for Commonality in Blood Banking Automation* (ICCBBA). These developments certainly will facilitate the global trade of medical devices, improve patients and user's safety and thus mark a mile stone for globalized standards.

2.5 European versus US-Regulations

2.5.1 Market Structures and Potentials

Seen historically, the United States formed already a unified commercial market with established laws and regulations while EU was not more than a vision. Consequently, the European regulatory landscape is still ways more heterogeneous and subject of efforts for harmonization, driven by the ideas of a unified and free European internal market. In the **United States,** legal boundary conditions for medical devices are defined by the *Federal Food, Drug, and Cosmetic Act* of 1938 and its amendments as federal law and are enforced by a federal agency, namely the FDA. It does form the largest unified regulated market by turnover with health expenditures of $2.800 billion[3] in 2012 (17.9% of GDP), expected growing to $4.700 billion by 2020 (19.6% of GDP). Once approved for marketing medical device may be sold in this entire market with all the opportunities and risks induced by its size. In **Europe,** up to the early 1990s regulatory laws were passed by every single of its member states independently

3. Like for any economic facts and numbers as well as their predicted development, many different sources with even many more figures are available. We decided to present mean values that are intended to give you a general image. This was done for all market figures presented for the United States, EU, and China.

with some at this time not having established any specifically for medical devices. Fundamental approach to harmonize the European regulatory market was done by agreeing on three directives which define a standardized process to approve medical devices for sales in the entire EU. These are *90/385/EEC Active implantable medical devices* (commonly known as *Active Implantable Medical Device Directive—AIMDD*), *93/42/EEC Medical devices* (commonly known as *Medical Device Directive—MDD*), and *98/79/EC In vitro diagnostics*. Within a year, these directives had to be transferred to national law by every single member state individually, whereas the directives particular result to be achieved were defined without dictating the means to do so. The result is a versatile structure of the European regulated market that features health expenditures roughly 8% of the GDP in 2012, expected growing 10–11% by 2020[4]. Additionally, every single state takes influence on its national health-care market and reimbursement system at significant different extent. While some spend less than 6% of their GDP, others invest more than 12%; a figure that considering the individual economic power of every single state underline the multilayer structure of Europe as health-care market. A device once approved for the entire EU still must be marketed country specific, increasing the costs for sales, but meantime allowing a multistaged introduction of innovative devices or drugs with less financial risk in case of complications. This is why several US-based medical device companies approve their products in the EU first and starting sales in defined small countries to generate stable turnovers and gain market experience at comparatively moderate costs, prior entering the US market.

2.5.2 Process of Approval

Basic legal requirement to produce a medical device (or parts of it) for the **US** market is compliance to 21 CFR 820, a regulation called *Quality System Regulations* (for medical devices). It is the company's responsibility to fulfill these requirements and compliance is monitored by FDA officers that may visit and audit the entire production process as representatives of the US executive. Prior marketing, it is mandatory to register the company at the FDA and any medical device needs to be approved via following the procedure to obtain a *510(k)* clearance (showing substantial

---

4. There is a confusing number of data and statements about the total health-care costs in Europe, depending on whether looking at the EU 5, EU 19 (those using € as currency), or EU 28. In consequence we decided not to give absolute numbers, but these are somewhere located lower than the United States but above China.

equivalence to existing devices), the procedure of *513(g)* (seeking support for classification), or the *de novo process* (for novel devices). The required documents must be provided by the company and will be reviewed and evaluated by the FDA with no further party being involved, making this agency the sole organization involved as regulating body. Once approved, devices will be listed in FDA's medical device database and their approval will not be rechecked on regular basis unless certain types of changes are applied to the product, e.g., design, way of manufacturing, intended use.

Prior-producing medical devices (or parts of it) for sales in **Europe**, it is necessary to install a quality system in accordance to the *Annex II* or *V* of *93/42/EEC* (MDD), whereas the most common way is getting certified according to the standard *ISO 13485* by an organization called notified body. These are third-party organizations (and thus may be for profit companies), that are accredited by their respective governments (acting as accreditation body) and entitled to assess compliance to established laws, standards, and regulations relevant for medical devices. Final market approval for the device must be obtained at least in one of the European states, and the conformity to all relevant European regulations is expressed by labeling it with *Conformité Européenne* (French for: European Conformity), usually referred to as ***CE marking***. The device is now free for marketing in the entire EU and some associated states. Companies not located in Europe additionally must appoint an authorized representative, abbreviated EC REP. Since 2011, all devices must be listed in a database called *European Database on Medical Devices*. Additional country-specific regulatory boundary conditions only may be given at minor extent, for example, reimbursement of the device or obligations for labeling and use instructions to be in national language. Any given approval must be rechecked by a notified body on a regular basis, usually in an interval of 6 or 12 months. It is worth mentioning that the process of CE marking of a plastic toy and a complex medical device like an artificial heart valve basically are the same, although the latter is affected by significantly more rules and regulations. Therefore, it is discussed to introduce a specific label for medical dives like CE med.

2.5.3 Global Harmonization

The GHTF, a voluntary group founded in 1992 by and representing the regulating medical device authorities of Australia, Canada, EU, Japan, and the United States, pursued a harmonization on global base (Figure 2.5). Major goal of the *GHTF* was to develop a worldwide standard for MDRs and to establish directives valid for every single member state despite their

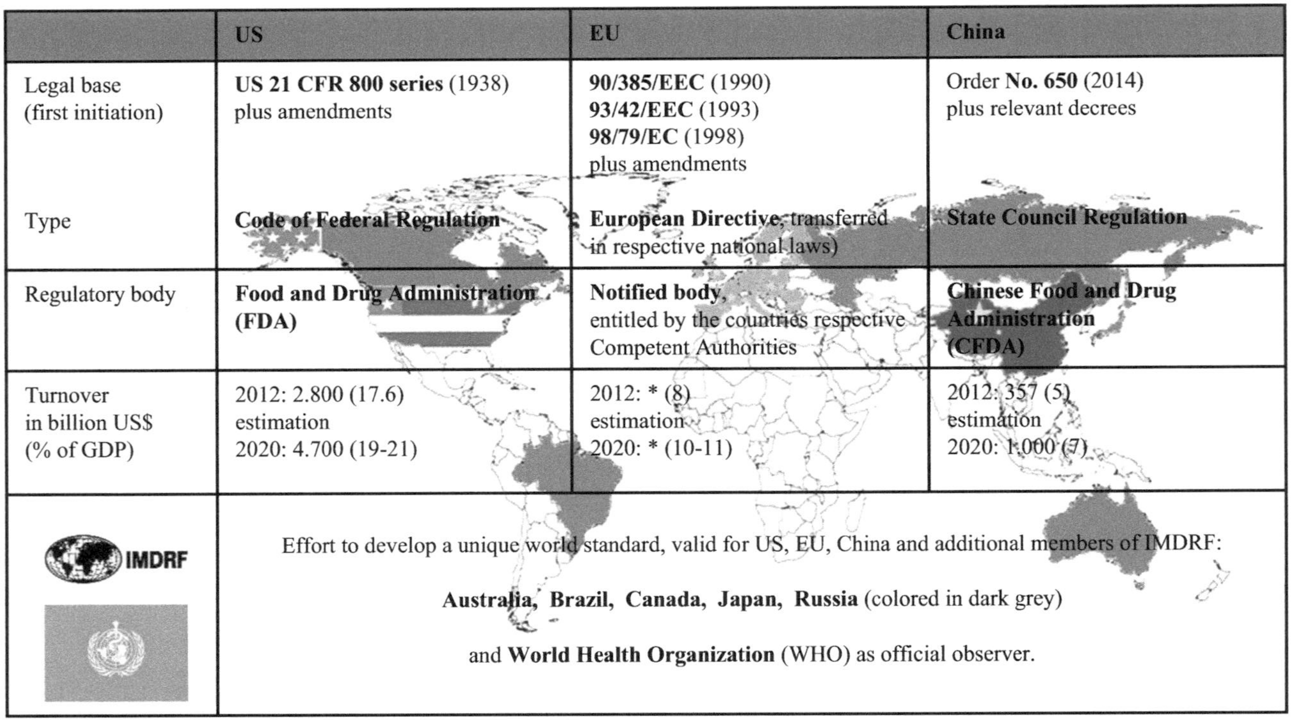

	US	EU	China
Legal base (first initiation)	**US 21 CFR 800 series** (1938) plus amendments	**90/385/EEC** (1990) **93/42/EEC** (1993) **98/79/EC** (1998) plus amendments	Order **No. 650** (2014) plus relevant decrees
Type	**Code of Federal Regulation**	**European Directive**, transferred in respective national laws)	**State Council Regulation**
Regulatory body	**Food and Drug Administration (FDA)**	**Notified body**, entitled by the countries respective Competent Authorities	**Chinese Food and Drug Administration (CFDA)**
Turnover in billion US$ (% of GDP)	2012: 2.800 (17.6) estimation 2020: 4.700 (19-21)	2012: * (8) estimation 2020: * (10-11)	2012: 357 (5) estimation 2020: 1.000 (7)
IMDRF	Effort to develop a unique world standard, valid for US, EU, China and additional members of IMDRF: **Australia**, **Brazil**, **Canada**, **Japan**, **Russia** (colored in dark grey) and **World Health Organization** (WHO) as official observer.		

* There is a confusing number of data and statements for total health care spending in the EU. So we decided to specify the percentage of GDP only.

Figure 2.5 Regulatory map of the world, displaying the three dominating markets US, EU, and China. The entire landscape faces strong attempts for global harmonization to develop a worldwide-standardized regulatory framework.

respective unique regulatory framework. It was disbanded in late 2012, but since 2011 its assigned task is continued by the IMDRF, a forum composed of the former *GHTF* members and representatives of regulating bodies of Brazil, China, and Russia as additional members and the *World Health Organization* (WHO) as official observer. The standards defined by *ISO 13485* are widely consistent to those that were developed by the GHTF and the IMDRF as its successor, slowly establishing it as the universal standard for design, manufacture, and marketing of medical devices on global scale. The last revision of the *US 21 CFR 820*, in effect since 1997, does reflect these developments and in consequence the law's content is close to be identical to the ISO standard, despite their significantly differing legal provenance.

In March 2012, the IMDRF initiated a pilot phase that is called **MDSAP**. Its major goal is to develop a uniform process to audit a medical device manufacturer's quality system that will satisfy the needs of regulatory authorities of all participating countries. Currently, these include Australia, Brazil, Canada, and the United States, and Japan expected to become full member in 2015. According to MDSAP this will give benefits to both parties, device manufacturers and regulatory authorities or third-party organizations, as these will face a less number of on-site regulatory audits when accessing multiple markets, thus reducing required effort and manpower. Starting in 2015, manufacturers of medical devices are invited to participate in this program. These developments underline the fact that all quality systems established by the respective regulatory authorities on worldwide base exhibit a convergence to a unique standard. Anyhow, the process of medical device approval itself is not subject to this approach. But as a review on the mandatory quality system does represent a crucial element for this, these developments may be seen as a nucleus for a uniform process for medical device approval that may find general acceptance.

Major influence on the regulated markets of Europe and the United States may be expected from the *Transatlantic Trade and Investment Partnership*, a combined free trade agreement and bilateral investment treaty, currently negotiated and intended to become effective in 2015 (as of mid-2015). One of its primary scopes is to reduce tariff and nontariff barriers to trade and thus to form a transatlantic free trade area that is unified at large extent. A high potential is seen in a mutual acceptance of product testing and market approvals. When thinking of regulated products such a step could imply far-ranging consequences that currently cannot be foreseen, ranging from a perpetuation of the current situation to a system where EU or US clearance for marketing would approve sales in the respective other market. Advantages and disadvantages currently a subject of controversial debates, fueled by the fact that content and coverage of the treaty are largely negotiated in secrecy. Anyhow, as an initiative of transparency, the EC revealed some documents concerning this issue in early 2015. It is the understanding of EU that both processes for market approval for medical devices are capable to assure patient safety sufficiently, and therefore should not be harmonized although very different in detail. Room for improvement rather is seen in approaches to optimize the access to the markets of EU and the United States. This should be done by a mutual acceptance of audits on the established quality systems, comparable to the approach of the MDSAP, although no member of the EU participated in this so far. Further, harmonized forms for application are intended in order to reduce bureaucracy for all parties involved and the UDI will be established in Europe to improve traceability and thus assure patient safety on both sides of the Atlantic. These developments strongly indicate an ongoing convergence of both medical device markets. It may be expected that a considerable reduced bureaucratic effort is combined with significantly increased market potential, and so will lead to a greater number of novel devices being developed and applied, generating more benefit of societies health, while consuming less value added.

2.6 China—The Future Major Regulator?

The past decades have seen rapid changes in the global stream of goods and economic role of individual countries. Among the group of *Emerging and developing economies*, as these are defined by the *International Monetary Fund* (IMF), a group of five members including Brazil, Russia, India, China (here referring to the People's Republic of China), and South Africa, abbreviated by using their respective first letters as *BRICS*, do exhibit a superior economic growth. The related increase in public wealth does expand their respective health-care markets, and a fast growing social group, usually referred to as middle class, can afford access to health system on industrialized countries level. In consequence, these developments fuel the evolution of their country-specific regulations. Reflecting the respective population among the BRICS states, the prospects of India and China as regulated markets become obvious.

Beyond its remarkable economic growth over the past decade, especially China did exhibit a comprehensive development in terms of regulating medical devices. In 2013, based on preexisting regulatory agencies with partially overlapping responsibilities, the Chinese State Council did form the *China Food and Drug Administration* (CFDA, Chinese: 国家食品药品监督管理总局) as an agency on ministerial-level, and thus highly resembling its US counterpart not only by name but also in terms of legal status and area of responsibilities. The process for approval of medical devices ministered by the CFDA may partially be seen as a combination to the approaches in the US or EU. Primary step is an application that does include a risk classification as defined by CFDA order No. 15, other required documents and for foreign manufacturers a notarized "proof of qualification of the manufacturer," a demand that usually is satisfied by ISO 13485 certification or FDA registration. Additionally, appointing a Legal Agent, serving as contact person for the Chinese authorities during approval, and an After Sales Agent, assigned to supervise marketing from a regulatory point, is mandatory. Both must possess Chinese citizenship or at least local business presence. The classification may be approved or adjusted by the CFDA, resulting in market approval, denial of approval, or additional requirements for testing. These tests must comply with relevant national standards, called Guobiao (GB, Chinese: 國標) and industrial standards for medicine, labeled YY. Preexisting tests performed according to other established standards will not be accepted automatically. Depending on its classification clinical trials may be mandatory, whereby these must be conducted frequently in China. Basing on a final review of all documents, the CFDA will, in case of success, grant market approval and list the device in its database. Foreign manufacturers will receive an *Import Medical Device Registration Certificate* (IMDRC), valid for 5 years. Some medical devices, in general those working with an electric current, require a *China Compulsory Certification*. This marking was introduced in 2003 and is highly comparable to CE marking in the EU. Approval of sale for a medical device in China gives access to a dynamic growing market of $357 billion in 2012 (5% of GDP) and that is expected to grow to $1.000 billion (7% of GDP) in 2020.

The regulatory landscape is still subject to a dynamic development, with a major revision of the regulations on *Supervision and Administration of Medical Devices* in 2014. This does outline China's ambition not to make a mere copy of existing Western systems but rather develop its own unique regulatory entity. Beyond cultural differences, this may induce issues during approval of medical devices as the assessment may vary even within the same agency. This may be interpreted by some as market protectionism, an impression frequently expressed when dealing with any highly regulated, foreign market. Since China became a full member of IMDRF in 2013, it actively participates in the effort to develop a worldwide universal standard for approval of medical devices.

With its considerable market power, and its expected development, this makes China one of the leading countries when it comes to influence on international regulatory standards that affect the medical device industry on national base. Setting and establishing new national and international standards usually give a competitive edge on both national and global markets. It is advisable closely observing the evolvement of China's MDR.

2.7 Medical Device Industry Goes Pharma?

2.7.1 Regulatory Issues

Although pharmaceuticals and medical devices have been essential tools for public health since their very first beginnings, both evolved with considerable differences in terms of regulations. First approaches to regulate pharmaceuticals can be found in sources as early as the classical antiquity. The oldest western world laws and regulations date back to the high middle age[5] and were consistently refined to the elaborated system of laws and regulations we encounter in today's industrialized countries. While the education and qualification of medical professional does exhibit a highly comparable history, regulations for tools and devices they apply were established considerably later with milestones like the US *Fair Packaging and Labeling Act* in 1966. As a result, the regulative boundary conditions for medical devices and pharmaceuticals are distinct and limited in interchangeability, although both play a vital role in the very same fields of modern medicine and health economy. When looking at the current trends in medical devices, the line to pharmaceuticals becomes more and more blurred. As state-of-the-art, established devices like coronary stents are coated with drugs to improve their biological activity, and biodegradable implants are used to store and locally distribute drugs, giving them the function as a drug delivery device. In parallel, pharmaceuticals that were traditionally distributed in glass ampoules or as tablets only are more and more often sold in ready-to-use application devices. Well-established examples can be found in prefilled syringes, giving the patient the opportunity for self-application beyond the attendance of a medical professional, as these are displayed in Figure 2.6. This is done for drugs like insulin to treat diabetes or heparin as an anticoagulant.

---

5. Among the first sources of the Western world are the "Consituations" decreed by Frederick II (Holy Roman Emperor) in Melfi 1231.

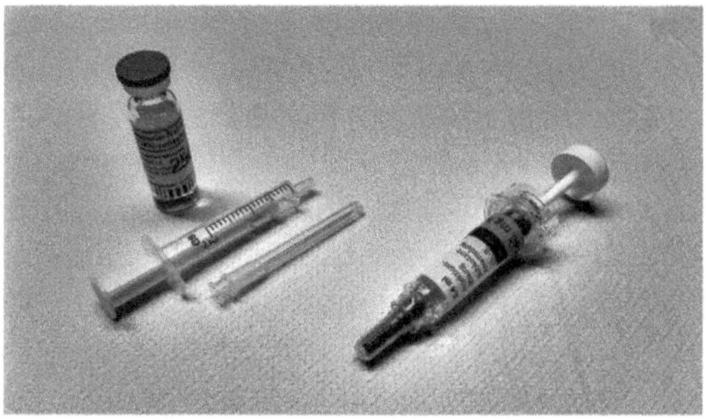

Figure 2.6 Same drug, two ways for distribution! Example for the convergence of medical devices and pharmaceuticals. Traditionally, drugs are distributed in ampoules and administered with a combination of syringe and hypodermic needle (medical devices), as these are displayed on the left. To simplify application, drugs frequently are provided in prefilled syringes combining all in one single product.

2.7.2 Combination Products

The merger of pharmaceuticals and medical device does open a wide range of new possibilities for therapeutical treatments but poses severe legal questions. Drugs are commonly defined as chemical in nature and are intended to interact with metabolic processes within the human body. Although very complex in development, their production and application follows well-established procedures and commonly are administered as pills, powders, or liquids (via injection). In contrast, medical devices rely by-and-large on a physical interaction with the human body and thus their design and way of application usually is determined by its intended use. Further, differing from administering a drug the application of a medical device frequently is highly dependent on training of the operator and its manual skills. This is why their respective process for market approval does follow different methods and in consequence does exhibit distinct differences.

Regulatory authorities did addressed this aspect by creating the term combination product. An accurate definition can be found in **US** 21 CFR 3.2(e) stating that combination products are therapeutics and diagnostics that combine two or more regulated products such as drugs, devices, and/or biological products. This does include two or more separate products packaged together in a single package or as a unit and comprised of drug and device products, device and biological products, or biological and drug products. As these components normally would be regulated under three different regulatory authorities (CDER, CBER, or

CDRH), they raise challenges concerning regulation, legislation, process of approval, and legal liability. One of the three health agency's evaluation centers for human medical products performs approval, while the others will be counseling. Since its creation, the first port of call is the Office for Combination Products. Anyhow, key properties for evaluation will be the Primary Mode of Action. The understanding of the **EU** competent authorities slightly differs, as well as terminology—and this may lead to confusions. A mixture of two different pharmaceutical substances in a single formulation is defined as fixed combination medicinal product, although no medical device is involved. Hence, the following resume will cover only those combining a medical device (as defined in Section 1.2.1) with a pharmaceutical. These are classified in three different manifestations. In case of a drug delivery device, used to administer a pharmaceutical, both are regulated under the respective legal provisions. If both form a single integral product intended for application in a given combination, it will be regarded as pharmaceutical, whereas it is a device if the medicinal action is ancillary only. As the term ancillary leaves room for interpretation, the definition of combination product within the EU sometimes is challenging. Still, medical devices feature a chemical substance as integral mode of action, but still are not considered as combination product.

2.7.3 In Vitro Diagnostic Devices as Special Case

A very prominent representative for this aspect can be seen in devices and systems that are summed up in a category labeled IVDs. The term in general does describe devices designed to perform diagnostics by analyzing a biological specimen, taken from the patient, in an artificial laboratory environment. As specimen may serve, any material harvested from the body and thus can range from tissue to any kind of body fluid (blood, sweat, urine, etc.). That way one gets a look into molecular–biological processes within a living body like through a window, what does explain the name, as in vitro is Latin for "in glass" and does refer to general laboratory work with glassy test tubes. Generally spoken, IVDs are utilized to gain information about

- physiological and pathophysiological processes within the living body

  For example, pregnancy test, blood gas analysis, or measuring blood sugar.

- derive and supervise therapeutic actions

  For example, verifying the physical presence of defined bacteria or viruses, controlling drug levels or determining metabolic panel.

- potential contraindications for considered actions

  For example, testing antibiotic resistance, determining blood type, or checking drug abuse.

IVDs have found broad applications for several decades within and beyond clinical environments like test strips to determine the blood type, measure blood sugar, check on pregnancy (application at home), and test on drug abuse (used in traffic controls). In Figure 2.7 some examples of those are displayed. Many of those systems are utilized by medical professionals for a quick analysis near the site of the patient, and thus are known as **bedside testing**, **point-of-care testing** (POCT), or **rapid diagnostic test** (**RDT**).

However, more complex examinations, like PCR-based verification on the physical existence of defined bacteria, regarding a potential antibiotic resistance of them still often are performed in an external biochemical laboratory, a time and money-consuming step. By automatically performing more complex and/or sequential processes, today's IVD devices enable medical professionals to analyze more and more elaborate aspects in less time and at reduced costs without involving a third party. Future developments will see interesting developments presented in Section 6.2.

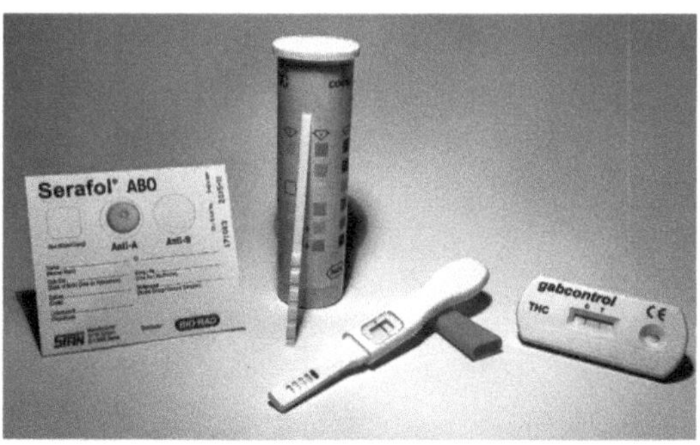

Figure 2.7 Examples of devices for bed-side testing, point-of-care testing (POCT), or rapid diagnostic tests (RDTs) that basically all are in vitro diagnostics (IVDs). From left to right: kit for determining blood type, test strips to analyze urine on the presence of sugar and ketones, pregnancy test for home application, test kit for checking on drug abuse as frequently utilized by the police. IVDs are not really new but rather found broad application within the clinical environment and beyond.

Sticking point is the fact that these devices necessarily imply the use of reagents that are by definition chemical in nature. This clearly does distinguish IVDs from classical medical devices as these commonly are defined as being physical in mode of action. On the other hand, IVDs do not directly influence the living body chemically, as the nature of pharmaceuticals commonly is defined, making them somehow a hybrid between medical devices and drugs. Most regulatory *authorities* asses IVDs as medical devices but enact additional regulations, like *98/79/EC* for the EU, defined parts of 21 CFR for the United States (parts 809, 862, 864, and 866) or *Administrative Order No. 5* for China. The amendment to the EU MDD (see Section 2.4.4) does reflect these aspects and consequently does involve the creation of a regulation labeled "In vitro diagnostic medical devices" 2012/0267(COD).

3 Design of Plastic Medical Devices

OUTLINE

Designing processes of plastic medical devices underlay the comparable regulatory demands as manufacturing processes. The actual functional design of these devices must comply with general engineering standards on the one hand plus specific medical device standards on the other hand. Hence, an old-school hands-on engineering approach is not suitable for medical devices. The design process itself has to be implemented within prior-defined product development process, which works with accepted methodical standards and includes

Emerging Trends in Medical Plastic Engineering and Manufacturing
http://dx.doi.org/10.1016/B978-0-323-37023-3.00003-8

the specific regulatory requirements for medical devices. Therefore, the whole product development process must be embedded into quality- and risk management systems as well as the applied manufacturing processes within medical device companies. The product development process, beginning with a product idea and up to series maturity, includes design phases, review phases, and risk analysis. The risk analysis is essential for medical devices and far-reaching: For example, imaginable and foreseeable misuses have to be considered and evaluated regarding risk occurrence probability and occurrence effects (as explained in Section 2.3.7). Many young engineers think about biomedical engineering as an ongoing designing, creation, and testing life, but regulatory affairs have an enormous impact on the actual engineering life, to be honest. Each major development step should be evaluated with generally accepted and comprehensible methods by an evaluation team, which has to approve each previously defined step within the quality management system finally. Similar product development, testing, and evaluation approaches are or should be implemented in most engineering fields (e.g., automotive or aerospace), but within the biomedical engineering business it is a general requirement, which has to be considered for each design or development of a medical device with the aim to reach market approval.

Legislatures, industry, and standardization organizations have developed a variety of measures, standards, or approaches to comply with the complex situation interacting with the human body (see Section 2.1), which actually helps current and future plastic medical device engineers during the development. The first step is to recognize the necessity of these approaches to reach the highest protection level for treated patients as reasonable as possible, beginning with a structured design and development process and ending with a validated manufacturing and packaging. The upcoming sections should give a quick introduction, how a product development process for plastic medical devices may look alike, which aspects are comparable to other engineering fields and which are unique for plastic medical devices, and which emerging influences may arise for future designing of plastic medical devices.

3.1 Product Development Process

The actual product development process for medical devices should be comparable to state-of-the-art product development processes within each engineering field. A classic hands-on engineering procedure, which bases mainly on the creativity and experience of engineers without methodical approaches, is not suitable for the development of medical devices. For medical devices, many different requirements may arise depending on the intended functionality, duration, and location of use. Class III medical devices (highest risk class, e.g., active implants) have to comply with more requirements than class I, but each device has its own specific requirements, which arise from existing legislations, standards, medical conditions, users' wishes, etc. Without a suitable, controllable, and evaluable product development process, medical devices may have implemented risks or malfunctions, which may lead to severe harm to operators and/or patients. As you see, it is not only important to ensure functioning quality and risk management systems within the production of plastic medical devices, but also within the design and testing phase as well.

But how to comply with the demanded quality and risk management demands may vary from jurisdiction to jurisdiction, but the major approaches are broadly interpreted risk analysis, which includes foreseeable misuses that not only should be addressed by mentioning their existence with an instruction manual warning. The goal is to achieve the best protection of patients and operators beginning already during the product development process.

With the upcoming subsection, we want to give an example how methodical engineering can be used as the base for complying with the general arising requirements for product development processes. We decided to work and explain the necessity and benefit of structured engineering with a recommended model for a so-called **technical file** or **design dossier** for medical devices, as these are state of the art within the European Union. Each jurisdiction may have slightly different demands, but the general meaning is the same. For the sake of completeness, a technical file or design dossier is called a **master file for devices** by the FDA.

Please be aware that requirements are subject to change by legislations and varying interpretations of existing standards and laws. It is our aim to give an introduction, how it may be suitable to establish working product development process, but we cannot give a fully working model for any product development for medical devices. Particular details may also be different for any type of medical devices, from electronic, mechanical, or software based.

3.1.1 Methodical Approaches

Technical files or design dossier, the actual wording depends on the applicable medical device risk class,[1] have to fulfill the notified bodies need to be able to evaluate the actual deriving risks of a medical device. Besides the

---

1. A technical file will be called design dossier within the European Union, if the described medical device requires a design examination based on the applicable medical device class for that product.

design process, including evaluation approaches and design histories, it is necessary to comply at least with the current state of the art to achieve standard conformity prior market approval within the European Union.

Within Table 3.1, a recommended style of such a design dossier is shown. Part A can be considered a quick overview of the actual device,

Table 3.1 Example Style Format for a Technical File or Design Dossier for the Approval Process of Medical Devices, Which Is Based on the Recommendations of the Global Harmonization Task Force and Has Been Adopted by Notified Bodies within the European Union

- Part A: Technical File/Design Dossier
  - Table of Content
  - Introduction
  - Design Dossier/Technical File Summary Information
- Part B: Annexes
  - Essential Requirements Checklist
  - Risk Analysis
  - Drawings, Design and Product Specifications
  - Chemical, Physical, and Biological Tests
    - In Vitro Testing—Preclinical Studies
    - In Vivo Testing—Preclinical Studies
    - Biocompatibility Tests
    - Biostability Tests
    - Microbiological Safety, Animal Origin Tissue
    - Drug/medical device combination
    - Blood Derivates, Human Tissue/medical device combination
    - Coated Medical Devices
  - Clinical Data
  - Labels and Instructions for Use
  - Manufacturing
  - Package Qualification and Shelf life
  - Sterilization
  - Conclusion
  - Declaration of Conformity (Draft)

the applied testing methods and standards, which are described more exactly within part B. The presented structure does not show the necessity to comply with generally acknowledged standards like ISO 13485, 10993, or 14971, (respectively 21CFR820 for the US) but it is definitely easier to argue conclusively and being accepted by notified bodies within the European Union, or other approval authorities, respectively. However, as already stated in previous chapters, the FDA offers its own guidelines, which generally may be comparable with standards, but differ in details. Working with a technical file it does not mean to comply with additionally deriving aspects from quality and risk management. You should see the technical file as the summary of your actual work, which should be as wide and exact as reasonable as possible to prove that you ensured the quality required and lowest risk possible of a newly approved medical device.

3.1.1.1 Methodical Demands by Quality and Risk Management

Quality and risk aspects have to be considered as early as within the product designing and development process. Many manufacturers as component suppliers advertise with implemented ISO 13485 and 14971 procedures, however, the aspects of product development may be excluded often.[2] Therefore, outsourced development and designing processes may be evaluated, validated, and verified additionally by the ordering party to comply with the evolving needs by quality and risk management, if the contracted company does not work according to accepted quality and risk management standards.

The current Chapter 7 of the ISO 13485 standard is structured as follows:

- Planning of product realization,
- Customer-related processes (customer requirements and communication),
- Design and development,
- Purchasing (supplier evaluation and verification),
- Production and service provision,
- Control of monitoring and measuring devices.

---

2. Within ISO 13485 as well as 21 CFR 820 regulation, it only is necessary to comply with those parts that are found to be relevant for the medical device quality. In consequence, many EU-based companies that only produce devices as contractor exclude Chapter 7 ("product realization") from certification.

The upcoming sections are focusing on the aspects of design and development and may help to understand the arising needs for the actual product development of plastic medical devices. As you have read already in the previous Section 2.4.3, the ISO 13485 standard is currently under review and a final update version is expected to be approved in 2015 or 2016. The update will clarify misinterpreted points, but it will be widely comparable with the current version. However, a major addition is the aspect of design transfer, which means the introduction and observation of transfer processes from the R & D department to the manufacturing entity of a medical device. Regarding the design and development requirements, it is and will be necessary to implement a working and documented process, which includes following points among others:

- Design and development steps with their own evaluation procedures, including defined management roles and documentation,
- Establishing, evaluating, and approving a list of requirements for the new or updated plastic medical device, possible sources are the following:
  - Intended use,
  - Arising topics by risk evaluation measures,
  - Costumer/patient needs,
  - Legislations and generally approved standards (e.g., biocompatibility),
  - Medical device classification,
  - Company and (future) product-related aspects (e.g., size, manufacturing, and marketing).
- Design and development verification,[3]
- Design and development validation.[4]

Each entity, which develops and markets medical devices, has to adopt working processes, which comply with the mentioned requirements for the quality and risk management during the product realization process. However, the actual entitled process can (and usually does) differ from entity to entity due to different management structures, evaluation approaches, and additional issues, which are addressed variously, like marketing, strategic, or financial evaluation aspects. A partial example process is shown in chart Figure 3.1.

---

3. Verification can be explained in this context as acceptable measures to confirm that the design and development results comply with the list of requirements (see Section 2.3.8).
4. Validation can be explained in this context as acceptable measures to confirm that the designed and developed (plastic) medical device fulfill the arising requirements of the previously defined intended use or application (see Section 2.3.8).

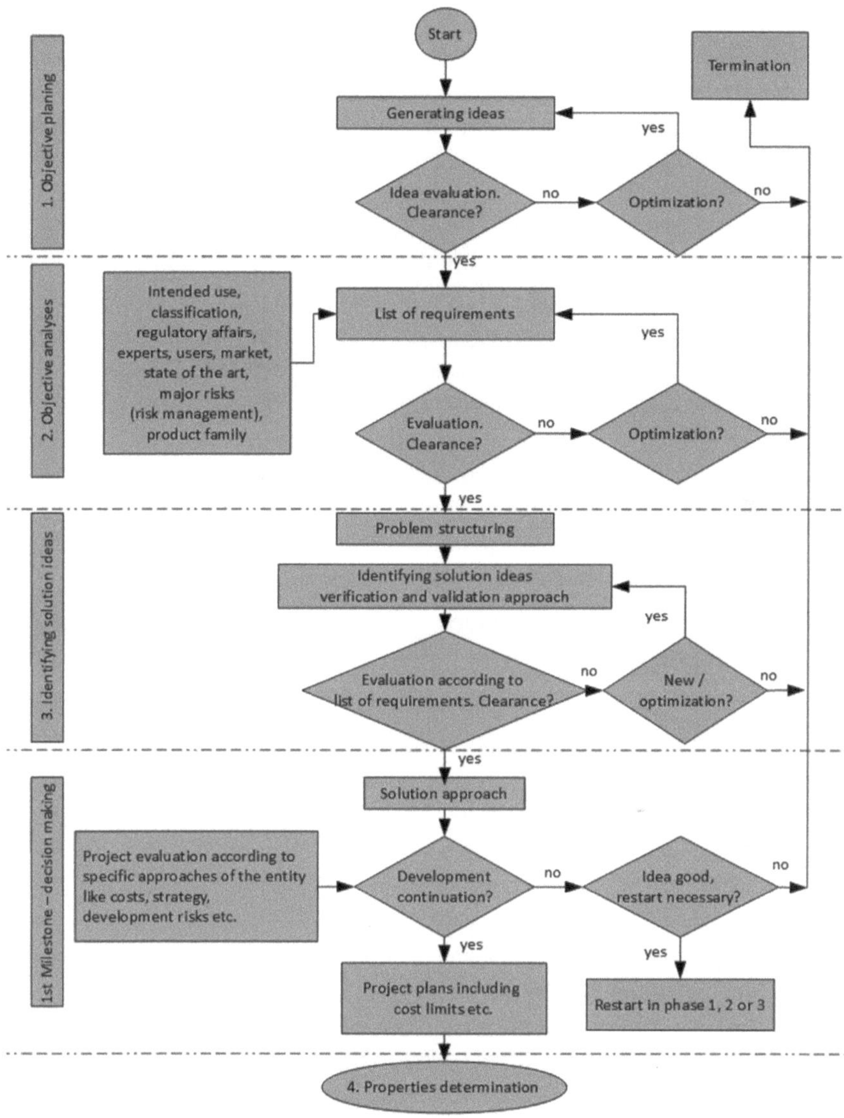

Figure 3.1 Example (section) of an operating procedure during development of a new medical device based on the requirements of ISO 13485 and fitted into product development workflow called the Munich Procedure Model, which is described within the next subsection.

You may have similar thought about such theoretic processes we had before working with it regularly: How can it be transferred within the actual engineering work during product design and development? Simply spoken, each aspect has to be translated into workable procedures and supporting documents, often implemented in some sort of product data management (PDM) tools,[5] which should guide the actual product development procedures by the assigned engineers without inhibiting their creativity. Many engineers have certain negative feelings about structured development processes. Sometimes, especially in start-ups or other smaller companies, the development process of novel (plastic) medical devices follows no structured procedure, as quickly as described previously, during the R & D period.

This unfortunate approach leads to subsequent enormous paper work, which has to be done without having actual benefits by working structured during the product development. The challenge is to implement a generally accepted system, which supports the engineering process and emphasizes the advantages without bothering the creativity and engineering potential too much. Think about the following aspects for you as engineer by working with such a system consequently:

- Avoiding cost-intensive product design changes due to missed requirements or subsequent risk management considerations,
- Evaluation steps may replace lonely decision-making process by team-oriented approaches,
- Clear development procedures lead to less misunderstanding between various engineering groups, often implemented during complex medical device developments,
- Detailed information about the product and its development, which helps to improve future developments by identifying additional requirements or possible challenges quicker.

A possible approach is to work with generally known product development processes, which are suitable and widely used in many fields of product engineering, and implement specific tasks arising by the medical device industry due to its regulatory boundaries. Many methods have been developed like V-model, lean product development, design for six sigma, or quality function deployment. All in common is to structure the actual product development, beginning with the more chaotic idea phase, over evaluation approaches, up to a final and approved product design, which is ready to manufacture.

---

5. PDM-software solutes, which are often linked with CAD-tools, help to manage, perform, and evaluate product development processes digitally. Often are necessary product development steps implemented, which have to be approved accordingly to the implemented quality and risk management system. However, if these are utilized, it is necessary to consider the regulation 21 CFR 11 (see Section 2.3.9).

In the next section, we choose a methodical approach, called the **Munich Procedure Model,**[6] which is based on the idea of using procedural patterns and works with rule-based and predictable methods to engage goal-orientated product development. Each described development step is backed by specific methods for generating ideas, analyses, and so on (described more deeply and fitted into the medical device world next).

3.1.1.2 Structured Engineering Approach to Fulfill Arising Demands

The overall mix of complying with the needs of technical files, quality, and risk management requires to ensure a structured engineering approach to avoid time-consuming (for ironing out) failures or forgotten aspects during the medical device design and development process, ending with the needs of the manufacturing process (the transition from product development to manufacturing is described in a separate, upcoming chapter). It is possible to work and comply simply with the arising demands, but it may be helpful to encounter these needs by adopting a more general structured engineering approach, often referred as methods for product development. These approaches can be fitted to comply with technical file, risk and quality management demands, plus help to ensure to find, evaluate and determine technical solutions in more comprehensible and probably innovative ways. As mentioned above, the methodical approach of the **Munich Procedure Model** is used to explain how to implement the requirements by laws and standards for the medical device development process into a structured product development system, which helps to encounter the overall problem including the specific tasks for (plastic) medical devices. The upcoming seven bullet points are the major steps during this approach. Each step can be addressed by applying workable and useful methodical tools, which are also suitable with minor updates for medical device developments. It is important to mention that these seven steps must not be followed in the listed order, it may be suitable to encounter steps more than once (e.g., decision-making or objective analyses).

3.1.1.2.1 Objective Planning

Aim:

Methodical approaches for identifying evolving development opportunities (let's call it ideas) by observing the needs of markets and

6. Derived from the better-known German expression *Münchner Vorgehensmodell.*

customers and comparing it to technical possibilities and/or existing products of the entity.

Applicable Methods:

Portfolio analysis, SWOT-analysis, trend analysis, scenario technique

Characteristic for Medical Devices:

In contrast to typical end-consumer markets, medical devices have to offer advantages not only to the actual customer (e.g., health-care facility or operator), but also to the patients, who may benefit from future developments. Therefore, it is helpful to address arising needs by observing trends within health-related aspects, which can be emerging regulatory challenges as well as emerging market chances (e.g., from standard surgical devices to minimal invasive devices) or upcoming financial restriction by the reimbursement systems.

3.1.1.2.2 Objective Analyses

Aim:

After developing first ideas, it is necessary to analyze the arising requirements for such an idea. An objective analysis is the base for the creation of a detailed list of requirements, which helps to address every necessary (e.g., demanded legal requirements, state-of-the-art considerations, applicability within existing environments) and desirable factors (e.g., ergonomic aspects, manufacturing opportunities).

Applicable Methods:

Requirement checklists, question techniques with experts, customers or any related persons, structuring techniques

Characteristic for Medical Devices:

The step objective analyses fit perfectly to address additionally the arising demands by quality and risk managements, intended use, and other medical device-specific requirements. Therefore, it may be helpful to supplement generally available requirement checklists with these specific topics to ensure far-reaching analyses as possible. The objective analyses should be updated regularly during the whole product development step (e.g., after meeting certain milestones) to comply with quality and risk management (think about the aspects of foreseeable misuse, which may evolve) on the one hand and to fulfill customer's need to the best way possible on the other hand. It is essential not only to update the list of requirements regularly, but also to evaluate and approve it by an authorized staff council, which leads us to step 6, decision-making, which is an aspect, which have to be addressed more regularly for medical device development to comply with the demands by the quality management (e.g., ISO 13485).

3.1.1.2.3 Problem Structuring

Aim:

After identifying an idea and establishing a list of requirements, structuring the problem helps to identify the major development aspects and the correlation between the single topics to gain a first theoretical model of the actual "problem," which is better explained as an idea with existing requirements but without an existing solution. A general "problem" should be separated in easier to solve partial problems, which can be picked up during step 4, identifying solution ideas.

Applicable Methods:

Relation-based function modeling, degree of freedom analyses, action planning, connection matrix in combination with the results of SWOT analyses, problem formulation

Characteristic for Medical Devices:

The problem structuring should be conducted by specifically addressing not only technical problems, but biological (see Section 2.1) and operator or patient problems as well. It helps to gain an interaction model to recognize possible correlations between these problems to avoid wrong guiding priorities.

3.1.1.2.4 Identifying Solution Ideas

Aim:

With step 4, identifying solution ideas, it is the aim to translate a structured problem ("idea") into possible technical solutions. This step is followed by the actual constructions and designing step, which is performed in step 5, properties determination. It is helpful to use the previously gained structure to provide partial solution ideas, which can be combined to an overall solution idea by using morphological boxes or similar evaluation criteria.

Applicable Methods:

Checklists, construction catalog, brain storming, bionic, effect collection, basic principle to resolve technical contradictions, morphological box, systemic variation

Characteristic for Medical Devices:

The aspect of identifying (partial) solutions can be supported by using bionic or effect collection, which are based on biological systems. Especially for medical devices, some aspects derived from natural approaches seem helpful to achieve better medical devices (e.g., specific surface variation, antimicrobial characteristics, lightweight structures, flow optimized cannula, or surfaces). Checklists, construction catalogs, and other basic principles help to address arising risks and requirements with at least state-of-the-art solutions, which should be used at least to address risk and quality management properly. This step should be completed by identifying necessary verification and validation methods to address the aspects of the upcoming step 5, properties determination, successfully. Before entering the actual construction, design and testing step 5, an evaluation of the identified partial ideas (according to step 6) should be performed and the most promising one (or more if it is not clear enough before step 5, which approach may proceed) may enter the next step.

3.1.1.2.5 Properties Determination

Aim:

The properties determination step is subsequent to identifying solution ideas and may be mixed together, however, during these step hard facts about the characteristics of the new medical device are determined by actual experiments or simulations. The results support the product designing, dimensioning, and material selection. Simply spoken, step 5 is the actual product engineering, how it is often expected or understood by new R & D engineers. As you know, it is a frequent problem that product development is started with this step right away, neglecting the previous steps of structured approach. However, as explained, doing so is prone to errors resulting from overlooked regulatory, technical, or biomedical boundary conditions. Step 5 can be supported by applicable methods to ensure a correct dimension, to avoid overburden experimental setups or simulations before the final design determination. It has to be considered state of the art and almost not worth mentioning that the designing process arises from CAD systems.

Applicable Methods:

Method of estimating and comparing, analytic computations, numerical simulations, empirically orientated experiments including design of experiments, rapid prototyping, plausibility analyses, checklists (property lists) deriving from list of requirements, similarity analyses

Characteristic for Medical Devices:

For medical devices, valid legal measures or standards demand regularly the properties determination based on any kind of computations on the one hand, but also on comparing with existing medical device products and its design, materials and manufacturing, and subsequent actual experimental testing regarding biological, hygienic, aging, or safety effects on the other hand. Existing experiences[7] are crucial for the (plastic) medical device development process in regard to product characteristic determination and product market approval. Design and development verification and validation are specific requirements for the actual properties of a newly developed medical device derived from the ISO 13485 standard among other measures. It is crucial to determine the whole set of properties (also in regard of a significant risk analysis) of a medical device and the actual deriving benefit (if the set goals are met). When using a CAD system to electronically document the history of design development, you must consider the regulation 21 CFR 11 (see Section 2.3.9).

3.1.1.2.6 Decision-Making

Aim:

Decision-making steps should be implemented at every major development step to ensure consequent development efforts complying with strategic goals of the actual R & D department and management level. Especially in

7. In the medical device context, experience for incalculable characteristics (like biocompatibility, sterilization behavior, or general aging effects) may be derived from research publications, market-approved medical devices, or actual experimental setups.

owner-led and small companies, the well-known gut instinct decision-making process is applied regularly and does work often; otherwise, the success of many of such engineering companies are not explainable. With an implemented decision-making procedure, comparability and traceability of development projects are easier done and approvable by (internal) reviews. Explicit methods may also help to crystallize comprehensible decisions how to proceed at certain product development steps, where crystal clear yes or no situations are not suitable due to the variety of factors to consider.

Applicable Methods:

Initial selection, selection list, point rating system, impact matrix (with weighting factors), goal preference matrix, cost–benefit analyses

Characteristic for Medical Devices:

Current standards and regulatory measures demand a comprehensible decision-making process to ensure strict clearance procedures to address deriving needs by risk analyses, biological interactions, or any kind of specific requirement adequately. The decision-making process has to be documented and approved correctly for actual market approval procedures, how it can be seen within technical files or design dossiers. Clear decision-making process helps to work with risk and cost–benefit analyses for new medical devices and vice versa.

3.1.1.2.7 Objective Achievement Protection

Aim:

Simply spoken, objective achievement protection can be translated into an applied and working risk and quality management.

Applicable Methods:

Cause–effect analyses, fault tree analyses, failure checklists, failure mode and effect analyses

Characteristic for Medical Devices:

The full application of the ISO 14971 standard for risk management within the medical device industry covers the aspect of objective achievement protection. The standard is accepted mostly and is often considered the state of the art of risk management within the whole engineering society. Although the FDA does not directly recommend ISO 14971, its understanding of risk management is highly comparable (see Section 2.3.7). In contrast to many engineering fields, a consequent performed risk management is inevitable for medical device developments. The previously described applicable methods can be found all in a certain extent within the requirements and recommendations of the ISO 14971 standard.

Methodical approaches applied during product development may help to ensure more structured, stable, and timely engineering, especially for more complex medical devices or teams with more than one person. However, such approaches have to be filled with life to achieve the presented advantages. Simply spoken: An introduced development procedure is only as good as the acceptance of the working engineers. For medical device approval processes, it is a no brainer to enact some sort of methodical development due to the deriving minimum requirements from standards or measures like ISO 13485. Therefore, an overall structured and supportive system is absolutely reasonable.

So-called innovative problem-solving methods are used to think one step ahead already: How to address a more coordinated and supported generation of new product ideas or solving of deriving problems. These techniques are relatively less known within the engineering community, but properly enacted they help to channel ideas on the one hand and to open new solution options on the other hand. Examples are the matrix of contradictions or substance field analysis, which are part of the theory of inventive problem solving (e.g., the TRIZ methods). Due to the highly interesting effects, we address this topic in an extra section, Section 3.2.5, as part of emerging influences for plastic medical device design.

3.1.2 Specific Requirements for Plastic Medical Devices

The previously introduced product development process and the deriving opportunities by methodical development approaches can be applied for medical devices in general, but naturally for plastic medical devices as well. Standard requirement lists for standard industrial devices do not fit perfectly into the scheme for the development of medical devices. Medical applications cause additional needs, which have to be complied with. On the one hand, the intended use of a medical device should have an enormous interest into a really good benefit-to-risk ratio to ensure the highest patient and operator safety as possible. The specific requirements can be summarized under the aspect **patient and operator protection**, which leads to following considerable needs:

- Unpolluted, decontaminated, or sterile products depending on the intended use,
- Acceptable form of biological response to product surface and its physicochemical nature,
- Identified and solved (as many and wide as possible) application risks.

These demands are the reason, why within the medical device industry considerable risk and quality management methods have been developed and standardized. Therefore, the medical device industry may be interpreted as a strict engineering field regarding the development procedure and deriving requirements and challenges, however, the modern understanding of structured development procedures with the ability to validate and verify the results are used widely in many engineering companies to ensure predictable product developments with the adequate triad of risk, quality, and functionality.

The introduced three needs for patient and operator protection imply additional requirements for plastics, which are manufactured and applied for medical devices. They can cause additional hurdles especially for polymers and shrink the applicable plastic materials widely.

The chemical industry has addressed these specific requirements for plastics used in medical devices by introducing polymer types named **medical grade**. Interestingly, the expression medical grade is not protected by certain standards or measures, which have to be complied with. Therefore, the actual medical grade polymers can differ widely with their granted-specific characteristics for medical device application. Following aspects should be addressed by the chemical manufacturer of medical grade plastics, but are not consequently:

- Long-term market availability and adequate change policy plus timely market notice

  Renewing the manufactured material specification or altering its way of synthesis may cause enormous trouble for medical device manufacturer. To update the material, it is necessary to reevaluate each linked step of the product development step and subsequently start validating and verifying the medical device properties. Depending on the device complexity, a material change leads to several months up to years of work until the change of a material in a medical device can be fulfilled properly.

A material change can be pushed by the medical device manufacturer itself, but the more common fact is a significant change of the chemical recipe or complete taking off the market of plastic materials by the chemical company. A major need by the medical device industry to receive a market notice as early as possible by manufacturers of medical grade graded plastic materials. Common expectation is a market notice of a significant change[8] of the polymer material 3 years prior the actual change takes place. Many polymer companies work with this period for medical grade plastics. It causes an enormous hurdle for a recipe change on the one hand, but a major change of chemical facility itself is definitely more demanding. Therefore, it should be not a big deal for chemical companies to introduce a working market notice system.

- Biocompatibility evaluation of plastic raw materials:

  Surely, biocompatibility depends on many factors like the material itself, the processing procedure and the medical device shape as well (see Section 2.2). Medical grade advertised plastic raw materials should be evaluated due to their biological interaction to a certain extent, however. Unfortunately, it is a common practice to reevaluate the material selection during a product development process for plastic medical devices due to unexpected biological material behavior even for previously positive tested types. But, a positive test result for the biological results of the raw material (besides your own experience with your own products) can be interpreted as the best hint you can get in regard of biocompatibility. More general, forecasts are not available and probably will not be soon. Bringing all the facts together, a minimum amount of biological testing should be done by the chemical manufacturers before using the expression of medical grade.

- Usage of unobjectionable ingredients in plastic raw materials for human applications:

8. What does significant mean in the context of a recipe change regarding the application and market approval of plastic medical devices? A plausible explanation can be done by using arguments of the ISO 10993 standard. The ISO 10993 standard describes approaches to evaluate the biocompatibility of medical devices depending on the intended use. Within these standards, it is defined how a material has to or should be evaluated (e.g., by comparing with state of the art or certain levels of experimental testing) for market approval. The ISO 10993 standard can be used for evaluating a change of a material manufacturing recipe due to its significance. However, many minor changes that happen in secret are not easy to be identified by the medical device manufacturers. Sometimes, deriving effects attract attention by necessary changes within the processing (like injection molding), but many times changes hardly may be detected.

We are always talking about processing of raw materials during the manufacturing of plastic medical devices. These plastics have to be manufactured in chemical reactions using many different ingredients. In addition to the standard backbone ingredients, so-called additives are added, which are applied to achieve certain characteristics of a polymer material. This can be softening agents, stabilizers (see Section 2.1), or even antimicrobial substances (see Section 5.3 for more details). Some regularly used additives have a biological origin, which is too risky for medical application for sure. But, some additives may also cause toxic reaction or other negative biological interaction. Many general behaviors are already well-known for single ingredients. These should be avoided for medical grade polymers. Surely, the combination of ingredients leads in many cases to toxic behavior as well, but toxic behavior of additives, which are often only partially chemically bonded within polymer chains, are not acceptable for medical grade polymers.

- Disinfectant and sterilization agent stability:

  Most plastic medical devices have to undergo some sort of hygienic processing prior application. Depending on the intended use, disinfectants or even sterilization procedures have to be performed. Most of these methods can be considered relatively aggressive regarding materials in general. Therefore, they induce some degree of aging in many cases within polymer materials, which is why the material manufacturers usually add compounds for material stabilization during sterilization. There is definitely no plastic material, which does not show any kind of aging for all available disinfection or sterilization procedures. Even the often praised polyetheretherketone (PEEK) can be degraded by high-energetic gamma radiation at a certain level. The question is not, if there is any aging, the question is, is the amount of aging acceptable for the intended use? Advertised medical grade polymers should have the option to be sterilized or disinfectant with at least one market available procedure.

The medical grade label offers a first hint for plastic medical device engineers about a general suitability of a certain material, but it cannot replace a specific material selection and evaluation procedure, a process called **materials selection**.

3.1.2.1 Materials Selection

Plastic medical devices can be and are made with a countless number of market available materials. It is often not easy to choose the best fitting plastic material just due to the huge amount of possibilities. Material selection depends on intended use of the device, process ability, and availability. Nevertheless, it can be broken into following aspects.

3.1.2.1.1 Technical Aspects

Although subject to many different requirements arising from biology and regulations, the selected material must comply with the technical boundary conditions resulting from its application. This may sound like a no brainer, but there is a risk that developing team distressed by complex medical aspects simply does neglect the basic engineering principles for material selection that are valid for medical devices, too. Therefore, you should at least consider:

- Appropriate **material parameters**, such as ultimate tensile strength or fatigue limit. This also may include the haptic perception of the material.
- Adequate **thermal stability**, especially for reusable medical devices, as these frequently are sterilized with hot steam or air. Thereby, the combination of heat and humidity usually induces an accelerated material aging.
- Especially **aggressive ambient media**, such as blood, sweat, urine, or disinfectants may significantly impair the materials properties during medical device application and thus should be considered thoroughly during material selection.
- Many medical devices are subjected to a **process of sterilization** prior application. Any sterilization will have impact on the material properties, especially the most frequently utilized sterilization with hot steam (autoclaving) or exposition to ionizing radiation (e.g., γ-radiation). Both will induce aging processes and may generate degradation products that are toxic to the human body.

3.1.2.1.2 Biological Aspects

The requirements to the material selection arising from the application within a biological system are presented more detailed within Sections 2.1 and 2.2. Therefore, you will find here a short listing only.

- **Biocompatibility**, biological safety, and (non)toxicity
- **Positive biological evaluation**, e.g., using USP (see Section 2.3.1) or ISO 10993 (see Section 2.3.4)

- Appropriate **material stability** within the biological system
- The **designated market** may influence the material selection as well, as the academic school of thought concerning the selection of biomaterials may vary from country to country.

3.1.2.1.3 Regulatory Aspects

As any action of medical device development, selecting the appropriate material must be compliant to the relevant rules and regulations. As you can imagine, this does include among others a risk management process for material selection and adequate biological evaluation. Moreover, it is legal requirement for any manufacturer to monitor the entire supply chain for its products, starting from raw materials to its decomposition after use. Thereby, it is strongly recommended to contractually assure that the supplier of the plastic material is aware of its intended utilization for a medical device. The agreement should include the following:

- **Approval** by the plastic manufacturer about knowing the application for a medical device
- A **quality assurance agreement**
- **Guarantee** for material availability and suitability

Most of these aspects are included, among other additional services and consents, as package when purchasing a **medical grade material**. Even more, many material suppliers try to proactively reduce risks that may result from legal liability if a medical device basing on their material fails in field. In consequence, when requesting a quote for a medical grade material, as first step you frequently will receive a form as part of the process of risk management performed by the material manufacturer. It is worth mentioning that although providing medical grade materials, material suppliers seldom are certified by ISO 13485 or fully comply with 21 CFR 820. After submitting the completed request form, the material manufacturer will perform a risk assessment of your intended application and eventually approve or disapprove your application. In case of disapproval, the manufacturer will refuse to sell any material. Moreover, even if the material was found to be appropriate during mechanical and biological evaluation, a disapproval of the intended application of the material eliminates the material as possible choice. Just imagine the device fails and during the legal review it is found, the material supplier disapproved upon application of its material. So, medical request forms, as displayed in Figure 3.2 are an emerging aspect during material selection for medical devices.

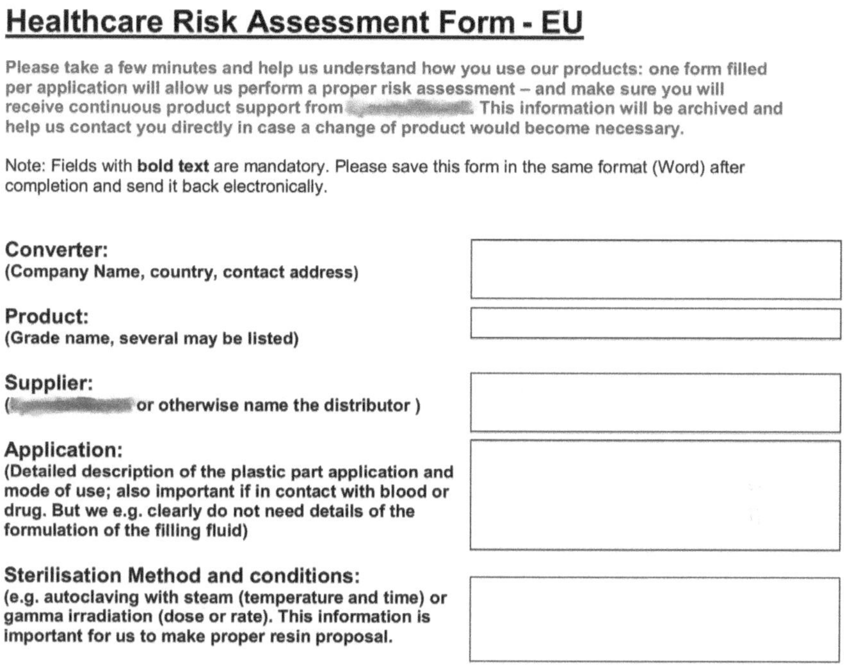

Healthcare Risk Assessment Form - EU

Please take a few minutes and help us understand how you use our products: one form filled per application will allow us perform a proper risk assessment – and make sure you will receive continuous product support from [redacted]. This information will be archived and help us contact you directly in case a change of product would become necessary.

Note: Fields with **bold text** are mandatory. Please save this form in the same format (Word) after completion and send it back electronically.

Converter:
(Company Name, country, contact address)

Product:
(Grade name, several may be listed)

Supplier:
([redacted] or otherwise name the distributor)

Application:
(Detailed description of the plastic part application and mode of use; also important if in contact with blood or drug. But we e.g. clearly do not need details of the formulation of the filling fluid)

Sterilisation Method and conditions:
(e.g. autoclaving with steam (temperature and time) or gamma irradiation (dose or rate). This information is important for us to make proper resin proposal.

Figure 3.2 Example of a medical request form as utilized by many material suppliers when trading medical grade plastics. The request form is intended to document consent upon the intended utilization of the materials for a specific medical device. An internal risk assessment performed by the materials supplier will result either in approval or disapproval of the request.

3.1.2.1.4 Commercial Aspects

Although usually at less extent compared to consumer products or home appliance, material costs are relevant for material selection for medical devices as well. For devices that are either complex and/or assembled from many subcomponents, the material price sometimes plays a subordinated role. But for many single-use devices purchasing the raw material contributes to the production costs at double-digit rates. Additionally, the material selection may have significant impact on processing and manufacturing costs. For example, PEEK exhibits superior mechanical properties and shows high biocompatibility for close to any applications, but may not be processed by standard machinery for plastic converting due to its melting temperature of about 300 °C (572 °F). A comparable correlation can be seen when considering liquid silicone rubber for an elastomeric component (see Section 6.4). On the other hand, the rather conservative nature of the medical device market should be considered too. The end-costumer of a device, usually a medic professional, shows a tendency to prefer devices basing on a material they are accustomed to. In consequence, selecting a novel material will lead to a fail in market, although coming along with technical and biological advantages. Important commercial aspects for material selection thus comprise:

- While for complex medical devices the purchasing price of raw materials plays a subordinated role, it may be a **dominant factor for single-use devices** rather simple in design
- The impact of material selection on the production costs resulting from purchasing price sometimes is **superimposed by** the **costs** for its **processing**
- Sometimes it is cheaper to select a material with rather **high purchasing price**, as this shows benefit on the process of risk management or improves the haptic perception of the product

3.1.2.2 Manufacturing

Besides the material questions, it is necessary to have certain knowledge about the specific requirements for the manufacturing process for design engineers for plastic medical devices. Honestly, the manufacturing has to follow certain rules regarding hygiene, packaging, allowed materials, or surrounding fluids (e.g., avoiding release agents in molds), but it is less miracle than many outstanding engineers may suggest and how it is often presented by medical device manufacturers. **Catchwords** like clean room, highest standards, FDA approved, certified, and many more are words thrown around regularly, especially by marketing departments. However, medical device manufacturing standards can be oriented somewhere between the demands of the pharmaceutical industry (biological contamination concerns), chip industry (overall particle concerns), and standard industrial requirements. Summarizing before entering the subsection more deeply: There is still some room for improvement for manufacturing plastic medical devices regarding quality standards, hygiene, and on the other side adopting new technological trends. The most promising trends are shown in Chapters 5 and 6, which may have a big impact on future plastic medical devices. In this chapter about designing plastic medical devices, it is our aim to give a quick introduction about **major manufacturing technologies** for plastic devices. We are using the word major with a reason: Plastic devices can be manufactured and assembled in countless ways with uncountable approaches or company-related innovations. Many innovations are not public or at least the key knowledge is kept hidden as far as possible. It is a way to combine device protection with property rights on the one hand and

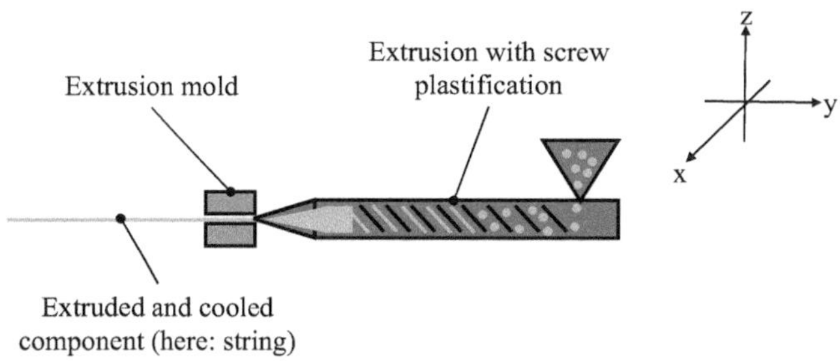

Figure 3.3 Extrusion principle: There are available quite a few extrusion materials and machine types. Basically, a screw extruder transfers plastic material through a die and an extrusion mold to form some sort of endless part, which is fitted into single parts afterward. For thermoplastic materials, the plastification unit with the screw plasticizes thermoplastic granules by applying shear stress and external heat to ensure liquid thermoplastic material while pressuring through the extrusion mold. Similar approach but opposite temperature curves are used for extrusion of thermosetting materials (e.g., silicones). It is the standard manufacturing approach for any kind of catheter, blow film, or tube, which are regularly finished with additional components (e.g., injection mold Luer-connectors).

highly innovative, difficult to cover, manufacturing approaches on the other hand. Nevertheless, most plastic medical device articles are produced with the standard plastic manufacturing equipment, such as extrusion and injection molding (see Figures 3.3 and 3.4 for their working principles).

Especially, mass and single-use articles are produced with standard equipment to keep the costs and risks as low as possible and the quality as high as possible. Validating and verifying a manufacturing is the key answer to that as well (as described in Section 2.3.8).

A quick overview of plastic manufacturing technologies for medical devices with no intention of completeness:

- Injection molding
- Extrusion
- Blow molding
- Thermoforming
- Three-dimensional (3D) printing
- Adhesive bonding
- Thermoplastic welding
- Milling, turning, grinding

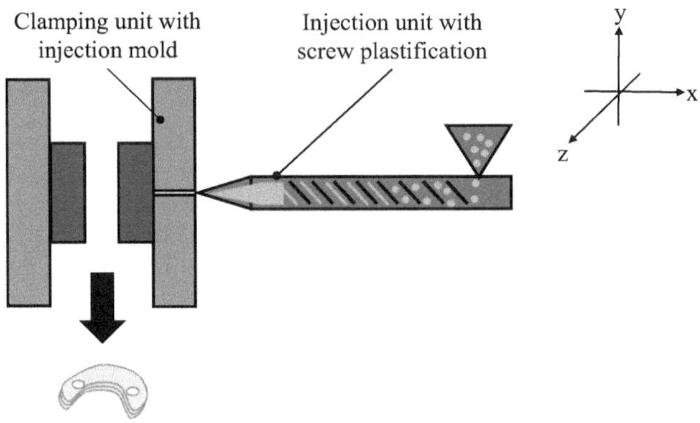

Figure 3.4 Injection molding principle: In contrast to the extrusion, injection molding is a discontinuously manufacturing approach. Per cycle a certain amount of injection-molded parts (from 1 up to 192 or even more, depending on size, mold-concept, handling, etc.). First, liquid plastic material has to be established similar to extrusion types, however, it is stored before the die prior injection by a linear movement of the screw. Most plastic parts are manufactured with injection molding due to the high degree of design freedom and wide range of available machine sizes, injection mold designs, and automation. A few injection-molded device parts examples are Luer-connectors, syringes, housings, three-way clock, and many more. Injection-molded parts can be ready to use after mold removal or may have some sort of postprocessing. Many approaches are thinkable like bonding, milling, drilling, surface treatment, and so on.

- Laser cutting
- Braiding machine
- Derivate of the core technologies and combinations of the above mentioned and many more

You can see the miracle behind manufacturing technologies for plastic medical devices: As long as the hygienic requirements and the need of validation and verification can be fulfilled any kind of plastic manufacturing technology may be used, but the major factor for standard technologies are often simply the manufacturing costs and availability of the equipment. Most plastic device engineers are not interested in using completely new or still in development approaches, simply because it is hard to forecast deriving risks and delays plus most engineers have the tendency to stick with well-known approaches until it is inevitable to change.

3.1.3 Safeguarding with Quality and Risk Management Tools

Many engineers understand the necessity of quality and risk management tools for manufacturing purposes to avoid costly and potentially dangerous manufactured (plastic) medical devices. Fundamentally, the same thinking should take place during a product development process. Safeguarding the development process is demanded by the ISO 13485 and 14971 or other regulatory measures. Simply spoken: The tools provided for a verified and validated manufacturing process can be transferred into a product development process. The approaches and regulations have been introduced in Chapter 2. Surely, the whole regulatory burden can be addressed at the end of an actual development by working out the necessary documentation, testing, validation, and verification, but this approach is likely to be extremely cost-intensive by additional work and risky due to potential development failures, which are addressed at the latest possible point during a development. However, it is still a complex matter when to start with the quality and risk management during a product development. QM-related personal often state that you have to start right away at the beginning, but this could be a burden for creativity and free-minded thinking without worrying about quality and risk-related topics. This topic gets even tougher, if you think about more complex, highly innovative developments, or even start-ups. Some further thoughts are presented in the Section 3.2.

3.1.4 From Design to Manufacturing

The design transfer is the logical step after finishing the actual medical device designing and development steps. Design transfer can be translated as a structured and documented procedure how to manufacture a (plastic) medical device, which keeps the previously defined characteristics constantly throughout the manufacturing processes within the acceptable range.

3.1.4.1 Design Transfer

The importance of structured and well-documented design transfers has been acknowledged by corresponding regulatory measures. Exemplary, the 21 CFR 820.30 section H states "Each manufacturer shall establish and maintain procedures to ensure that the device design is correctly translated into production specifications." The FDA regulations give some hints, which are summarized as follows:

- First, the design and development procedures should include a qualitative assessment of the completeness and adequacy of the production specifications.
- Second, the procedures should ensure that all documents and articles which constitute the production specifications are reviewed and approved.
- Third, the procedures should ensure that only approved specifications are used to manufacture production devices.

The FDA regulations refer to the international quality management standards ISO 9001 and 13485 how to implement a well-working design transfer system within a medical device entity. Currently, the revision of the ISO 13485 (see Section 2.4.3) focuses on an updated design transfer and changes recommendations (among other update aspects in other sections) due to the fact that the current version does not rate high the importance of the fact of a well-implemented transfer of development results into the actual production. Both partial systems (development and production) are elaborated well and the connection of both (often seen singularly in companies) will get an additional attention. The draft version of the revised ISO 13485 published in 2014, which is under discussion right now, states following aspects, which should be considered in an adequate way:

- Quality and suitability of suppliers,
- Qualification and technical ability of employees, advanced training,
- Manufacturing process, process validation,
- Materials,
- Tools for production, manufacturing methods,
- Manufacturing environment,
- Installation,
- (Preventive) maintenance.

Probably, you may think that all these measures should be clear in a certain way. Medical device engineers are always easy to implement, if you work with a modern understanding of adequate engineering. Many other engineering disciplines should work similar to the medical device world, however, within the medical device industry it is not only recommended but also a duty to comply with the needs of a structured and documented (!) design plus transfer and of course also how to handle design changes.

3.1.4.2 Design Changes

Medical devices should be constantly under review, if they still comply with the initial need and benefits. Medical device companies have to review market situations adequately and have to react to unexpected device situation with appropriate design changes. Additionally, most companies update their devices regularly to comply with the state of the art, market wishes, and so on. These design changes of existing and market introduced medical devices have to be considered similar to the market launch of a complete new market product. Design changes can be considered a combined process of design update and design transfer. Exemplary, 21 CFR 820.30 section I states "Each manufacturer shall establish and maintain procedures for the identification, documentation, validation or where appropriate verification, review, and approval of design changes before their implementation." The FDA regulations give two acceptable approaches to consider:

- Document control-enumeration of design documents, and tracking their status and revision history. Throughout this section, the term "document" is used in an inclusive sense to mean all design documents, drawings, and other items of design input or output which characterize the design or some aspects of it.
- Change control-enumeration of deficiencies and corrective actions arising from verification and review of the design, and tracking their resolution prior to design transfer.

3.2 Emerging Influences Plastic Medical Device Design

Designing plastic medical devices follows standard validation and verification procedures, as these are published by many competent authorities, to ensure the best possible benefit-to-risk ratio for patients and operators. Trends and needs for new or updated plastic medical devices are tough to forecast correctly as it is in most cases. However, the medical device industry may have some little advantages in comparison to high volatile end-consumer markets (e.g., electronic devices):

- Many plastic medical devices are subject to an actual need, without these devices many clinical procedures are unthinkable.
- Intense validation and verification requirements for development and manufacturing (shall) prevent quick and maybe overhasty market launch of newly developed devices.
- Regulatory hurdles harden quick market entries of competitors or manufacturers.

The best evidences of these theses' provided the last big worldwide economy crash and financial crises, beginning in 2007 with the subprime crises. End-consumer manufacturers felt an enormous drop in their revenues due to quick landing of the economy. Especially, plastic device manufacturers for the automotive industry had to struggle with melting profits. Many of these manufacturers thought about entering a more stable and less volatile market: the medical device world. The major appeal was the steady growth of the health device market for decades and clearly less impact of the financial crises on the revenue to the actual need of medical devices in most cases. The vast majority of manufacturers, thinking about entering the medical device market, dismissed these plans. Reasons are sure; the quickly less struggling economy on the one hand, however, the tough regulatory hurdles still play a role, which should not be scoffed at. However, it is worth mentioning that most nonmedical plastic manufacturers meet most of the necessary regulatory efforts by following the rules of the automotive or air and space industry. There is a distinguishing difference between being the manufacturer and being the actual distributing company in this fact, as you should already know.

Nevertheless, even the medical device market is tightening up regarding the achievable rates of growth. This is caused by a few more competitors in the market, which managed to entry the market during the financial crisis for sure, but the major factor is caused by the general health-care situation in most countries: Demographic changes, increasing costs of treatment, and many more reasons force most health-care insurers or systems to restrict the annual increases in costs. In the meantime, the advances in medical sciences enable to treat more and more diseases, which is why the number of treatments and therapies grow faster than the available health-care budget. This situation affects the medical device industry as well, which causes a considerable share of the overall health-care costs.

Any treatment or therapy must be performed at less cost, either by cheaper devices or by accelerated process of healing.

These facts lead us to some emerging influences on plastic medical devices, we choose to present exemplary based on our knowledge about the health-care environment, beginning with the most obvious after reading the last paragraph: cost and time reduction within development processes.

3.2.1 Cost and Time Reduction within Development Processes

"Time is money" is an old saying, which becomes truer for the medical device industry as well. The reasons for cost concerns have been introduced already in the previous subsection. But, what does that mean for the design and development process for plastic medical devices? Many approaches are thinkable, let's stick with some examples:

3.2.1.1 Development Cost and Time Reduction

The budget for developments is regularly under scrutiny regarding cost-saving potentials, especially for public-traded companies. A common approach in the medical device industry is to outsource development steps to engineering service companies or component suppliers, which is definitely state of the art in many big player industries like automotive and air and space. Partial and even whole developments for new medical devices are getting outsourced or at least internal development departments are in cost competition to these engineering services. The advantage is that engineering services can be specialized in certain aspects within the whole development and design procedure (e.g., material selection with hygienic considerations or state-of-the-art sterile barrier packaging). Especially for smaller companies, which are usually less known for outsourcing due to expertise reasons, might even acknowledge the necessity of buying in additional expertise for specific (partial) development. This might seem to be more expensive on the first look, but these specific experts may ensure less risky, quicker, and therefore less expensive development in comparison to a whole in-house development team and approach. Think about vascular implant company, which has about 350 employees, and is a market-known expert in providing well-suited vascular implants for aneurysm treatment. This company needs some sort of applicator, which helps to insert these implants into the patients in a minimal invasive manner via the arterial system. Such an applicator is crucial for the success of future implant developments, but the engineers of the company are experts in designing implants and not in designing a plastic single-use applicator. The company's overall size is too small to build its own applicator engineering expert team. In this case, it is a combined question of cost and time saving to outsource these developments to specialized expert teams, which have long-term experiences in designing plastic single-use devices for medical applications. Overall, reducing necessary development time ensures an earlier market launch of new products, which is commonly known, but which gets more important by the minute for medical device companies as well to ensure future competitiveness.

3.2.1.2 Device Design Focusing on Manufacturing

Additionally, outsourcing development steps to market-accepted experts, focusing on manufacturing cost reduction while designing a new device should be well known, but it is getting more attention recently for sure. Of course, there is always the trend of automating the production to decrease necessary labor. Within the medical device world, product update cycles are definitely longer than in most end-consumer markets due to the high amount of regulatory efforts to ensure device quality and patient benefits. Therefore, it takes clearly more time to adopt well-introduced manufacturing trends within the medical device world. Manufacturing opportunities (more detailed trends are presented in Chapters 5 and 6) trigger changes in the design of medical devices, which were unthinkable couple of years back. The device design departments should always have an eye on emerging manufacturing trends to translate these potentials into future developments.

3.2.1.3 Error Margin Reduction

Every engineer has learned the cost effects of errors during the product development process: The later and closer to start the production of development errors has to be handled with, the more it costs to fix the resulting problem(s). The availability and increased usage of (FEM)-simulation and rapid prototyping/3D printing (refer Chapter 4) help design engineers to reduce the error margin of ongoing developments before entering the prototyping stage with the actual intended manufacturing procedure. However, the major aspect to reduce error is to work with actual experts for the single-development step. This can be dealt with an own expert team or outsourcing specific task, as described above. The major challenge is to ensure the availability of well-educated and regularly trained engineering staff.

3.2.2 Employee Education and Liability Factors

Keeping up the overall employee skills is and will be a major hurdle within all development departments around the world. It is definitely not a challenge just for the medical device industry and it is not limited to the area of development solely, but it has to be addressed specifically within the medical device industry to keep up with the state of the art and working well with the tasks of liability. Medical devices are regularly under scrutiny regarding their actual benefits and existing risks. Besides that, the regulatory boundary conditions are changing permanently. New measures, harmonized standards, or even legal disputes may influence the daily work of medical engineers around the world. We do not want to express the feeling that medical engineering consists of continuously checking current regulatory changes, but most medical device engineers are facing at least about a quarter of their actual working time preparing some kind of regulatory documents. Most employers have or let's say should have introduced some kind of procedures to keep the workforce up to speed regarding regulatory on the one hand and of course it is necessary to keep development engineers at least on the state-of-the-art level on the other hand. It is not adequate and will not be successful with notified bodies to develop and design new (plastic) medical devices, which do not meet the minimum requirement of the state of the art.

Universities or professional schools have tried to address the need of skilled engineers for the medical device industry by establishing more and more courses of study with melodious names like biomedical engineering, medical technology engineering, bioinformatics, etc. The question is now, if these studies are the right answer for keeping up with the need of well-trained, highly innovative, and efficient design or development engineers? It is a not provable impression, but in most cases it would be better to have an engineer, who is perfectly trained within his preferred and therefore own discipline (mechanical, electrical, and so on engineering) during tertiary education. It does not mean that there couldn't be some introductory courses about the specific regulatory and biological burdens for medical devices, but the focus of most course should be on the specific engineering field. These fields are developing so fast and it is not adequately addressable by interdisciplinary course works in most cases. However, it does mean as well that necessary precautions have to be implemented within the medical device company to ensure a well-working regulatory, biological skill environment without forcing the actual design, and development engineer in too many different roles, which won't be addressed each with the same attentions. This fact is combinable with the aspects of the previous subsection of outsourcing specific tasks to consultants or companies with these specific expertise.

An additional factor has to be taken into account, especially within the well-developed and industrialized countries: aging population with demographic changes, which may lead and already has lead in some areas to a looming shortage of skilled workers. A lack of engineers will impact the success of each medical device company. Maybe, some economist won't agree with this aspect, but the creativity of engineers held constantly, if there are not enough engineers available. Every job should be worried to become unnecessary, if it is replaceable in some way by machines, computers, and so on. Think about taxi drivers, who will be needless at the point, when autonomous car driving will be available commercially. We will end this section with a simple question: Will big data/computers make medical device engineers and their creativity needless?

3.2.3 Individualization of Medical Devices

The medical device industry has invented and developed uncountable amounts of medical devices, which are used daily for also uncountable types of medical treatments and therapies. Medical devices are available in a wide range of sizes or are size adaptable to match with most patients' needs and anatomical differences. Nevertheless, there is still enough room for patient-specific medical devices. Especially in cases, where anatomical situation have to be addressed most adequately (e.g., specific dental implants), an individualized device has to be taken into account. Formerly, individual medical devices could be understood as the need of manually performed labor. Working with standard plastic manufacturing methods is not suitable due to the fact of enormous fix costs to create a manufacturing lane. Some aspects of individualization have been addressed by using medical-adapted CNC-milling machines, especially in the dental world, for quite some years. But, the field of application of these milling machines is limited to 3D-geometrical boundaries.

In the last years, one technology has experienced a rising attention: 3D printing. The basic technologies have been in development for quite some time. Major invention was realized in the 1980s. The fast-driving changes within the possibilities of the IT world have broadened the 3D printing into the focus of many industries, even private end-consumer markets. With some modification, 3D printing offers an extraordinary opportunity to address the needs of patient-specific medical devices. With these devices, it will be possible to close the last gaps within the product range of medical devices, which were not producible cost efficiently and anatomically adequately with state-of-the-art plastic manufacturing technologies. Individualized medical devices mean additionally that whole digital process chains arise: beginning with scanning a patient's anatomical data, virtual device planning environments, and 3D-printing technology, respectively. The whole aspect of 3D-printed medical devices is highly interesting regarding the wide opportunities, some already market implemented, some palpable and concrete, and some appearing on the horizon. It is a perfect match to the scope of this book: emerging technologies regarding plastic medical devices. In our opinion, this is quite a perfect reason to address 3D printing in general and patient-specific medical devices in specific in an extra chapter (see Chapter 4). The whole topic is a question of design and new design opportunities, the whole possibilities are definitely not yet seen, and the fitting manufacturing technology to transfer the digital into the real world.

3.2.4 Complex Design Validation and Verification

It is generally acknowledged and demanded that plastic medical device have to be designed and manufactured in a verified and validated manner (further reading in Section 2.3.8). According to the development process of new medical devices, it is the big question when to begin with a validation and verification process. On the one hand, it might be useful to start as early as possible to ensure the best possible list of requirements by checking the status of the current development regularly with a full extended design verification and validation. On the other hand, it is doubtful to achieve reasonable and forecastable results in early development stages with not yet finally designed devices and it drives the actual development costs up. Just to be on the same page, a quick heads up: Verification means to ensure the compliance with the previously established device requirements, and validation means to ensure the compliance with the previously established intended use of the new device. An example: A new endovascular application device should be developed with a highly innovative safety feature to ensure a manually performable backup by a quick dissembling functionality. It is likely to need some sort of soft-component materials. There are some requirements due to the functionality, and of course requirements like sterilization resistance and biocompatibility regarding ISO 10993. Summarizing, the simply looking choice of materials is a complex question of functionality, mechanical-optical-haptic characteristics, sterilization resistance, and biological interaction with the human body. Currently, a validation and verification procedure needs for approvable test results some sort of physical test specimen. Think about biocompatibility: Material behavior is not only a question of the chemical structure, but as well a question of processing conditions and product geometry (mainly surface). The actual shape of the device correlates with the processing conditions (changes in the injection mold, for example) and therefore has an enormous impact on the biocompatibility, plus additional effects regarding surface interaction or volume-to-surface ratio. The material question, especially if you have little or no experience with the needed material, can be an enormous burden or risk factor for simple plastic devices but especially for even more complex or multicomponent representatives. Design validation and verification is already some sort of statistical analytics regarding risks, likelihood and the actual patients' benefits.[9] Currently, design verification and validation cannot be fully implemented before the first design freeze.[10] Only partial testing and engineers' experiences ensure a certain level of security for positive design verification and validation results. You can probably imagine, it is more likely to achieve with less complex and less innovative medical devices. This affects mainly the innovation levels: It is definitely a costly risk factor during the development of highly new devices, because it is not possible to date to forecast design verification and validation results based on the first drafts with some sort of experience-based medical device validation and verification database. This is definitely speculative, but it would help to ensure quicker and less costly product development processes for medical devices to a certain extent. However, it is absolutely less likely to have such fully covered databases implemented due to competitor protection, confidentiality agreements, and other strategic reasons. Actually, regulatory bodies like the FDA or the European Union have implemented already some sort of database, which may help to ensure a broader database about possible problems deriving during the development of new device types or working with a different kind of materials: medical device failure databases.[11]

What we can say right now: Complex design validation and verification is getting more important due to the rising complexity of new

9. A life-saving medical device with no existing alternative may have a higher acceptable failure risk than a standard medical device with plenty of available alternatives.

10. The development is majorly accomplished and approved positively by the development team, however, design verification and validation may cause new reason for optimization, which may open the actual development phase again.

11. The FDA has implemented an openly achievable database called MAUDE—Manufacturer and User Facility Device Experience. The European Union integrated data upon incidents or near-incidents which occur during the use of a medical device in its EUDAMED database.

medical devices to ensure novelty, costs savings, and increased patients' benefits. It would be an enormous help to have some sort of design verification and validation simulation environment to keep the costs down. This idea is based on the mainly introduced technologies of computer-aided engineering, which are common during designing phases like mechanical structural simulation, manufacturing process simulation, and many others. A solution for device design validation and verification simulation would be the logical next step within the medical device industry.

3.2.5 Innovative Problem-Solving Methods

Innovative problem-solving methods are typically under suspicion to undermine the creativity of engineers during identifying processes for new product or solutions. To the surprise of many old school, or let's call it standard engineers, there have been developed some highly interesting approaches support problem-solving processes during product developments without damaging someone's development creativity. These methods may be more understood as channeling principles, which help to connect existing experiences or creativity facts within the engineers' heads. Summarized, well-experienced but still open-minded engineers do exactly the same, combining solutions in a channeled way, without the need of supporting methods of these so-called innovative problem-solving methods. Well-experienced but still open-minded for new solutions may not be easily achieved by all engineers. Therefore, these approaches may help to increase the creativity outcome during product development processes. Probably, you might now think about this subsection: "What are the authors talking about?" Exactly, this subsection started completely out of a regular order by a quick stating the deriving pros and cons of innovative problem-solving methods without having a proper introduction. We choose this way of introduction to show that there are always many ways to achieve a goal or let's say to travel to Rome. But let's get back to the idea of innovative problem-solving methods. If you know these approaches already, which are often named TRIZ or TIPS,[12] you may see this chapter as a quick refreshment. Interestingly, not so many medical device engineers have heard about TIPS so far. On the one hand, medical device engineers do know the aspects of structured, documented, and evaluated work really well due to the needs by regulatory measures or international standards.

---

12. TRIZ is a Russian acronym for "Teoria reschenija isobretatjelskich sadatsch," which is regularly translated to "theory of inventive problem solving," TIPS.

On the other hand, innovative problem-solving methods are used rarely, which may be caused by the average size and ownership of (plastic) medical device companies. Most of these companies can be considered as medium-sized, often referred to the German word *Mittelstand*. We don't want to say that these companies are not innovative at all. It is actually the case that these companies have highly interesting and innovative solution for existing problems and many of them are labeled hidden champions within their respective market. This is caused often by the enormous quality and experience of the resident engineers and highly sophisticated ownerships. But the bigger the company, the tougher it gets to achieve overall innovative problem solving without a well-defined structure.

TRIZ or TIPS is a basic principle to combine structured and creative engineering work. It might not be the ultimate approach for every product development, especially for newly started companies or creating absolutely new ideas with less existing experience (e.g., like the idea of social media). But, especially for product improvements or having an actual problem (like a surgical treatment with need for device support) the TRIZ approaches should be considered. However, the use of the methods should be evaluated regarding the proper implementation and the deriving benefit. The best methods do not work well without acceptance within the workforce. In this subsection, we focus on the basic principles of TRIZ and how derived methods can look alike. Many extended methods have been developed in the last 20 years, which are all based on the classic TRIZ approaches. But, it is worth having a look into standard TRIZ, which is still highly interesting, though the first ideas were published in the 1950s, and is getting more and more into the focus of current product development and research groups, respectively.

3.2.5.1 TRIZ—Theory of Inventive Problem Solving

The question is how the theory of inventive problem solving has been developed and how it actually works. Surprisingly, the basic approaches are not a result by big and concentrated research efforts in the last couple of years. The basic ideas were developed in the 1950s by Russian scientists or engineers, headed by Mr Altschuller,[13] who recognized first basic principles of guided creativity during his employment with the Soviet patent office. Three major regularities were detected by observing countless patents and technical documents:

- Most inventions are based on a relatively small amount of solution principles,

13. Genrich Saulowitsch Altschuller (*1926, +1998).

- Eliminating root contradiction allows innovative inventions,
- Evolution of technical systems follows determined patterns and regularities.

Based on these regularities, Altschuller and his companions developed several tools, which should help interested engineers during the daily work. Especially in the last couple of years, the interest in TRIZ has risen, which has become visible by numerous updates of existing tools and development of new methods based on the three theses. TRIZ methods and tools have been developed to comply with any field of engineering. In the case of medical device engineering, it should be openly discussed, which methods are likely to work and which not. However, this should be the case in any engineering field. Due to the relatively small size of engineers, there are not specific medical device TRIZ methods available. This might be an interesting approach for future updates to focus more on the specifics of engineering fields, which have to comply with interdisciplinary situations like technical background and human interaction.

Innovative problem-solving methods may sound a little bit abstract, but how to explain it better than introducing some general examples. It is our aim to stimulate some sort of interest in such approaches, which may help to increase performances of development departments and may lead to better or at least faster achieved plastic medical devices. But, we have to make clear: These methods have been developed to establish innovative solution to existing problems or let's better call it product or device ideas. They do work and fit perfectly into product enhancement, structured, and more forecastable development procedures. However, there has to be any kind of idea or problem detection, which is the fundament for the innovative problem-solving. To be on the same page, these methods may trigger new ideas, but generating basic and completely new ideas is and will be always the mission of creativity, knowledge, and experience of (future) engineers.

3.2.5.2 TRIZ Solution Path

Innovative problem-solving methods help to find innovative solutions for existing specific problems with less trials and errors phases and to become less vulnerable to lucky punches of the engineering department. These methods do not make any engineer unnecessary. They would not work with nonengineering-related professionals properly. It is always fascinating and productive having a second or third opinion by experienced operators or designers, who are not typical engineers, but even method-based development processes will not work without engineers. As shown in Figure 3.5, the TRIZ approach is based on following path:

1. Having a specific problem
2. Abstraction to a typical problem (contradiction)
3. Applying and working with Altshuller's principle methods
4. Having a typical solution
5. Concretize the typical solution
6. Having a specific solution

Knowing this path alone it does not help at all during a (medical device) development. It was Altshuller's major achievement to abstract this path on the one hand but to also provide applicable methods, which support the engineer to follow path of innovative problem-solving.

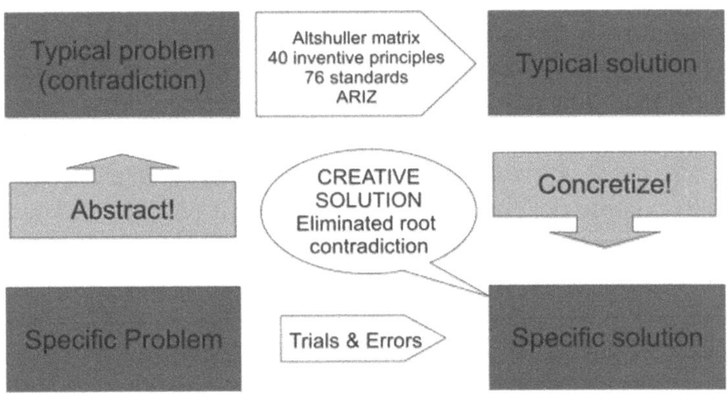

Figure 3.5 The TRIZway to work creatively with specific problems: In contrast to the classic experience-based approach of trials and errors, TRIZ works with abstraction of the actual problem in therein based contradictions. The theory is that any problem can be solved by terminating these contradictions to a certain extend. After detecting contradictions TRIZ solution methods help to find typical solution by working with inventive principles, innovation checklists, or list of effects. After all there should be a specific solution to specific problem with less trials and errors phases but with more structured and less time consuming methods. *Figure courtesy of "TRIZway" by AndriuZ/Wikipedia.*

3.2.5.3 TRIZ Methods Overview

Based on Altshuller's first methods, many updates, extensions, and completely new approaches have been developed for the last decades. Additionally, each development department may have its own specific implementations. Current research is doing its best to concretize and improve these methods as well. Therefore, it is not possible and absolutely not the scope of this book to provide you with every possible and available solution. We added subsequently a few examples to get you a better understanding. Hopefully, you got some interest in these approaches. Many good introduction books are available on the market.

3.2.5.4 TRITZ Methods (Selection)

- Ideal final result and ideality approach,
- Functional modeling, analysis, and trimming,
- Zones of conflict,
- 40 inventive principles of problem-solving,
- Matrix of contradictions,
- Substance field analyses,
- Separation principles,
- Laws of technical evolution and technology forecast,
- 76 standard solutions.

The daily work with these methods is the crucial step for implementation within development departments. The most common way is to work with some sort of templates (as shown in Figure 3.6), which are easier to implement into the daily work routine by using common office solutions, or more advanced solutions, so-called computer-aided innovation tools.

3.2.5.5 Open Innovation—Idea Generation

Innovative problem-solving methods help to identify solutions for already known problems. Problem is a typical engineering expression, which should be better called ideas. Most developments within the medical device industry are based on the aim to improve or copy existing systems or devices. Less than 1% of the actual developments are absolutely new inventions, but even little inventions can have a huge advantage for future operators or patients. The big question is, how to identify existing

Current situation

1 *Name or short description of the technical systems:*

Minimal invasive surgical instrument

2 *The most important, primary function of the technical system:*

Allowing minimal invasive surgery

3 *Description of operation, environment, and working conditions of the technical system.*

Operating within patients with minimal incisions, sterile conditions, plastid medical device, ergonomic considerations, long surgical treatments, sterile and non sterile medical professionals, operator with sterile gloves, incisions as small as possible, ...

4 *General description of the innovation task or problem.*

Formulate the anticipated results: what is to be done or achieved. Describe if necessary the undesired harmful effects in the system to be blocked or eliminated.

Problem analyses

Super-System:	*Useful Function*	*Undesired Property*	*Substance*	*Field Resources*
Operation theater with video system	Helping patient with surgical problem, broadcasting video signals	Hygienic need for sterile conditions, high preparation effort before	patient sterile coverage, monitors, theater	hygienic air stream, electrical energy, electrical signals,

↑

System:	*Useful Function*	*Undesired Property*	*Substance*	*Field Resources*
Minimal invasive surgical instrument	Allowing minimal invasive surgery	High training effort for acceptable results necessary	Plastic materials, steel materials, handle, forceps, gripper, cutter	electrical, mechanical forces during operation

	System: ↓	*Useful Function*	*Undesired Property*	*Substance*	*Field Resources*
1	Handle	Translating operators motions into surgical instrument motions	Unergonomic handling during surgical procedure	Plastic materials, steel materials, handle, surfaces, joints	mechanical forces by the operator
2	Gripper	Performing the intended motions by the operator to interact with the patient's surgical problem	Low freedom of movement, restricted field of vision, size limitations	Steel, riffle surface, joint	mechanical forces on the gripper
3					

Figure 3.6 Problem analyses example based on the TRIZ approaches to abstract a specific into technical problem: First, the specific problem is divided into useful function, undesired properties plus correlated substances and field resources. Second, the specific problem (system) is considered in correlation with a supersystem and partial systems to abstract necessary functionality and to find essential contradictions, which are the bases for typical solutions (e.g., with 40 solution principles and a matrix of contradictions). With engineering knowhow, these typical solutions can be fitted for the actual specific problem and an innovative solution can be found.

problems for operators and patients. Simply spoken, it would help to listen to them most of the times. Or another example: Manufacturing employees can be a useful tool to identify cost-intensive problems within a running medical device. Sometimes aspects of better assembling approaches, but also solutions for more product benefits, are within the heads of the employees. It is not possible for development departments to keep in touch with every manufacturer, operator, research groups, and so on. Additionally, it is quite the same way around: Which operator has the time and the resources to think about existing problems with devices more deeply? Consequentially, there is a hidden huge potential for future devices or at least improvements. A quite interesting approach is the open innovation methods: Companies are building interaction communities, where future solutions can be discussed, evaluated, and selected. The idea of open innovation was introduced in end-consumer-related fields, where innovation contests animate end-consumer to think about future development of existing problems or products. Transferred to the medical device industry, many different approaches may seem possible: medical professional innovation communities or at least innovation communities within a business entity (e.g., company) to bring the minds in the cloud together by placing a virtual platform of idea exchange. Bringing interdisciplinary thinking together seems to be more forward-looking than educated interdisciplinary engineers, who do know everything a little, but nothing at the best possible level.

4 Generative Manufacturing Technologies—The Future?

OUTLINE

Emerging Trends in Medical Plastic Engineering and Manufacturing
http://dx.doi.org/10.1016/B978-0-323-37023-3.00004-X

Lately, generative or rapid manufacturing technologies, in common better known as rapid prototyping or three-dimensional (3D) printing, have gained more and more public attention. This trend is mainly fueled by alarming newspaper articles like “Tools of Modern Gunmaking: Plastic and 3-D Printing” (*NY Times, 2013*) or “Danger in 3-D: The Rapid Spread of Printable Pistols” (*Spiegel International, 2013*). But, what is the origin of growing interest in a specific technology? We are talking about an approach for manufacturing, which had been developed as early as the 1980s. Do you know somebody not engineering related, who takes stock within any other comparable production techniques, for instance, injection molding? A two-way explanation seems plausible: availability and pricing. The digital revolution has induced a progressive technical evolution that generates very powerful digital-based prospects, just think about the amazing digital modeling methods as example. These software solutions are often freeware or even open source with a growing supportive community. Think about a typical young teenager 20 years ago, who loved to spend his time with creating handmade car or aircraft models in hours, let’s say days of dedicative work. Now, imagine the same type of teenager nowadays: computer, game console, or just the smartphone are the number one amusement. This young person still loves to create something for his own good and it hasn’t been easier to perform it digitally. The logic subsequent step is to combine real-life modeling with its digital counterpart. And here we are: 3D printing. Try to imagine how somebody felt about the first two-dimensional (2D) printer in the office community. Nobody thought about the possibility, that everybody would be able to buy such a machine. Nowadays, it is state-of-the-art to print your own holiday pictures in photo grade quality. The same process now occurs with the 3D-printing machine market. Surely, the industrial grade machines are still cost-intensive and have a wider range of freedom, material selection, or printing quality (mainly resolution and surface properties). It’s like comparing your desktop printer with a full-scale printing machine. Nowadays, it's no big deal anymore to buy a simple 3D-printing system with your local electronic market. But, where's the relevance for emerging technologies for medical devices? The medical device industry is quite conservative (refer to Chapter 1) in adopting new manufacturing approaches due to liability concerns, lack of process know-how and materials, or just because a lack of regulatory boundaries (yet!). Without satisfying regulations, it could be an extreme risk to utilize these new approaches, but it must be seen as an amazing chance for medical engineering (or any Life Science) offering the potential to improve health and wealth and to accelerate enormous growth and economic success. Besides the huge engineering capability that is implied in rapid prototyping technologies, they come with certain disadvantages, however. In the upcoming chapter, we have tried to address the chances and risks for medical device applications. Due to the growing interest and the enormous amount of newly developed machines and applications, with some already being established in medical engineering, we have decided to dedicate the 3D printing within the medical device industry with a whole chapter.

Within this chapter, the expression **3D-printing** is used as synonym **for generative manufacturing technologies** with **plastic** materials.

But, why isn't the 3D printing a standard manufacture procedure already, though the development has been intensified for 30 years? It is worth to have a second look at the stated articles about 3D-printed guns at the beginning: The technologies are fare from being easy to use mainly due to, e.g., printing process, design, cheap systems that offer poor quality or the reduced set of applicable materials compared to standard plastic machining tools. A couple of years ago, some major patents were phased out due to maximum guarding periods, which have blocked technology transfer and cost reduction for 20 years. Since the discontinuation, many new manufacturers of rapid manufacturing machines have entered the market. The described effect fits perfectly in a Gartner's hype cycle. In Figure 4.1, a qualitative analysis of the enterprise 3D-printing hype is shown.

Additionally to lower prices, new competitors will trigger new approaches, higher technical quality, and additional teaching efforts about the technology. For instance, as state of the art within the rapid manufacturing industry, a material is linked to a specific type of machine and vice

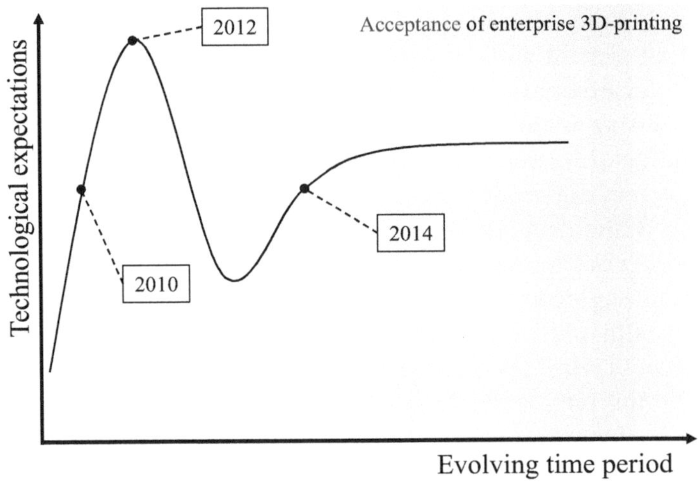

Figure 4.1 Qualitative analysis of enterprise three-dimensional (3D)-printing acceptance from 2010 to 2014: The enterprise 3D-printing development has developed faster than projected since 2010 with a technical expectation peak in 2012, just 2 years after a strong expectation rise in 2010. After another 2 years, the overall 3D printing reaches soon acceptance within the worldwide engineering community.

versa. Translated to the injection molding technology: The machine type XYZ is only suitable for processing polyamides (PAs) and ZYX may be used for polyolefines only. Other batches aren't applicable, because it is necessary to receive a clearance code from the supplier for each material, which often happens to be the machine manufacturer too. Additionally, most rapid manufacturing machines are locked: Only a few parameters are adaptable to impede usage of extraneous material(s) that might be cheaper. However, the rapid prototyping market is changing with new machines, even totally different technologies, entering the scene, which can be used with less restrictions and will definitely lead to lower production costs. Lower machine prices combined with new technologies will trigger development of new materials; some especially designed for the biomedical application with its specific challenges (refer Chapter 2).

The conservative medical device industry already exhibits some interesting approaches for rapid manufacturing, but it's far from being a blockbuster technology due to existing disadvantages like material selection, lack of regulatory boundary conditions, and surely the lack of the hit application. The 3D-printing technologies can be used to individualize implants and devices or to manufacture small lot sizes, which would be highly cost-intensive with traditional methods. Imaginable individualized medical devices can be classified into two ways: displacement procedure for labor-intensive handmade products (e.g., pontics) or individualized standard devices (e.g., masks for sleep apnea syndrome). However, most of them are only premarket and research based. The hearing instrument and dental industry can be seen as the major exceptions. Due to the often labor-intensive adaption procedure required to improve patient's comfort while wearing or applying such devices, both industries are leading in adopting new rapid manufacturing trends within the medical device landscape. Some people may address, this is based on the fact, that there exist more a try-and-error approach in both field regarding 3D printing, especially if you look at the current regulatory framework. For issues as in what way to authorize or how to handle liability, quality, and risks, only very few regulations specific for patient individual medical devices do exist. However, to address the upcoming market opportunities that are triggered by the evolving of rapid manufacturing technologies for medical devices, including any kind of digital process chain, will show considerate impact on the regulatory landscape. Current explorative interest of the Food and Drug Administration (FDA) in this particular field can be considered a trend-setting signal. It announced to give guidance on 3D printing in 2015, especially focusing on the point, that individual-made medical devices are currently less regulated than any industrial standard devices. Additionally, the Association of German Engineers has taken special interest in developing standards for digital process chains for individualized medical devices.

The prevailing chapter implies the provocative question, if the generative manufacturing technologies will be the future of the medical device industry. This book is focusing on the emerging plastic technologies. Therefore, we are trying to give adequate answers within the world of plastic manufacturing and engineering, which may include different forecasts for the future of rapid manufacturing approaches. Nowadays, the manufacturing procedures of standard plastic devices are predominantly designed to achieve high-volume output. However, even the injection molding market is moving toward more specialized, less throughput devices, due to more individual application approaches. The major question is, if the use of rapid manufacturing technologies is suitable regarding possible degree of individualization, production speed, or even available material selection. The upcoming sections give a quick overview about the state of the art; however, the focus is on showing future potential of rapid manufacturing technologies for the production of medical plastic devices.

4.1 Fundamentals of 3D Printing

The application of rapid manufacturing technologies does not consist of usage of a 3D-printing machine only. It rather does require a fine-balanced chain of several technologies to achieve the desired printed devices. A schematic process workflow for a rapid manufactured medical devices is illustrated in Figure 4.2, with a dental drilling template taken as thinkable example.

> **3D-printing** consists of a whole processing work flow including **data acquisition**, **pre-processing** of the **geometric data**, **preparation** of the **printing machine**, **printing sequence** itself and **post-processing** procedures.

A standard rapid manufacturing process can be separated in the following steps with the need of certain tools or techniques.

4.1.1 Acquiring Geometric Data

Compared to those for traditional techniques like injection molding, geometrical designs for 3D printed are less subject to manufacturing-related boundaries. Of course, not every geometry is printable due to machine resolution and spatial restrictions, the need of support structures, material limitations, and so on. The knowledge of suitable designs is indispensable for future medical plastic engineers, who are interested in specializing in 3D-printed medical devices.

Basically, the standard well-known CAD systems can be used to generate the desired geometry, whereas especially systems capable of free-form surface modeling are from particular interest for 3D-printed applications. The major advantage of 3D-printed devices is the high degree of freedom in design that may be challenging to handle with standard CAD software. Think about possible 3D-printed individual adapted dental implants: The geometrical shape has to be adapted to each single patient individually. Therefore, it is necessary to obtain individual geometrical data, usually based on optical methods like X-ray, ultrasonic, or laser scanning. These techniques can also be used for copying existing solid bodies with rapid manufacturing technologies. The upcoming chapter contains an outlook of possible future developments for device design. There are already many applications available on the rapid manufacturing software market, e.g., those to design individually printed dental braces.

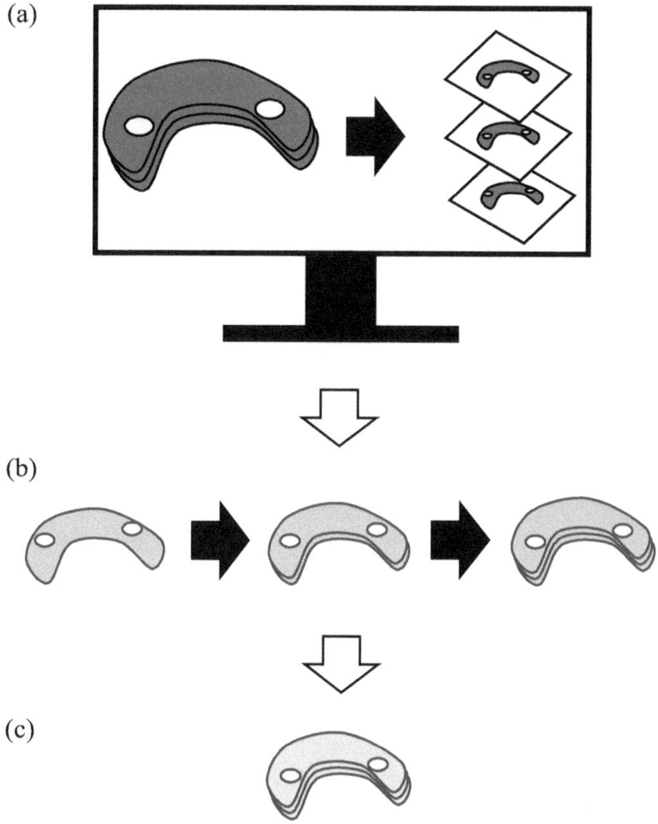

Figure 4.2 Schematic process workflow for rapid manufactured medical devices (here: dental drilling template): Prior the manufacturing procedures, it is necessary to generate the three-dimensional (3D) data, e.g., with CAD or (laser) scanning an existing structure (a, left) or using X-ray-based data acquisition. The data can be modified by adding additional functions like drill holes. The 3D geometry is sliced digitally into layers and, if necessary, support structure information is added (a, right). The 3D structure is printed layer-by-layer with the chosen rapid manufacturing method (b). Afterward, a finishing process has to be added typically, e.g., curing, surface treatment, or support structure removal (c). Ideally, all process steps after the data generation would be automated, which cannot be considered as state of the art.

At this point, it is worth to have a short outlook in the emerging dental medical device market regarding the effect of 3D-printing technologies. Currently, the preparation of individual implants (e.g., tooth crowns) is regular in a labor-intensive process, which has to be performed for each patient individually. Standard technologies like milling do not show satisfying results.

Therefore, the preparation process is still mainly manual work, which correlates with extensive labor costs. The classic approach to diminish these costs has been shifting labor to less costly countries like Eastern Europe or China for the last decades. Interestingly, the dental market is highly innovative in adopting new technologies. It can be seen as the leading market for new technologies, accompanied with the hearing device industry. This innovation adopting environment leads to a highly interesting trend within the dental device market: In the upcoming years, the introduction of new virtual planning software in combination with new 3D-printing materials and processes is expected to shift back the individual dental implant production to labor cost-intensive countries. Additionally, business forecasts do see potential in decreasing market prices for these medical devices.

4.1.2 Preprocessing Geometric Data

The step of preprocessing the data is linked to the chosen 3D-printing technology at certain extent. The following section should be considered as a general overview. Most generative procedures use a layer-by-layer method, which is the major reason for the usual need of support structures within many complex 3D designs. The CAD data have to be fragmented digitally into 2D layers by the printing software, often referred as slicing. The stereolithography (STL) language established itself as the standard file format for 3D data with additional layer information. The major printing approaches for complex 3D geometries with overlapping projectures are shown in Figure 4.3. The need of support structures for undercuts depends on the chosen plastic material properties (liquid or solid precursor), the manufacturing method, and the complexity of the generated geometry. Exemplary, fluidic methods with photopolymer droplets require more often support structures, as within powder-melting-based laser techniques, the unprocessed raw material itself may serve as support structure. Especially, approaches that cure the 3D shape within unprocessed material tolerate more overlapping angles than droplet or string methods like fused deposition modeling (FDM). Generally, support structures imply the disadvantages of an increased material consumption and postprocessing effort, as these structures must be removed. Additional surface treatments have to be included to avoid superficial imperfections. The 3D-printing industry knows about the difficulty and strives to establish new ways to avoid support structures to a certain extent or even fully. Quite interesting is the method using a 3D-turning baseplate, which is explained figuratively in Figure 4.3(d). The baseplate is mounted on a multiaxis robotic system (comparable to a gimbal lock), which turns it depending on the current droplet position required within the 3D space of the printing geometry.

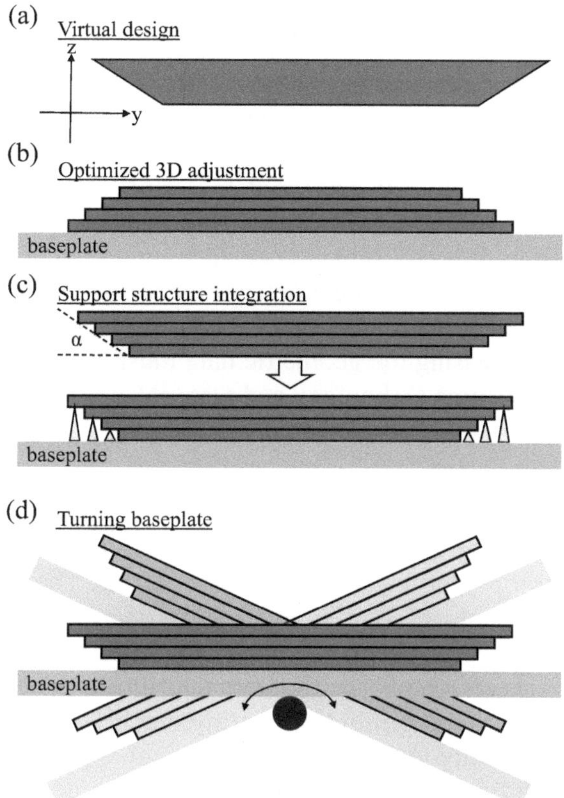

Figure 4.3 Complex three-dimensional (3D) geometries with overlapping projectures in y–z-levels determine additional printing approaches for most technologies. The major approaches, which are often combined as well are shown figuratively. The easiest procedure is to adjust a virtual design (a) 3D for the printing task (b) by, e.g., turning the z-direction through 180°. A standard approach as well is to use removable support-structure-material (c, here gray triangles), often water-soluble. The need of support structure varies for each printing technique, material, and overlapping angle α. Support structures imply additional printing time and finishing work. A newly introduced approach to diminish their need is the use of five-axle-guided baseplates (d), which allows to decrease overlapping angles individually for each printed space 3D by continuous moving of the baseplate.

The basic idea behind is to decrease locally the overlapping angles to diminish drainage or warpage of not yet solidified material. The locally diminished angle must be allocated until the printed material part (e.g., droplet or string) is solidified and aligned. As you can imagine, the mentioned approach requires a powerful software and hardware technology, which is able to plan, calculate, and perform the 3D printing and plate-moving procedure. Therefore, the technique is far from being state of the art; however, it shows interesting potential within the industrial 3D-printing market, especially caused by market entrances of well-known mechanical engineering companies. This development will help to improve the manufacturing quality and will enhance the R & D capabilities of the respective industrial sector.

Before printing, it is advisable to consider additional aspects like optimal spatial utilization or printing order. For individual printed devices, it is indispensable to integrate some kind of unique part number. Moreover, all options for preprocessing the geometric date must be considered respecting the selected printing technology and material.

4.1.3 Printing Machine Preparation

After finishing the geometrical data preparation, the next step is to provide a working printing machine and material. The actual printing data, mostly referred as STL file, is often transferred via IP-based networks. The printing machine software calculates the most promising and efficient traverse path for the actual printing process. The used material has to be filled within the printing machine: This step depends on the chosen printing technology. For medical application, aspects of hygiene and risk of contaminations have to be considered while preparing and printing the device. Furthermore, additional requirements like biocompatibility or some sort of contamination after printing have to be kept in mind. Especially for laser sintering application, it is very uneconomical to use only brand new powder. Now, think about a laser sintering process, which uses 20% recycled powder, which has not been shaped but was already heated to a certain extent in a prior printing. All these factors have to be taken into account for validation of a 3D-printing process according to the relevant regulatory landscape. However, these questions have not been fully investigated (see Chapter 2 for a deeper look).

4.1.4 Printing Sequence

With manufacturing periods up to several hours, the actual printing sequence is the most time-consuming process and does depend on the material utilized as well as size and chosen resolution of the geometry. The printing machine performs the printing sequence automatically with usually no human interaction required.

4.1.5 Postprocessing

The majority of current 3D-printing applications require postprocessing steps to a certain extent. Typical postprocessing steps are the removal of support structures, postcuring for ultraviolet (UV)-based technologies, and surface treatments. For medical application, the postprocessing has to be extended often due to hygienic requirements, which correlates with the specifications in other polymeric manufacturing methods. Examples are rinsing, disinfection and sterilization procedures, or packaging. In addition, typical validation and risk management procedures, obligatory within the medical field, have to be considered.

4.1.5.1 Generative Manufacturing Technologies

The catchphrase *3D printing* is utilized regularly in this chapter as the synonym for additive, generative manufacturing, or rapid prototyping, though the nomenclature is not absolutely correct, historically seen. For easier understanding for nonexperts, we choose to stick with *3D printing* as the major expression for rapid manufacturing technologies. There exist many different printing approaches and even more available plastic materials. All approaches have in common, that polymeric materials are joined with different techniques to generate 3D objects with a layer-by-layer process in contrast to subtractive methods like CNC milling. 3D printers ranging from small end-consumer to large-scale machines for industrial purposes, whereas the size usually correlates with the printing quality, complexity, and of course costs. Our aim is to provide an overview of possible printing technologies regarding 3D-printed medical devices. Therefore, this chapter contents exclusively industrial grade 3D-printing technologies, which are or likely will be used within the medical device field. It is a short overview about the technologies, with their existing (dis-)advantages regarding the medical application. The different plastic 3D-printing methods can be summarized within the following three major approaches:

- 3D printing with polymer powder,
- 3D printing with melted polymer,
- 3D printing with liquid polymer.

Plastic **3D-printing** technologies can be categorized with the applied **polymer type and phase**: polymer **powder** (thermoplastic based), **melted** polymer (thermoplastic based) and **liquid** polymer (curing system).	!

Interestingly, the often seen effect of interconnectional new techniques has been seen in the development of actually improved and new printing machines. Therefore, we have decided to present shortly major techniques consecutively without further classification (see overview Table 4.1).

It is worth mentioning that most (industrial) 3D-printing machines are sold under the **razor-blade business** model: You may buy a machine at moderate prices but then only can use the printing material, which is certified by the printing machine distributor. In the past, this lead to relatively high material prices, especially if compared to standard thermoplastics. But, the whole 3D-printing market is currently subject to change. Expired patents allowed the introduction of new printing machines with less restrictive material selection, which lead to an increased effort in new material development and price reduction. Additionally, long-established mechanical engineering companies have entered the 3D-printing market with new highly innovative technologies, which are focusing on diminishing current or old problems like expensive materials, lack of materials, and other market restrictions. As you can imagine, this trend will help to establish 3D printing within the medical device world due to the development of new biological-tested materials or processing technologies, which are capable of using already certified materials from other technological fields like injection molding or extrusion.

4.1.5.1.1 Stereolithography

The development of the STL approach started in the 1980s. Under the supervision of Charles W. Hull, the printing principle of the STL was developed, that is often considered the first commercial 3D-printing technology. It uses polymers that cure by applying UV beams, often referred as UV laser, which is why these commonly are called photopolymers. Nowadays, countless types of photopolymers are available, some already acceptable for use in medical devices for a certain extent. The procedural principle of STL process is described in Figure 4.4. Summarizing, a UV laser slips over the parts of a pond filled with a photopolymer that has to be cured. The applied wavelengths have to fit the requirements of the used photopolymer, which depends on its chemical structure. This procedure is repeated for each layer to be printed. The Hull group developed the standard layer-by-layer file format, which is known as the STL format. It allows creating layer models of a 3D (CAD) file.

The **stereolithography** technology works with **UV-lasers**, which cures **photopolymers** in the previously defined geometrical manner layer-by-layer.	⚠

Table 4.1 Major 3D-Printing Approaches

	Stereolithography (STL)	Digital Light Projection (DLP)	Multijet Modeling (MJM)	Selective Laser Sintering (SLS)	Fused Deposition Modeling (FDM)	Arburg Plastic Freeforming (AKF)
Printing duration	++	+++	++	+	+	+
Minimal layer thickness (resolution in z-direction)	10 μm	10 μm	16 μm	100 μm	200 μm	100 μm
Material selection	o	++	o	o	++	+++
Process stability	++	++	o	++	o	++
Acquisition costs	o	o	+	o	++	o
Surface quality	+	++	++	o	–	+

Several 3D-printing technologies have been developed for the past decades. So far, no technology can be considered to be a definitive market share leader. Some technologies are similar to a certain extent, which is often rooted in workarounds for existing patents. The mentioned properties are subject to change and should be considered a general overview of a whole technology family. For instance, the minimal layer thicknesses in stereolithography machines can range widely.
+++, best; ++; +; o; –, worst.

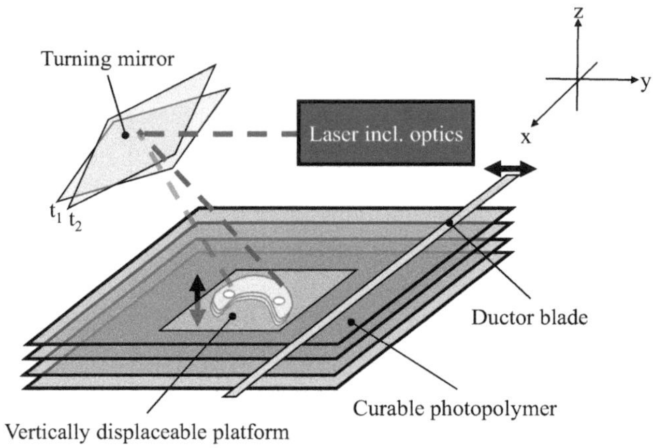

Figure 4.4 Procedural principle of stereolithography: A laser beam slips over certain parts of a pond filled with liquid photopolymer, which correlates with a layer of the printed device. Photopolymers are curable by applying UV beams with specific wavelengths, which have to be fitted to the actual material. After finishing a layer, a vertically displaceable platform is lowered (typically about 10–20 μm) and not-cured photopolymer is spread regularly across the pond by using a ductor blade. The next layer of the device is cured by the slipping laser beam.

The STL process is characterized by a relatively fast printing speed with good surface quality and process stability. With STL, it is possible to print highly accurate models, with layer thickness down to 10 μm (xy resolution down to 5–10 μm, regular machines slightly more). The accuracy of the layer thickness correlates with the chosen printing speed: More accuracy means more printing time. STL machines are designed to print with one or even more lasers a single material component. Current technology does not allow including additional components or even the use of any kind of inserts (e.g., metallic conductors). Therefore, support structures for complex 3D elements have to be printed with the same material. It is indispensable to attach postprocessing steps to remove the additional material, to improve surface quality, and to add a subsequent UV-curing process. This process is necessary due to the short UV application during the printing procedure to achieve the fastest building speeds possible. However, each printing and curing process leaves 3D-printed devices with a certain amount of uncured monomers. This leads us to the current major disadvantage of photopolymers: Uncured monomers frequently are toxic and thus responsible for less biocompatible properties of UV-cured photopolymers. It exits already in batches, which have approval for short-term application in contact with the human body. It is a topic of current research to improve the biological key properties of these photopolymers in order to widen the range of possible fields of application. This material limitation is common for all 3D-printing approaches basing on photopolymers. STL is already used in hearing devices, dental drilling templates, or printed copies of human bone structures for planning of surgical intervention.

4.1.5.1.2 Digital Light Projection

The digital light projection (DLP) approach is similar to STL. Comparable photopolymers with its (dis-)advantage, especially regarding the medical device application, are cured by applying ultraviolet beams (e.g., an LED source). The positioning of the beams ("where to cure") is realized with a technology called digital light processing, which is mainly used in projectors and is eponym for this 3D-printing technology. The procedural principle of DLP 3D printing is explained in Figure 4.5. Selective micromirrors, including microlenses, do focus single beams either on the position within the photopolymer-pond where curing is desired, or track them toward a position somewhere outside. Thereby,

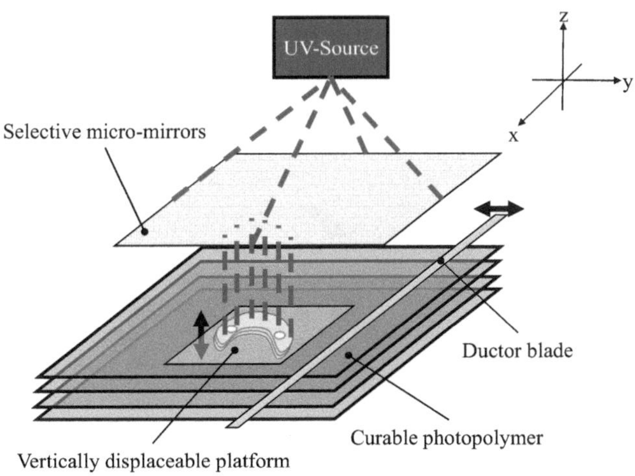

Figure 4.5 Procedural principle of digital light processing (DLP): The layer-by-layer curing process with photopolymers is comparable to the stereolithography approach. The DLP technology uses selective micromirrors to guide single UV beams (often an LED source) only at the required areas to the photopolymer pond. The micromirrors are switched per layer. All necessary parts of a layer are solidified at once. Thus, the DLP approach is known for its relatively high building speed.

the minimal curing size is determined by the number of micromirrors, whereas current systems feature arrays with up to 4160×2080 single mirrors, resulting in a resolution in the range of 30 μm. Due to the fast-evolving technology, the actual maximum amount of single mirrors (and thus minimum resolution) certainly may be expected to improve even more.

> The **digital light projection** technology works with **a UV-source and micro mirrors** (DLP-technique), which cures **photopolymers** in the previously defined geometry layer-by-layer.

As a whole layer is cured at a time, the DLP technology is known for its relatively high printing speed. However, the photopolymers currently available induce same disadvantages like necessary postcuring processes or noncured monomers.

4.1.5.1.3 Multijet Modeling

Similar to the ink-jet printing, the multijet modeling (MJM) technology uses a printing head that literally sprays the printing material into the desired shape. It can be seen as actual 3D printing in the truest sense of the word. The creation of 3D structures is possible by using self-curing resins or photopolymers (see Figure 4.6).

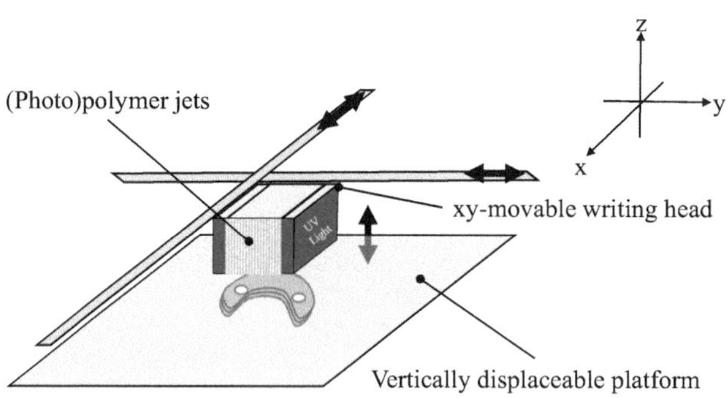

Figure 4.6 Procedural principle of multijet modeling: Uncured material is spread via so-called jets on the built device surface layer. The jet nozzle consists of one or several photopolymer jets, which provides the uncured material on the surface, and UV beam spots, which induce the curing process right after the photopolymer was applied. The jets can consist of different materials, e.g., for support structures.

The **multi jet modeling** technology works typically with a 3-dimensional movable **printing head**, which provides **photopolymers** jets and **UV-light** in the previously defined geometrical manner layer-by-layer.

This technology can be described as a drop-by-spray approach: The uncured material is sprayed at a certain position with a certain layer thickness and directly afterward cures automatically (e.g., cooling or drying) or is cured usually by applying a UV beam. However, different curing approaches with glue-based systems do exist, especially for metal or ceramic printing. The printing head can consist of several parallel jets, allowing increased printing speed or enabling to simultaneously print with different materials. This can be helpful for easily removable support-structure-material, which is added directly within the printing process. The problems involved when using photopolymers are similar to the approaches mentioned above, especially concerning noncured monomers in medical application.

4.1.5.1.4 Selective Laser Sintering

The selective laser sintering (SLS) technology uses thermoplastic polymers as powder, which is bonded locally by applying pulsed energetic laser beams (see Figure 4.7). Prior each step of curing, a thin layer of powder is filled within a container that may be moved vertically. Even and smooth distribution is achieved via a ductor blade moving across the working space. Subsequent the laser beams melt thermoplastic powder at the desired positions, which induces the local bonding up to a solidified layer. SLS is a typically layer-by-layer technology, which needs less supporting structures than other printing approaches due to the solid state of the powder. The applied laser beam has to be fitted to the used thermoplastic powder. Therefore, it is usually not possible simply to grain standard thermoplastic material and start using SLS machines.

The **selective laser sintering** technology works with mostly surface modified **thermoplastic powder**, which is **locally melted** with high energetic **laser-beams** and causes a **bonding process** in a previously defined geometrical manner layer-by-layer.

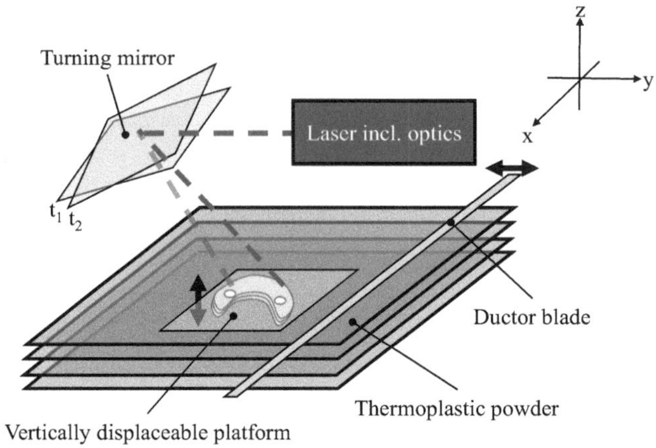

Figure 4.7 Procedural principle of selective laser sintering: In contrast to the stereolithography approach, the laser beam is not used to induce a curing process within a photopolymer layer. Instead, thermoplastic powder is used. An energetic laser beam (about 50–100 W) melts locally thermoplastic particles, which bond together to a solidified layer. After finishing a layer, a vertically displaceable platform is lowered (typically about 10 μm) and thermoplastic powder is spread regularly across the pond by using a ductor blade. The next layer of the device is solidified by the slipping laser beam. Due to the solid state of the powder, supporting structures are mainly not necessary in contrast to other printing approaches (especially the liquid approaches).

However, wide ranges of thermoplastic powders like PA, polyetheretherketone, or polystyrene are available. Due to the razor-blade business models frequently found, the powder often must comply with the machine technology utilized. In order to improve local laser bonding, suppliers often preprocess the materials with a special coating. Selective laser sintered medical devices are investigated for drilling templates, partial cranium implants, or printed copies of human bone structures for surgery planning. A problem often unmentioned is hardly or even nonbonded thermoplastic grains on the built surfaces. Due to their specific volume-to-surface ratio, these microscopic grains may induce a severe immune response and inflammatory processes within the human body and thus may cause issues concerning biocompatibility.

4.1.5.1.5 Fused Deposition Modeling

Due to its simplicity, the FDM is probably the most spread 3D-printing approach. Since the end of the protection period of major patents, FDM has emerged with open-source projects, which provide detailed instructions not to build and open-source software (e.g., firmware) for operating a machine.

The **fused deposition modeling** technology works with melted **thermoplastic strings**, which are deposited in a previously defined geometrical manner layer-by-layer.	

Via a heated nozzle, a thermoplastics string is melted and extruded, thus providing the melted thermoplastic filament (see Figure 4.8). This filament is deposited layer-by-layer in the previously programmed shape. Often, a second nozzle with a different thermoplastic type is used to provide support structures.

Due to its lack in surface and printing quality, FDM is mainly utilized for classical rapid prototyping or private printing projects. As generally of minor suitability for medical applications, this approach primarily is mentioned for the sake of completeness.

4.1.5.1.6 Arburg Plastic Freeforming

Additionally to the main generative manufacturing principles presented, the Arburg plastic freeforming (AKF) is the final technology, we want to introduce in this chapter. The nomenclature of the technology may be confusing to some, as it includes the company name of a German

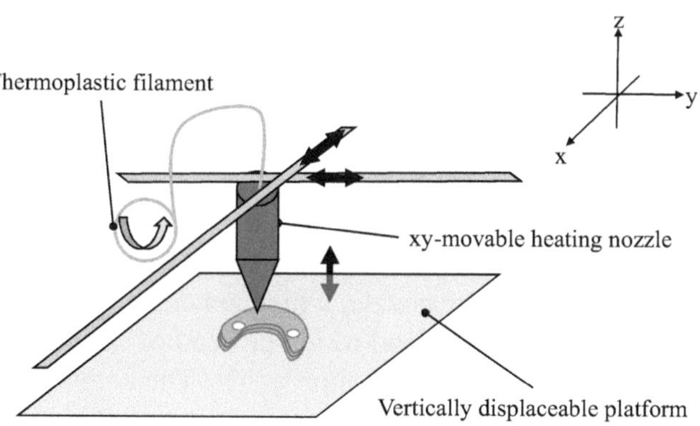

Figure 4.8 Procedural principle of fused deposition modeling: An xy-movable heating nozzle provides melted thermoplastic string by extruding and melting a thermoplastic filament, which is deposited on a layer regarding the shape of the printed layer. After finishing a layer, a vertically displaceable platform is lowered during the running printing process. Additional nozzles with (support) materials are regularly used.

manufacturer of classic injection molding machines. Within this book, we try to avoid any bias concerning emerging technologies only based on a company or regional background. However, the AKF technology is such a groundbreaking technology, which has already and will have a huge impact in future developments within the generative manufacturing world since the market launch autumn 2013. But, what is the extraordinary feature provided by the AKF approach? Simply said: For the first time standard thermoplastic resins can be processed without any special treatment like graining or by adding additional compounds to cure a 3D system. As basing on standard thermoplastic resin, this opens an enormous potential due to the highly evolved thermoplastic material market. The chemical industry has developed uncountable different types for the classic polymer processing technologies like injection molding or extrusion. Even for the medical technology, comparatively small with its 5% market share, many dozens of suitable materials are available. The major chemical industry companies are triggered on markets with big volumes. Therefore, 3D-printing materials are mainly developed and processed by medium-sized companies, often with close ties to the printing machine manufacturer. As you can imagine, this effect heavily influences the price of such materials and meantime narrows down their availability for medical applications enormously, as the so far small market volumes is not worthy to invest. As mentioned above, the AKF technology breaks through the vicious circle of small market volume that leads to little material selection, especially concerning our favorite: plastics for medical application. This effect will bring us to interesting thoughts about 3D printing as an emerging technology for the medical device world in the upcoming chapters.

The AKF technology is described in Figure 4.9. It can be divided in a material-melting section with a typical screw plastification and a printing head consisting of a heated piezo nozzle, which provides fully melted single droplets (current diameter range: 100–300 μm). A 3D displaceable platform is moved around the nozzle, which generates the 3D device layer-by-layer. This technique may lead to lesser need of supporting structures in comparison to other 3D-printing approaches. The combination of two or more screw plastificiation plus printing nozzle is within the future's range and allows to print multicomponent models.

The **Arburg plastic freeforming** technology works with melted **thermoplastic**, which is plasticized with a regular extrusion screw and is deposited in a **micro droplet** shape by a **piezo nozzle** in a previously defined geometrical manner layer-by-layer.

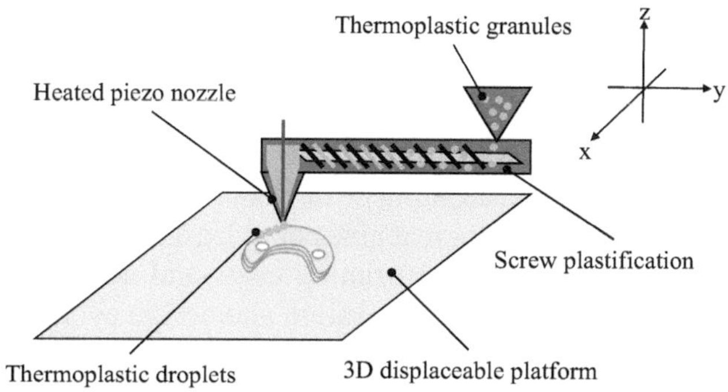

Figure 4.9 Procedural principle of Arburg plastic freeforming (AKF): The AKF approach is currently unique using standard thermoplastic granules, which can also be used in injection molding or extrusion processes. Granules are plasticized with a regular extrusion type screw plasticization, which provides thermoplastic melt to a piezo nozzle. The piezo nozzle is used to deposit microdroplets of the melt on three-dimensional (3D)-printed layer. By using a 3D displaceable platform, the AKF approach is suitable to work with less or even no support structures in comparison to other technologies. Additionally, more component systems are available.

Due to the ability of processing standard thermoplastic resins without the necessity of a special treatment, the AKF technology may be used in a wide range of plastic medical devices. There exist already many medical grade thermoplastics, which could be most likely processed in a certain biocompatible way. The hints and clues are described in the chapters before. However, the AKF technology leaves some room for improvements, due to existing issues regarding production speed, material aging, and component quality.

4.1.5.2 Trends and Potential for Improvements

Identifying generative manufacturing trends can have the same difficulties like a 1-year-long weather forecasts. The market is currently highly innovative with several dozen new approaches, technologies, or business ideas. It is not our aim to present single technological effort, which are definitely worth mentioning, but can be misleading by identifying the major trends within the generative manufacturing environment. The expected major trends can be sorted into device design, industrial manufacturing, and technological trends. However, each cannot be considered without mentioning others due to the strong mutual interdependences. End-consumer trends are skipped due to a lack of connection to the scope of the book.

4.1.5.2.1 General Trends and Potential for Improvements

Generally spoken, the current focus within the 3D-printing world is to bring down the costs for machines, materials, and production. This includes increasing manufacturing speeds and improved process stability, which leads to a reduced number of deficient products. The increasing availability of 3D-printing machines or at least available print services in combination with decreasing printing costs and adapted design software will lead to faster product innovation and design cycles, which is the actual, well-known rapid prototyping. The engineer can focus rather on the actual functionality of a designed product than dealing with trouble to generate prototypes prior transfer to serial production. The increased availability leads to a more broader understanding within the engineering world of the opportunities and restrictions of 3D printing, existing materials, and boundary conditions. This vicious circle leads to improved software solutions, which helps to create more design fascinating products with less standard modules. Especially for small batch productions, it is currently highly cost-intensive to create manufacturing tools. Therefore, small batch products are either pricy or based on standard modules. Increased manufacturing and better material selection allows upcoming device designs to focus more on the actual design with less worrying about the manufacturing conditions, if the actual costs of generative manufacturing technologies keep coming down. Thanks to the development of high-quality digitalization tools like laser scanning; it is conceivable for future engineers to integrate natural shapes digitally, which are difficult to handle with traditional standard CAD approaches.

3D-printing technologies offer still enormous **development potential** regarding the **process** and **material selection**.

Overall, if the printing costs and available materials are acceptable, an increased use of 3D-printing technologies will lead to faster idea to product cycles. As already mentioned, it can help within the design creation process ("rapid prototyping"), but an often forgotten fact is, that building up a production line including typical manufacturing tool, e.g., an injection mold, needs a certain period up to several months, depending on complexity, costs, and availability. It is worth mentioning frequently that it is not expectable to have a future manufacturing in general and especially within the medical device world only depending on 3D-printing technologies.

As already described, on the one hand the manufacturing costs for standard plastic single-use products or any high-volume device are unlikely to match with 3D-printing technologies in comparison to established plastic manufacturing techniques like the numerous times mentioned injection molding or extrusion. On the other hand, there exist still many limitations within the 3D-printing world, which can be considered state of the art with other technologies. The increased efforts to improve technologies including available materials have brought better manufacturing machines and printing approaches in general. But, if you compare the current 3D-printing standards with the current injection molding standards, it will be an easy task to see the upcoming trends. Just think about the following points (no guarantee for completeness), which are addressed to a certain extent by current developments or start-ups:

- fully automated, robotics-based production,
- high-speed and high-volume manufacturing,
- multicomponent production,
- material selection or material refinement (e.g., with compounding),
- carbon- or glass-fiber-reinforced polymers,
- additive integration (e.g., antibacterial, antistatic, color masterbatch),
- minimization of passes,
- integration of functions,
- miniaturization,
- manufacturing tolerance,
- process stability and monitoring,
- sensor or metallic insert integration,
- ultraclean room facility,
- surface quality,
- precision-optical components,
- waste material fraction,
- recycling/regranulation (thermoplastic vs resin system).

It is definitely not the aim of 3D printing to comply with all of the mentioned points within one technological approach. Some are definitely state of the art in different plastic manufacturing technologies, so the list might be helpful to recognize possible future development trends, let's say for an ideal 3D-printing technology including available materials and general variability. Some points of the list above are already addressed by current developments. Exemplary, the AKF technology is suitable to work with standard thermoplastic granules, which easily can be modified with additives. In contrast, no standard 3D-printing technology is able to work properly with carbon- or glass-fiber-reinforced polymers or allows simply to integrate metallic inserts or sensors, which is state of the art in plastic engineering and manufacturing to minimize work passes.

The general improvements addressed are mainly based on the comparison of the current 3D printing with the well-established state-of-the-art plastic manufacturing technologies like injection molding with all of its subcategories (e.g., micro-, multi-, fluid-injection molding). As comparatively new, 3D-printing processes themselves have still considerable room for improvement without adding further technological aspects or creating new material formula. Especially the process stability and automation, as well as surface quality, offer enough improvement potential. For example, the position of a printed device within powder bed can interfere with the quality of the generated part in SLS machines. This effect may be explained by different thermal flow conditions within the thermoplastic powder close to boundaries in comparison to a position right in the middle of the powder bed. Standard machines do not address different conditions of cooling by varying the laser power level. The conditions of cooling are yet not fully predictable for all techniques, which uses thermoplastic melt to a certain extent. Also the photopolymer-based technologies may have some problems with process stability throughout the printing space. Varying UV beam intensity can lead to different degrees of cure. Surely, DLP- or MJM-based processes exhibit less intensity problems than focused laser beams. However, it is still worth considering the possible effects regarding potential for improvements. This leaves us with the wisdom that the position within the building space has to be considered for validating 3D-printing processes, which is a crucial point for medical devices, especially those for high-risk applications (further addressed in Section 4.2.2).

Typical 3D-printing materials have evolved drastically in the last years; but the variety of material properties are still worthy of improvement. Some mechanical properties or limitations are caused certainly by the layer-by-layer building principles, which lead in general to relatively brittle component behavior. More elastic materials are tougher to process due to stability constriction of the cured parts to ensure 3D shape accuracy. In general, an increased material availability is a function of market interest or volume and technological improvements.

4.1.5.2.2 Improvement Potential for Medical Device Manufacturing

The above mentioned improvement potential should be considered as well regarding the application of 3D-printing technologies for medical devices. As design and manufacturing of plastic medical devices generally is a subset of classical engineering, any advances in technology will show more or less impact. Additional requirements should be considered for the design and manufacturing of plastic medical devices, which are caused by applications close or within the human body: It is worth looking into the existing world of medical plastic engineering and manufacturing, which leads us to the major tasks of hygienic manufacturing, stability during disinfection, or sterilization processes and bio-/hemocompatibility. Although these aspects already are addressed by current research and development, commercially available machines and materials leave enough room for improvement regarding the mentioned facts.

When considering hygienic manufacturing, it is again worth looking into the conventional plastic manufacturing technologies. About 20 years ago, leading injection molding manufacturers acknowledged the medical manufacturing as independent market with its own special requirements, especially concerning hygienic considerations (e.g., low-particle production, easy-to-clean surfaces, or thermal interferences with clean room air flow). Prior standard machines had to be adapted for clean room applications where possible. Then, triggered by regulatory demands and the emerging medical device markets especially adapted machines were developed. It seems well-conceivable that parallel changes will be necessary or even worthwhile soon for 3D-printing machines due to their evolving utilization for medical device manufacturing. These machines will help to establish easier to validate and certify manufacturing processes regarding regulatory requirements.

> Current and future developments of **3D-printing technologies** and **applicable materials** will have enormous potential for future plastic medical device applications.

Material stability during disinfection or sterilization processes and bio-/hemocompatibility is a question of demand and established know-how regarding these points. For plastic materials, there do not exist plausible forecast models concerning the effects of disinfectants, sterilization, or human interaction. Materials have to be tested for each acceptable condition of these points. Exemplary, any change in material supply will require to repeat all tests necessary to patient safety. This burden is also an explanation of the relatively slow adoption of new technologies or materials within the plastic medical device world. Additionally, the individual processing conditions for different medical devices can lead to different results concerning material stability and biocompatibility. Material manufacturers can provide biocompatibility testing for the raw material only. Probably due to the lack of demand, material manufacturers haven't had a focus on developing medical grade 3D-printable materials, yet. Surely, new technologies like the AKF can use standard thermoplastic materials, which is also helpful for selecting materials for stability and biocompatibility. Especially, the field of the often-used photopolymers, but also the thermoplastic powders, has enough room for future developments concerning the three of material stability, bio- and hemocompatibility. Medical devices, 3D printed with photopolymers, always exhibit certain remains of uncured monomers and other agents necessary for the curing process, like initiators or stabilizers, necessary for the process of UV curing. These agents may elude during medical device application and that way show negative influence on biocompatibility (see Section 2.1.1). Most of the existing 3D-printed medical devices accept compromises regarding the trias. However, this generally disallows usually long-term or implant application.

As mentioned in Section 2.2, the biologic reaction to a medical device is not only determined by the raw material utilized but also by its design and process of manufacturing. 3D printing enables to create extraordinary 3D shape of plastic medical devices. The shape, including surface conditions, has to be taken into account while estimating the biological effect. Currently, no methods exist to estimate these effects, even for standard design. It would be a tremendous help to generate device design methods, which helps to increase the likelihood of bio- and hemocompatibility and is not solely based on design experience and elaborate experimental tests.

The mentioned missing possibilities with 3D printing currently limit the spectrum of applications in comparison to state-of-the-art plastic manufacturing technologies concerning the utilization for medical devices. However, the application of 3D-printing technology allows already the development of completely new approaches for medical devices or at least faster small batch productions for simple medical devices, if the demands of regulatory affairs can be met. But you should always keep in mind the conservatism within the medical device world regarding the introduction of new manufacturing technologies, which is often related to a certain anxiety of new regulatory burdens. In the upcoming chapter, we show and discuss general prospects of 3D printing for medical devices to put possible anxiety into perspective of the arising opportunities.

4.1.5.3 Opportunities of 3D-Printed Medical Devices

Right now, you should have gained a certain knowledge level about generative manufacturing technologies. Based on our experience, some possible engineering opportunities are selected, which can be transferred to a broad range of prospective medical device applications. Surely, the chosen concepts can be considered as a forecast with no guarantee to prevail effectively. It is our aim to broaden future engineer's horizon concerning the opportunities of rapid manufacturing technologies within the medical device engineering and manufacturing field. Increased knowledge about potentiality allows to develop so far unthinkable techniques, manufacturing approaches, or designs.

> **3D-printed medical devices** may provide opportunities for future engineers concerning **cost saving** potentials, more **complex geometrical** designs, improved **device design** and **rapid tooling**.

4.1.5.3.1 Opportunities for Engineers

New technological approaches can be considered worthless, if there is a lack of sufficient trained research and development engineers within the related field. Many engineers have heard about the 3D printing, several are familiar with the basics of the technology; however, only few engineers are fully aware about its potential for the medical device industry. Existing knowledge about plastic engineering for medical devices can be considered helpful, but it is not directly transferable to 3D-printing approaches. To explain why, let's stick with the thermoplastic injection molding technology. Injection molding is a cyclic operating manufacturing method. An exact amount of previously plasticized thermoplastic polymer is injected in the provided cavities of the molding tool. Afterward, the molded device has to be ejected. The major engineering questions are often: Which material is suitable, which geometrical limitations are present, and which manufacturing costs are acceptable. These three bullet point questions are transferable to the plastic 3D printing, but that's quite all. Injection molding comes along with certain design limitations that may be reduced by constant technological evolution, yet not fully be resolved. An engineer has to consider maximum flow paths for high-viscous plastic melt correlating with the injection pressure, which also correlates with the filling capacity, tool temperature, and so on. With rapid manufacturing technologies, an engineer doesn't have to examine those confinements caused by the necessity of a part shaping tool. In contrast, there are many limitations within rapid manufacturing world, which are tried to be diminished as well. Rapid manufacturing is often referred to be the ultimate technology to create 3D geometries without boundaries. However, supporting structures set the first drawback, which are often indispensable due to the layer-by-layer built up principle. Therefore, comprehensive understanding of the manufacturing principle is crucial devices to push the boundaries toward highly innovative, extraordinary engineered devices. As you can see, rapid manufacturing engineers have to dismiss certain standards, they learned as principles of manufacturing orientated design within classical engineering. This can be considered as a barrier or a challenge. Therefore, the content of the upcoming sections should be seen as a guideline for future medical device engineers in which new related topics may emerge. It is not our goal to identify every detail of possible opportunities within the 3D-printing world to achieve respectable results for the medical device world. Major topics are abstracted and placed in context how they do affect upcoming medical device engineers.

4.1.5.3.2 Cost Reduction Opportunities

Classic approaches for cost reduction are faster product development, streamlined manufacturing, or ideally a combination of both. The utilization of 3D printing as rapid prototyping technology enables to reduce development costs by less time for prototyping, functionality control, ergonomic topics, user feedback, etc. Moreover, although a relatively slow manufacturing procedure when compared to high-volume technologies, 3D printing offers some opportunities for cost reduction when manufacturing plastic medical devices. This may sound paradox, as manufacturing speed usually correlates with cost of production. But as approaches for 3D printing manufacturing are not intended to copy or replace established technologies, a simple transferring of an existing manufacturing approach is not expedient and thus a direct comparison of time for actual manufacturing is misleading. Surely, technologies like AKF may help to ease a transfer from classic plastic engineering toward the use of generative manufacturing. However, it is not the aim to show the limitation, but rather explain possible opportunities regarding cost reduction with the assumption that possible restrictions are solvable.

Actually, there are foreseeable some possibilities for cost reduction issues (selection):

- small batch production,
- reduction of processing steps,
- substitute of manually performed labor,
- complex geometries not feasible with classical injection molding.

Production costs per single piece can be itemized by material and manufacturing costs. Further, manufacturing costs can be separated in variable and fixed costs. Variable costs are mainly driven by material and energy costs and thus only little influenced by the volume of production. Fixed costs are mainly driven by the acquisition costs of machinery and tools. Concerning the comparison of production costs between classic production technologies and 3D-printing approaches, it may be cheaper to use generative technologies due to less fixed costs like injection mold manufacturing. The last passage is just the attempt to explain in a simple manner for the highly complex world of business economics-concerning decisions for manufacturing approaches. Generally spoken, it is most likely to see more 3D printing within small batch production for plastic medical devices (if questions concerning material selection, process stability, etc., are addressed properly) due to cheaper fixed cost plus possible faster implementation of a production lane. 3D-printing machines do not need additional tools like injection molds, which are usually custom-made in a time-consuming and expensive manner.

Moreover, using generative manufacturing methods enables to reduce the number of processing steps required for highly complex designs with integrated functionality. Due to the layer-by-layer setup, it may be possible to integrate features within a plastic medical device directly during the printing process. Especially, multicomponent 3D-printing technologies can lead cheaper multicomponent devices. Multicomponent (multifeature) devices can be manufactured by multicomponent injection molding or by assembling of parts as well, but it may be cheaper to manufacture with a 3D-printing technology, especially when combined with a small batch production. Costs for injection molds are considerably higher for multicomponent injection molding in comparison to standard molds, and additional processing steps may result in higher level of automation or increased labor costs.

Labor costs can be considered the driving force behind the next opportunity of 3D printing within the plastic medical device world: the substitute of manually performed labor. Within the medical fields of dentistry and otolaryngology, the accelerating use of 3D printing may have started already an enormous change within the manufacturing of patient individual medical devices. Currently, the major cost for individual-created devices such as occlusal splints (often acrylate polymers) for bruxism therapy is the actual labor costs for the dental technician. Shifting the manufacturing of these devices in low-wage countries may reduce these costs, but may induce issues regarding the possibly lower standards regarding regulatory affairs in these. 3D-printing technologies in combination with digital data generation (e.g., laser scan, digital X-ray) and suitable virtual planning software will most likely lead to less labor-intensive manufacturing of patient individual medical devices thus are expected to trigger a relocation of manufacturing facilities closer to the actual patient. At least the introduction of virtual planning and 3D printing can be already considered as an actual trend, not only an opportunity, within the medical fields of dentistry and otolaryngology. This trend may induce comparable developments in other, more conservative medical disciplines. However, it should be considered that both mentioned fields are more driven by costs for therapy than other fields, often caused by limitation concerning medical insurance reimbursement or even potential lack of insurance coverage, especially when considering prosthetic dentistry.

The cost reduction approach might not appear at first sight due to the limitations in manufacturing speed, but we see opportunities regarding costs within 3D printing. Because of an existing lack of experience regarding the actual cost-saving potential, it is necessary to develop methods and to collect data sets for actual cost comparison studies. But the cost-saving approach is already within range for some plastic medical devices, especially for patient individual treatments, and may lead to so far unthinkable products caused by more lucrative small batch production for highly complex devices, for instance.

4.1.5.3.3 Complex Geometrical Design

Typically, the geometrical design of plastic medical devices follows certain design guidelines due to limitation within manufacturing tools. Five axis CNC universal milling machines plus eroding procedures allow to build manufacturing tools for injection molding and co, which significantly have increased in its geometrical complexity for years. Free-form surfaces are well known within CAD software solutions and allow designing relatively complex 3D shapes. Laser structuring or etching methods can generate surface structures within manufacturing tools, which may help to produce specially fitted surface parameters, like hydrophilic properties. However, prevailing cost of manufacturing correlates with the geometrical complexity. Prime examples are undercuts that usually require moveable slides within the injection mold. Although rather simple in geometry, this design feature significantly increases tool complexity and thus manufacturing costs, giving 3D-printing technologies a decisive advantage. In contrast to standard manufacturing technologies, 3D printing has little limitations concerning the 3D shape of device. Naturally, building space, necessary support structures, and minimal resolution—always in combination with the chosen technology and material—have an impact on geometrical boundaries. Using 3D-printing technologies may allow medical device engineers to correlate their design more with actual situation within human bodies, thinking about personalized implants. It is possible to integrate patient's personal anatomical data prior the manufacturing of certain medical devices or at least add a complex geometrical surface finishing on standard manufactured blanks. Or, it may be interesting to integrate hidden functionality, like building a structure with a damping effect behind a closed surface. Generally spoken, it is possible with 3D printing to shift the geometrical thinking for medical devices away from manufacturability (thinking about drill holes, even surfaces, rounding) and easily geometrical description to more complex, but may be more patient friendly 3D designs. This possible approach is naturally not the gold standard for high-volume single-use products, which have no or only little contact with a patient, but may be interesting for implants or long-term application within the dental or otolaryngology field. Classic CAD tools, even with added free-form modeling, are usually based on the typical abrasive thinking with drilling and milling. It seems plausible to have different tools for creating more complex 3D shapes, which are already known in other technical fields like computer game design.

4.1.5.3.4 Device Design Opportunities

Within the prior section, general implications with complex geometrical designs have been discussed. The logical next step is to take a closer look into device design opportunities. With some randomly selected examples, we try to show opportunities for innovations to increase the **ideality** of plastic medical devices. The term of ideality is defined as the ratio of useful functions and the sum of costs and harmful functions. Regarding the improvement of plastic medical devices, it may be a useful approach to increase the amount of useful functions, to decrease manufacturing costs, and/or to eliminate harmful functions. The consideration of ideality should be done for each product individually. The following examples are merely intended to show different approaches to address the idea of an increased ideality by new device design opportunities.

4.1.5.3.4.1 Application Optimized Devices

Additionally to the actually patient benefits, acceptance and usability of medical devices depend on the empirical values of medical professionals. The aspect of ergonomic considerations is often underestimated regarding the effect on possible economic success. Industrial manufacturing methods facilitated an increased ideality due to lower production costs in accordance with evolving development processes and modern materials, which allow more functions that are useful. The next industrial developing step for plastic medical devices may be a combination of positive effects of industrial grade development and manufacturing with personal demands of future operators. Especially, ergonomic features may play a greater role for future acceptance of medical devices. Today, medical device engineers for surgical instruments address different requirements depending on the anatomical conditions of the operators simply by offering various sizes. It is most likely not profitable to address individual ergonomic issues for single-use devices; however, it may be a likely task to increase the ideality of medical devices for reusables. Virtual example of an ergonomically optimized instrument handle is shown in Figure 4.10. It is a simple illustration for application optimized devices, which seem only realizable concerning efforts and costs with 3D-printing technologies (plus a data generation and virtual planning environment).

4.1.5.3.4.2 Patient Individualized Medical Devices

As you can imagine probably, not only application optimized devices are a great opportunity evolving with 3D-printing technologies for plastic medical devices. The next step is individualized therapies with individually adapted medical devices, which do exist to a certain extent especially in the dental field with manually, labor and cost-intensive devices. This may include therapeutical know-how, which is implemented in the design of the medical device. From the patient's perspective, this opportunity may be the most astonishing and for engineers, it opens a new field with great opportunities to improve patient's treatment and more idealistic medical devices. We see amazing possibilities with individualized medical devices. Therefore, we addressed this major topic with an extra chapter (see Section 4.2).

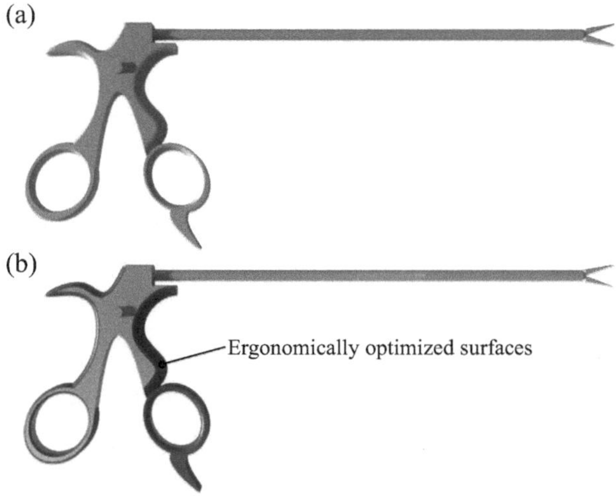

Figure 4.10 Virtual example of an ergonomically optimized instrument handle: Laparoscopic surgical instruments can be designed with a reusable handle to control single use, e.g., clamping or hemostatic cauterization units (a). With rapid manufacturing methods, it seems possible to manufacture handles with ergonomically optimized surfaces individually for a surgeon (b). This is certainly just a model for further discussions, but it may help to rank the ergonomical potential for individual medical devices.

4.1.5.3.4.3 Tissue Optimized Medical Devices

The biological response on implantation of medical devices depends mainly on the biological system, contaminations, their chemical configuration, and their surface texture (see Section 2.1). A biological system (here the human body) cannot be altered for better interaction with medical implants. Contamination issues can be considered as a solvable problem during manufacturing processes. Chemical configuration is designed by chemical engineers and can be altered minor by adding additives. The medical device engineer has to focus on material selection, the design itself plus the surface texture to improve biocompatibility issues. Tissue and its cells can be challenging regarding surface interaction. Different tissues prefer various surface textures. For example, bone tissue favors craggy, sharp-edged surfaces while hepatic tissue requires a smooth, cavernous surface. This should be considered while designing and manufacturing the surface.

Establishing tissue optimized surfaces for medical devices may be challenging. If the preferred texture cannot be implemented during the actual production process itself, additional processing steps will be necessary. Some of the current 3D-printing technologies enable generating with printing resolutions down to 10 μm or less. This dimension is indispensable to alter surfaces in advantage to tissue response. The metallic laser sintering process is already used for production of porous hip joint prosthesis (improved biointegration) due to less cost-intensive manufacturing steps. It is likely to have these facts be transferred to plastic 3D printing for medical devices with long-term biological interaction. Generally, it is worth considering the opportunities of 3D printing for surface treatment in challenge with existing postprocessing surface treatment methods.

4.1.5.3.4.4 Lightweight Construction and Medical Devices

In contrast to the automotive sector, lightweight construction is not a matter of reducing the weight to decrease energy consumption during the application of medical devices. In fact, the biological reaction of the human is only little affected by the implant density, even though some exemptions do exist. However, nonimplantable medical devices may have ergonomic aspects, which correlate with their weight. Think about respiratory masks for treatment of sleep apnea syndrome that patients wear regularly during night sleep. Every option to increase convenience may increase the patient's acceptance. The opportunities of individualized medical devices have been discussed already. An additional step may be to change the medical device design toward lightweight construction to increase the patient's compliance. Especially, the combination of individualization and lightweight design offers highly interesting opportunities of 3D printing for plastic medical devices.

A second aspects for lightweight constructed medical devices are material costs. Lightweight construction may be helpful to bring material costs down for special materials like medical grade biodegradables. These groups of materials are utilized for drug delivery systems or biodegradable implants (see Section 6.5). Due to strict specifications, high production costs and small market volume, these materials can cost up to several thousand euros per kilogram granules. Often not avoidable sprue gates for injection molding are already expense factor, if working with biodegradable materials.

These types of medical devices are often small volume batches due its relatively high costs and often small number of cases. It may be an interesting approach for prospective device design and manufacturing to think about 3D printing with its arising possibility of less material consuming design or at least manufacturing procedure. 3D-printing technologies have to be fitted toward processing biodegradable materials, but basically prepared technologies are already developed and previously mentioned.

4.1.5.3.5 Rapid Tooling—3D Printing for Faster Mold Construction

Rapid tooling is an interesting technological solution, which shows the great opportunities with applied 3D-printing components and may help to widen the horizon of future developments for plastic medical devices. Direct 3D printing of medical devices may have disadvantages. For plausible reasons, 3D printing will not be the one and only approach of manufacturing medical devices. Existing technologies are consequently evolved and provide in many circumstances better results concerning device quality, manufacturing costs, and material selection. Therefore, by far the most medical devices will be processed (partially) with standard or *classic* manufacturing technologies like injection molding and extrusion. Most challenging for small batch production with these technologies is the fact of expensive mold plus its time-consuming creation with CNC milling, erosion techniques and drilling, among other things. Rapid manufactured injection molds may be the solution for these small batch productions. Small batch can be caused by a small market volume for specialized products, but can be caused also for spare parts considerations. Think about long-term medical devices like computer tomography systems: These machines are often in operation for many years plus the overall market volume is relatively small. Spare parts for these products must be deliverable for many years. Replacement injection molds can have an extreme share on the overall manufacturing costs, if used rarely. The solution might be the use of 3D-printed injection molds, especially made from plastic materials (a 3D-printed test mold for an injection-molded tension bar can be seen in Figure 4.11). Plastic materials are usually less resistant to abrasion in comparison to typical steels for injection molds. This fact is of minor importance, if the 3D-printed injection mold is only used for small batches. The major advantages of 3D-printed injection molds are the easier and most likely cheaper creation of the mold itself, especially for relatively simple mold designs. However, moveable parts such as slides are challenging to implement.

The thermal conductivity of plastic materials is smaller than for metal-based systems. That is the major reason, why polymer melt cools differently, slower, in plastic molds compared to metallic molds. A metallic mold is tempered on a certain temperature, depending on the processing conditions of the used thermoplastic. Within a plastic mold, it can be possible

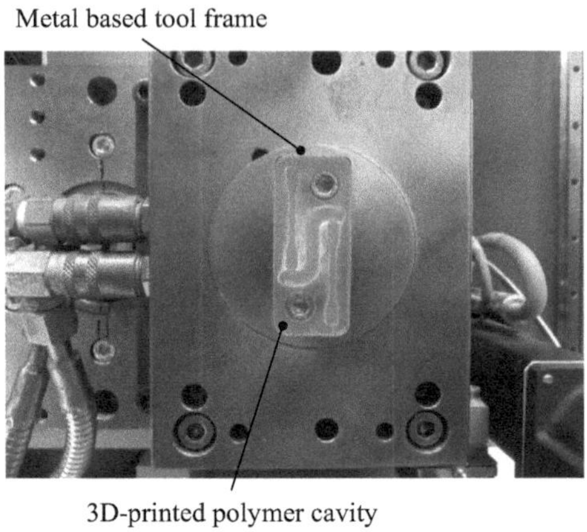

Figure 4.11 Three-dimensional (3D)-printed polymer cavities for small batch injection molding: Per cycle two tension bars are produced within a plastic mold. The mold is manufacturing with 3D printing (multijet modeling) with a UV-curing photopolymer. Research experiences show good results with acrylic butadiene styrene plastics, polyoxymethylene, and polyethylene. Further materials may be possible as well.

to run the injection molding process without any tempering system or at least less energy-consuming tempering system due to its different thermal conductivity. This will help to keep the manufacturing cost down in addition to the faster mold creation time with 3D printing.

4.2 Manufacturing of Individual Medical Devices

Medical devices had been manufactured individually for many hundreds of years until the industrial era. With the industrialization, standardized medical devices became reasonable and less cost-intensive in comparison to handcrafted counterparts. Standardized plastic medical devices are and will be state of the art for many medical applications, where individualized treatments will have no or minimal evidence-based advantages in comparison to standardized products. Still, even today many individual medical devices are regularly utilized in some medical fields. Examples can be found within dentistry, e.g., occlusal splints for bruxism therapy, or within otolaryngology, e.g., earmolds for hearing aid devices. Technician regularly makes these devices in a labor-intensive matter. Especially, these labor and therefore money-consuming individualized medical devices may be manufactured with increased quality level and lower production costs with suitable 3D-printing environments, which includes individual data generation, virtual planning, and the 3D-printing process itself. First approaches have been developed since the introduction of 3D-printing materials, which fits the biocompatibility standards to a certain extent. The medical fields of dentistry and otolaryngology are definitely progressive regarding adoption of new medical device techniques including new treatment approaches. However, first individual 3D-printed medical devices have been introduced in further medical fields. For instance, laser sintered sawing templates are applied during surgical operations to ensure more exact orthopedic surgery results. These templates show the amazing opportunities, which may be possible with individual 3D-printing environments: Better outcome due to more individualized treatments seem possible or even 3D-printed devices, which include treatment know-how and allows further distribution of highly specialized therapies.

> The opportunities of 3D-printing will have an enormous impact for the development of new approaches regarding individualized medical devices.

Individual medical devices will be a synonym for 3D-printed medical devices in the future. Surely, the given opportunity aspects in the prior chapter will produce additional fields for 3D-printed plastic medical devices, which are not fitted for the individual patient. The treatment possibilities and enormous cost-saving potential will be extraordinary for these devices; however, as it can be seen in some already realized, and partially mentioned, examples. But especially the individualized manufacturing causes several open questions, which have not been addressed properly. Within the regulatory market of the European Union, individualized medical devices, which are made for a specific patient, are exempt from the obligatory conformity declaration (also known as approval process) for medical devices. This rule was included within the regulatory framework, when individualized manufactured medical devices were considered to be handcrafted by professional trained technicians, and the potential of 3D printing was not foreseeable for patient individualized devices. Today, it is actually a regulatory loophole. It is not clear, if a patient individual medical device, which is manufactured within an industrial facility, has to comply with regulatory affairs, like the necessity of a quality and risk management system. Due to its importance, these legal questions are addressed separately in an upcoming chapter to discuss necessary regulatory clarifications and normative adaptions to ensure high-qualitative medical devices, which are manufactured individually with industrial standards regarding quality, risks, durability, and hygienic issues. Especially, the liability question ("Who is liable for which malpractice during the individualized manufacturing process: the prescribing medical practitioner, manufacturer or both?") will become more and more important, if the reach of individualized 3D-printing environments is getting more popular.

The whole 3D-printing world is a nonunified industrial field with many different development trends, research projects, and ideas in general. It is not possible to address each single development step within these engineering worlds. With the upcoming section, we try to address the impact and probably importance of 3D-printing technologies for patient individualized medical devices. Beginning with our personal biased overview over current applications of these devices, it is our aim to give hints for future developments for upcoming medical device engineers, true to the motto "knowing the existing world, to innovate the new world." It is helpful to understand the opportunity of individualized plastic devices, under which circumstances these products may increase the patient's treatment, respectively outcome, and which medical fields are mainly in focus. Based on this, existing challenges for these emerging designs and techniques are evaluated to show necessary developments for a wider integration within the medical device industry. As you should have learned so far about the medical device world, the development of new treatment approaches is not only a technical matter, but it is also a regulatory question. Rarely known or absolutely new treatment opportunities are often considered skeptical by regulatory bodies or faces tough challenges regarding verification process. Due to the lack of existing regulations or normative standards, possible legal challenges of individual manufactured devices are discussed with regard to the utilization of 3D-printing processes. The term 3D printing may be used in this context more widely and includes a whole process chain to produce individualized medical devices under industrialized standards regarding product quality, risk management, and biocompatibility.

4.2.1 Current Applications of Individual Medical Devices

It is worth looking into current applications of plastic 3D-printed individual medical devices to understand the occurring development and predict emerging trends and necessary improvements within manufacturing and materials. As you have learned already, utilization of 3D printing implies uncountable opportunities. Surely, it has to be considered under which circumstances its application is suitable and worthwhile. Within the upcoming chapter, we will show evolved application with increased integrated know-how. The chosen devices are extraordinary examples, which help to understand the possibilities for future applications. All applications have common thinking in a whole process. Simplified, a 3D-printing machine cannot produce useful individual medical devices without adequate individual anatomic data and virtual planning environment adapted to the specific application along with an appropriate product management system to guarantee a correct classification of anatomic data and printed devices to the actual patient. We have to make sure, you understand the opportunity of 3D printing by showing these examples, but due to the fast growing and changing market it is not possible to provide a complete overview about all available individually printed devices. Especially in university medical centers with a strong research approach, uncountable 3D-printing research takes place with minimal regulatory boundaries, but always under supervision and approval of ethics committees during application. The European Union regulations allow to an exclusion of the regular approval process for so-called in-house developed medical devices (an example is also shown within this chapter).

4.2.1.1 Manual Treatment Planning or Device Production with 3D-Printed Casts

It is a common ground within the world of medicine that the correlation between treatment time and costs is absolutely relevant. Cost reduction for single treatments is, in most industrialized countries, a major topic due to general increases caused by demographic aging or new expensive treatment opportunities, which includes highly specialized drugs. Therefore, it is understandable that cost reduction was and still is a strong force behind the implementation of 3D-printed plastic devices. Think about the cost incurred during a surgical procedure with several medical professional (from anesthesia to the operator) necessary: reduction of surgery time leads to lower operation costs. During complicated surgical procedures, e.g., major facial fractures with tremendous work of reconstruction, it is extremely helpful to have a planning opportunity before surgery. Surely, imaging methods like computer tomography provide excellent virtual planning possibilities. However, it is favored by an increasing quantity of surgeons to plan tricky operations with actual 3D-printed models based on the generated anatomic data with imaging methods. In this case, 3D printing is utilized as a planning tool for elective treatment procedures. An example treatment is shown in Figure 4.12. It takes a certain amount

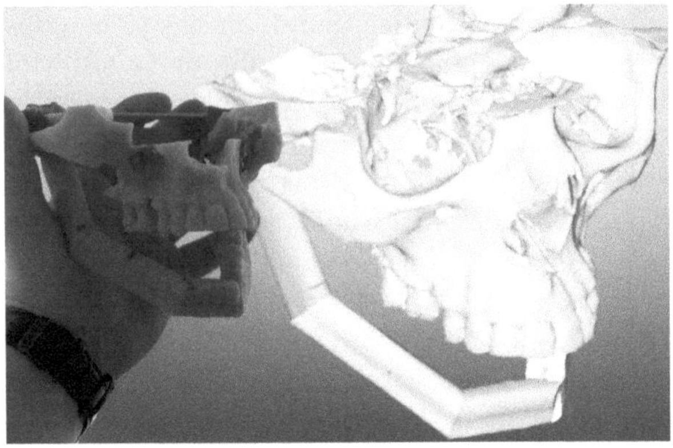

Figure 4.12 The Department of Oral and Maxillofacial Surgery of Mainz University (Germany) uses virtually planned and three-dimensional (3D)-printed models for jaw, facial, or head reconstruction surgery based on an initial CAT or MRI images. The printed models help to understand more patient friendly treatments regarding operation time including anesthesia, traumatic impact, and healing outcome. In addition, the 3D-printed model helps to adapt necessary implants or templates before surgery. *Figure courtesy of Peter Pullkowski.*

of time to manufacture these casts, mainly due to the lack of 3D-printing machines in treatment facilities and caused by the duration of the printing process itself, making it not suitable for urgent surgical intervention so far. Specialized fast track printing machines with less concern of surface quality, long-term resistance, or mechanical properties, may be helpful to increase possible fields of application, especially in short-term applications, for such planning or individualized supporting devices (described in the next section).

3D-printed models cannot only be helpful within highly elaborated surgical procedures, but especially within dentistry these 3D-printed casts are already in application to reduce time-consuming manual labor steps in some dental laboratories. To understand the possibilities of 3D-printed plastic casts, let's have a look into the state of the art of manufacturing individual dental bridges. Based on a dental imprint, a model of the jaw and set of teeth is modeled with plaster cast materials. After these initial steps, dental bridges are modeled on the plaster cast and fitted toward the individual needs. These steps are time-consuming to the actual labor work plus the waiting times for curing processes. The implementation of a 3D-printing environment including digitalization unit and virtual planning can help to decrease the manufacturing costs. Additionally, quality monitoring approaches may be easily implementable within such a

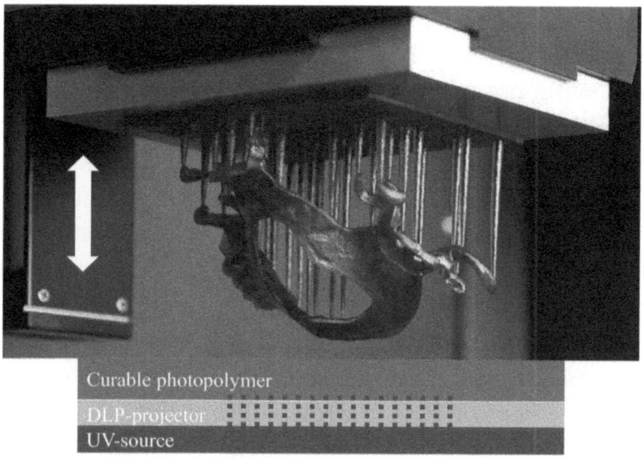

Figure 4.13 DLP-based model casting for dentistry: The patient's anatomical dental information is digitalized three dimensionally (3D) with X-rays or intraoral scanners. Manually produced dental casts require several labor-intensive modeling steps. With a suitable data generation and virtual planning environment, it is possible to decrease the actual amount of labor steps by digital planning plus a 3D-printing procedure. In this case, a DLP technique is used to cure a photopolymer material. The UV beam is applied from below, and the cured layers are drawn upward. This technical arrangement works without additional ductor blades. Uncured material is spaced out evenly by forces of gravity. *Figure is modified, figure courtesy of Martin Klare, pro3dure medical GmbH.*

3D-printing environment and software solution than in a typical mainly labor-based work. Due to the lack of appropriate 3D-printing plastic materials for dental bridges (which have to be considered long-term medical devices), current 3D-printing applications for individual modeling focus on 3D-printed model casts as shown in Figure 4.13. The 3D data are generated usually by laser-based intraoral scanners or X-ray. With improved long-term applicable materials, completely virtually planning and 3D-printing processes are likely and may lead to decreased manufacturing costs for these medical devices. Currently, many patients worldwide cannot afford accurate dental care.

4.2.1.2 Surgical Treatments Supported with 3D-Printed Devices

Well- and long-trained surgeons should perform surgical procedures. For the last decades, support technologies have been developed to improve general quality and therefore patients' outcome. A major technological step was the introduction of navigated surgical systems, which allow accurate implant positioning basing on virtual planning. These techniques work usually with optical tracking systems including time- and skill-consuming linking process of the actual patient with the virtual data to allow accurate navigation. Additional trackable landmarks have to be fixed on the patient's body in most cases. As you can see, navigated surgery can be well-blessing, especially for less experienced surgeons to avoid faulty positioning of implants. However, the navigation technologies on the contrary require comprehensive training of medical professionals and their application during surgical treatment is often quite time-consuming.

Why not using 3D printing as a chance to decrease the necessary operation time even for navigated purposes, additional to the prior mentioned planning approach? These 3D-printed devices, which increase the surgical performance during the actual procedure, can be considered the next development step for individually 3D-printed plastic devices. They are actually used during operation instead of preliminary planning only. Some individually 3D-printed and intraoperative used devices have been developed so far; however, the overall approach has not yet developed as state of the art in many surgical fields. Therefore, it implies huge possibilities for future developments and application under the slogan of 3D-printed devices for **assisted surgery**. The necessary development input, especially in beneficial virtual designing environments, increases with the complexity of a surgical procedure.

Relatively simple approaches have found their way from research and development into some operation theaters. One of them is shown as an example in Figure 4.14, which describes a PA-based, laser sintered sawing template for knee arthroplasty. Basing on anatomic, the precise positioning of the implant has to be planned before surgery. With software, optimal positioning is allocated regarding mobility, forces, and operational impact, among other parameters. Based on the positioning, a sawing template is generated virtually, which will be fitted easily with pins on the surgical area before the implantation procedure. The 3D-printed sawing template easily may be fixated on the patient during the surgical procedure, allowing faster treatment compared to traditionally assisted surgery approaches.

The approach of integrating a certain amount of functionality in an individually 3D-printed device in combination with a simple handling during the application offers a wide range of opportunities for future developments of individually 3D-printed medical devices. The next introduced application field with integrated treatment shows again, how much know-how can be transformed from medical professionals' experiences into highly specialized and individualized 3D-printed medical devices.

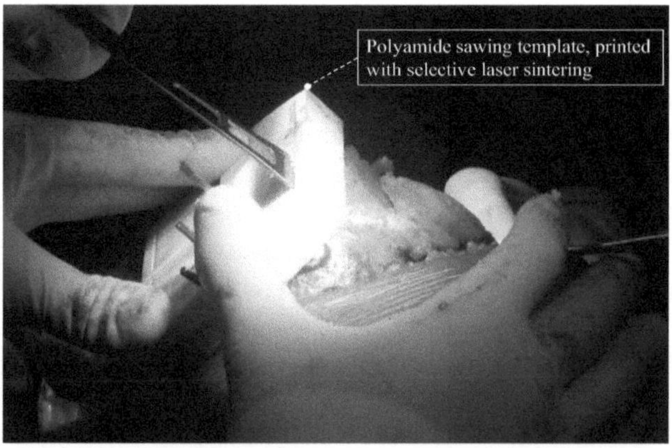

Figure 4.14 Laser sintered polyamide sawing template: A correct positioning of knee implants is essential for the patient's outcome. Positioning is a question of surgical experiences. Therefore, support systems have been developed for many years and are often referred as navigated surgery. Optical tracking approaches are relatively complex for operators and therefore time-consuming. A new approach is to plan the actual necessary bone cutting previously in a virtual environment based on the patient's anatomical data. Based on the planning, individually adapted sawing templates are printed and applied during the surgical procedure. In contrast to existing navigated systems, sawing templates can be attached to a patient with pins less time-consuming. *Figure is modified, figure courtesy of Maurice Scheer, 3D-LABS GmbH and Aesculap AG.*

4.2.1.3 Virtual Planned 3D-Printed Devices with Integrated Treatment

The chosen examples should widen your imagination about the arising opportunities caused by the combination of individualized medical devices, virtual planning environments, and 3D printing. Each application field, from the relatively simple cast printing up to devices with integrated treatment functions, implies many so far not considered or even unthinkable new development opportunities. It is worth mentioning at this point, that it is not our aim to evaluate all these examples and opportunities regarding economic considerations or patients' outcome on a long-time frame, but to create knowledge about emerging technologies and their possibilities. The upcoming example of a virtual planned 3D-printed device with an integrated treatment functionality has caused already many discussions about the (dis-)advantages of such devices. However, it can be considered a successful approach, which may be considered in future years as the groundbreaking development for such devices. We are talking about the 3D-printed aligner medical devices for teeth adjustments. The planning and printing procedure is described in Figure 4.15. Beyond only supporting it, they actually perform the treatment. First, the desired arrangement, and thus appearance of the teeth is virtually planned. The necessary teeth adjustment is broken into several displacement steps. Therefore, the needed displacement forces are provided by 3D-printed aligner samples. Each sample fits to the next wished substep of the whole adjustment process, and it induces the displacement forces until the single displacement step is finished (up to 0.3 mm per aligner). The aligner principle

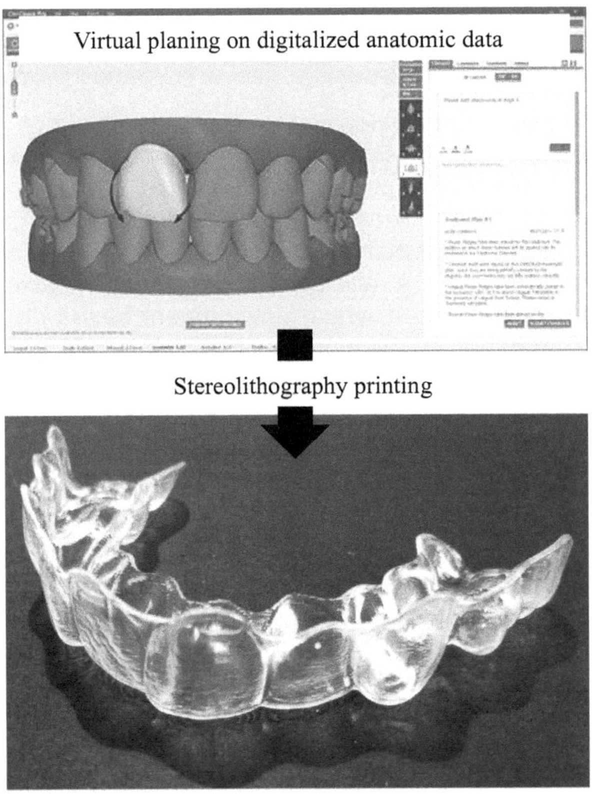

Figure 4.15 Incremental aligner device for teeth adjustment, printed with stereolithography: Based on digitalized anatomic teeth data, a patient individual treatment is planed virtually. Each printed aligner should induce a teeth adjustment up to 0.3 mm per 1 or 2 weeks (overall treatment period up to 14 months). This aligner concept is an amazing, Food and Drug Administration approved, example for a fully established patient individualized device manufacturing process based on three-dimensional printing opportunities. The used materials are subject to criticism due to low-biocompatibility results, in addition to the outcome results itself. *Figure is modified, figure courtesy of Smikey lo, Wikipedia Commons.*

tries to copycat the know-how of dental retainers without the manual adjustments and the permanent fixation within the oral cavity.

The aligner principle is applied frequently around the globe and can be considered as among the first major FDA approved 3D-printed individualized medical device. Due to its tremendous change in comparison to classical teeth adjustment treatments, the technology has faced many critics for the last years, mainly regarding the actual adjustment effect. However, medical device engineers should have a deeper look into criticism concerning the used 3D-printing materials. Although approved by the FDA, the aligner technology uses materials that exhibit some issues concerning patient safety. Reports show allergic reactions and research groups discuss negative effects on human cell growth. Technologically spoken and as mentioned repeatedly, 3D-printing materials generally are still a huge concern regarding long-term application and biocompatibility. Due to its groundbreaking approach, the technology is and will be approved, but possible future application with included treatment functionality need to have a bigger focus on materials, besides further quality and risk management issues. This quick debauchery may help to understand the correlations within the whole medical device world.

The final example fits perfectly to emphasize the major fact of this chapter, which you should keep in mind: Get to know current applications, stay informed about upcoming developments and existing problems, combine ideas and you can develop highly innovative approaches, which will have an impact on future medical devices and their application. The RapidNAM technology is such a product combining these aspects with the opportunities of 3D-printing processes for individualized medical devices. Young patients with cleft lip and palate can be treated with so-called nasoalveolar molding devices to induce a cleft reduction and nose alignment prior first surgical procedure. This allows reducing the number of surgical inventions required, while improving the results. However, conventional production of these molding devices is time-consuming and combined with a certain impact on the young patients (mostly 1 or 2 weeks old). Based on the knowledge about the previously described aligner technology, a research group, has started efforts to develop a virtual molding device planning environment to decrease the production times with 3D printing plus to increase the distribution of these highly complex treatments for young, strongly affected patients. First clinical trial shows promising results that exhibit at least equivalent results on comparison to the state-of-the-art treatment. The application of local forces to adjust a body part is comparable to the aligner principle, however, adapted strongly to the different medical task. The major technological consideration is the implementation of natural growth within these individual design and manufactured devices on the other hand. The included treatment functionality is therewith on a completely new level. This example should show that previously existing thinking boundaries may be reviewed critically by medical device engineers and may create extraordinary new medical devices, which are adapted within a 3D-printing process to patients' special needs (Figure 4.16).

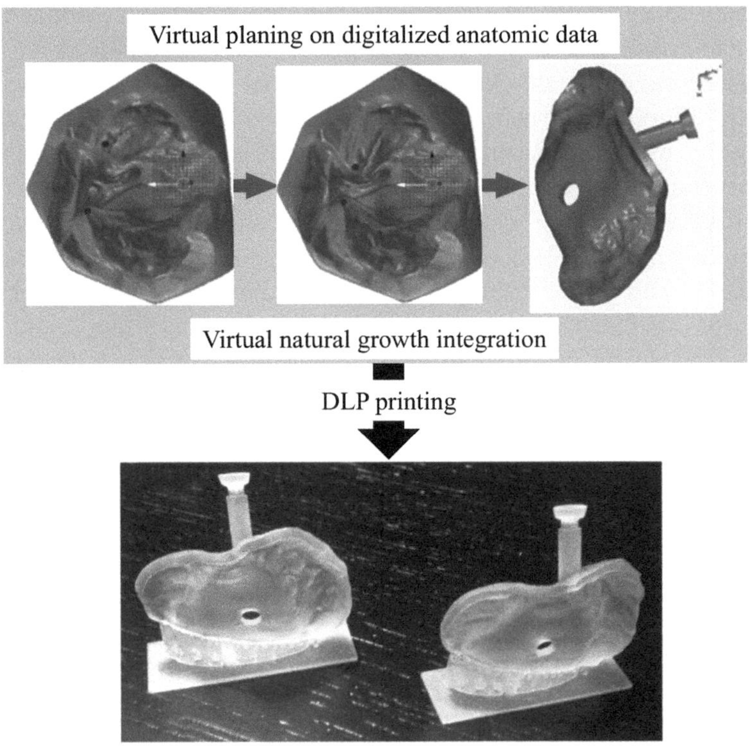

Figure 4.16 Virtual planned nasoalveolar molding devices for presurgical treatment of infants with cleft lip and palate: State of the art is to create these devices manually by the medical practitioner, who need a high level of experience for device production. The induced decrease of cleft size and nose deformity depends on the applied deformation pressure. It has to be avoided too much pressure due to possible formation of necroses. Before implementing a fully functional three-dimensional (3D)-planning and 3D-printing environment, the experience of medical practitioner has to be implemented within a working planning tool plus addressing effects of the existing general growth of infants. After planning, these devices must be producible within 24h to avoid treatment delays. The used 3D-printing materials should imply ergonomical issues regarding the young patient and must have a high biocompatibility level due to treatment period of about a week per device, up to 14 devices in a row. *Figure is modified, figure courtesy of Markus Schönberger and Martin Klare, pro3dure medical GmbH.*

4.2.2 Emerging Design and Technical Challenges for Individual Devices

During the introduction of 3D-printing fundamentals and current applications of individual medical devices, some challenges have been mentioned already. To establish a broader understanding about existing technical challenges, which can be translated with improvement potentials regarding individual medical plastic devices and their manufacturing, the design, engineering, and manufacturing process of such devices are analyzed and further discussed. It is definitely not our aim to point out every possible technical challenge or likely problem, but to create a general understanding and show major facts. Following subsections are chosen, inspired by typical development processes and translated into a possible engineering workflow for individualized medical devices with 3D printing:

- treatment options versus market volume,
- designing of individual medical device solutions,
- material selection,
- testing of individual medical devices,
- 3D printer and hygienic design,
- process stability and hygienic handling,
- liable process chain and virtual environment.

4.2.2.1 Treatment Options versus Market Volume

For many diseases, the development of specific medical devices hasn't been lucrative with conventional manufacturing technologies. Surely, 3D printing offers new approaches with acceptable cost levels, but it is still a question of possibility and lucrativeness. As you can imagine, many treatment options with individualized medical devices seem to be realizable, but do not offer enough market volume. Especially within university medical centers, many research groups are looking into the development of individualized devices for any kind of illness (e.g., tracheobronchomalacia treatment with 3D-printed splints).

It is easily understandable, why research groups are interested in developing individualized 3D-printing approaches: Major work is caused by the development of virtual environments, availability of 3D-printing technologies, and a lack of regulatory boundaries. Industrial engineers and product developer may have such freedoms as well, but most times the major fact is about the market volume prediction, possible revenue, and return of investment. Due to lack of sufficient data, it is not easily predictable under which circumstances an individually 3D-printed medical device will be a blockbuster or covered by health insurance systems. Currently, many highly specific 3D-printed applications work with regulatory exemptions or live within a gray area. Therefore, it is necessary for future engineers to establish acceptable evaluation methods regarding emerging possibilities with 3D-printing environments, acceptable market volume, and possible reimbursement rates. It is a typical chicken and egg problem: On the one hand, sufficient data help to decrease portfolio and development risks while on the other hand you need developed 3D-printing products to generate these data. Hopefully, current high-risk developments within research facilities will lead to increased interest within existing industrial entities for individualized plastic medical devices and to more sufficient treatment options, even for less attractive patient portfolios.

4.2.2.2 Designing of Individual Medical Device Solutions

The design or better-called engineering process for conventional medical devices requires the consideration of mechanical properties, resistance questions, or hygienic points, among other things. Therefore, process parameters for manufacturing are defined, test samples are produced, and existing test procedures, e.g., accelerated aging, are applied. All these aspects are necessary to develop medical devices that comply with the relevant regulations. Now, let's try to adapt the existing conventional designing and engineering process for patient-specific 3D-printing environments. Mechanical properties of plastic devices depend on the parameters of the manufacturing process, the material behavior, and environmental influences. Patient-specific devices may imply different material curing, melt periods, or varying aging vulnerability. For example, the occurrence of environmental stress cracking, a major aging process in thermoplastic polymers, is highly influenced by the actual processing parameters during manufacturing. With relatively constant manufacturing parameters, it is no problem to address these potential aging problems, but how is it possible to observe potential aging problems before finishing approval processes. Aging effects have to be discussed a priori to evaluate necessary mechanical properties in combination with basic materials properties. Transferred to individual medical devices, it means every single product has to be observed regarding patient safety issues, if you follow the existing approval process for standard plastic devices. This question has not been addressed properly in current individualized devices, which are commercially available.

As already mentioned (and therefore described within an additional chapter, "Legal Challenges of Individual Manufactured Devices"), existing approaches have been approved within a certain gray area of the regulatory world (e.g., defining the device for short-term application use instead of the actual intended application period) or received exemption status due to extraordinary conditions, like the FDA-ruling humanitarian use device: "humanitarian device exemption for diseases or conditions that affects or is manifested in fewer than 4000 individuals in the United States per year." In addition, some 3D-printed devices already gained 510(k) approval by the FDA. Not only mechanical properties depend on chosen manufacturing conditions, but also bio- or hemocompatibility issues as well. Think about individually designed orthopedic implants for hip joint replacement: In addition to individual biomechanical properties, the significantly differing biological response should be considered. This might be caused by individually different surface conditions, which could lead to different biocompatibility results.

Future approval processes and adopted regulations are likely to be passed within the next couple of years. A thinkable option for future approval processes for patient-specific 3D-printed materials might be the switch from a product-based approval to a manufacturing process approval. Therefore, it would be necessary to establish manufacturing threshold values based on the design boundaries of the individualized medical device. If the individually manufactured device is within previously defined manufacturing limits, it will be granted approval due to an approved manufacturing process or to put it another way: Engineers of industrial-based-individualized medical devices like the Invisalign technology must define acceptable boundaries, in which the individual device must be processed. It means that the individualization of medical devices implies certain limitation regarding availability to patients; exceptionally, anatomical patients may not fit into the previously approved manufacturing boundaries and therefore cannot receive the treatment. However, the more process and manufacturing orientated approach allows to have approval concepts for individual 3D-printed medical devices, which are comparable to the existing approval processes for standard medical devices. This might be also transferable to biocompatibility questions. As you should know already, it won't be financially acceptable to regard every possible surface design and processed material within the chosen manufacturing boundaries. Biocompatibility and related topics should be observed with a worst-case thinking by defining the worst-possible manufacturing and surface conditions regarding the biological response and fitting the test environment accordingly.

4.2.2.3 Material Selection

Virtual planned patient-specific plastic devices must be translated into a real-existing product at a certain time to start the patient's treatment. Besides the later discussed challenges with 3D-printing machines, the material selection is the major defiance concerning the nonvirtual processing for individualized devices. Engineers have to consider available materials for the chosen printing technology and the intended use of the device, which can be a short-term noninvasive up to a long-term invasive plus vascular application. In contrast to state-of-the-art manufacturing technologies, the availability of medical approved 3D-printing materials leaves considerate room for improvement. Thermoplastic granulate-based printing technologies might be excluded, because using standard plastic materials without 3D printing-related optimizations is feasible. Future developments regarding 3D-printing materials should focus on issues like reduced residual monomer content, improved resistance to disinfection or sterilization, applicable forces, and reducing material costs. The material costs are often not caused by the actual costs for synthesis procedures, however. Most 3D-printing materials are fitted to a certain machine type and vice versa certain machine types are only workable with specific materials, often artificially restricted. It is comparable with the razor-blade business: The actual costs arise with the consumable materials.

If you are looking on the material issue in a classical plastic engineer manner, you might think about material modifications with additives or functionality integration. These are additional topics, which should be discussed within future developments within the materials for 3D-printing world. The design freedom on the one hand is restricted by material limitations on the other hand.

4.2.2.4 Testing of Individual Medical Devices

The quality and risk management issues have been referred within the previous sections. The general concerns can be summarized by the statement that the product approval process for 3D-printed-specific medical devices should be altered to a manufacturing approval approach. It would be a more statistically performed procedure, which would require specific testing operations to ensure a worst-case testing and for definition of the necessary boundary conditions. It is worth having a look into sterility testing. It is not possible to examine each product regarding its sterility profile. Therefore, statistical approaches have been developed, like the decimal reduction time, to evaluate sterilization process instead of the product. The logic behind these approaches is that a product is sterile if the sterilization process is within the boundaries to guarantee sterile products. Similar thinking might be useful for 3D-printed patient-specific medical devices, especially implants, in the future. The approach to test one product type, manufactured under a certain condition, is not helpful to evaluate biocompatibility issues for such patient-specific devices, for instance. Applicable test protocols to evaluate parameter matrices (e.g., short-, middle-, long-curing periods with corresponding residual monomer contents in combination with applied stresses) should be in focus for future testing. The major challenge is to define useful and approvable parameter matrices for necessary testing, be that for biocompatibility, mechanical properties, resistance to aging, sterilization, or disinfectants. The challenge is to generate enough data to address these questions properly in combination with statistical tools to guarantee certain likelihoods. These approaches are well-known within the manufacturing world and might be adopted for product testing of patient-specific 3D-printing environments, including the virtual planning, material, and the 3D-printing process.

4.2.2.5 3D-Printer and Hygienic Design

3D-printing machines have been developed for some decades already. Regarding the application for medical device manufacturing, there are some development opportunities left for sure. Despite an individualized or small batch manufacturing future 3D-printing machines should be reconsidered concerning hygienic design for future medical device applications. Current developments are focusing in increasing printing speed or accuracy, but not with the same effort on hygienic considerations. Hygienic design, including clean room facilities, in combination of an automated handling is a key role within conventional manufacturing methods. If 3D-printing machines are getting more into the focus for medical device production, regulatory bodies will have a closer look into hygienic conditions. Comparable to the injection molding world, this may lead to specific 3D-printing machines, which are optimized concerning cleanability or integration capability into clean room environments.

The business model for patient-specific medical devices may include a device manufacturing by service providers or within the medical facility as well. Invasive medical devices have to be applied in a sterile manner to patients. Sterilization methods are often time-consuming or imply limitation regarding suitable printing materials. In combination with the increasing printing speed, it may be a great opportunity to have patient-specific 3D printer within medical facilities or even within surgical theaters to optimize patient's treatment on the flow. Surely, this vision fits only for some applications. But even, if the 3D-printing procedure is done with service providers or before operations within the medical facility, sterility will be a major concern for 3D-printed individual devices or, being more accurate, for the utilized 3D-printing materials. A thinkable solution of the sterilization issue is the so-called autosterile production approach,[1] which can be considered state of the art within the pharmaceutical industry. Autosterility means to manufacture and package under extra clean conditions, which allows to put such devices into market without a subsequent sterilization step. Transferred to 3D-printing machines, their design may be altered regarding more hygienic manufacturing opportunities to get rid of the disadvantages of subsequent sterilization procedures.

4.2.2.6 Process Stability and Hygienic Handling

Serial production is usually based on the premise to achieve constant processes quality, independently to the applied manufacturing technology. Most development approaches have in common to achieve higher-quality levels by more accurate process stability. Summarized for plastic parts, this goal can be translated of having constant part dimensions, therefore volume, and mass. Even for serial production, it is not easily achievable due to various regulated parameters like melt temperature or production speed. However, there exist excellent statistical methods to prove certain production stability regarding tolerances, which are getting tougher and tougher every year. These methods can be applied by testing produced parts in correlation with machine parameters. Some machines, especially injection molding ones, have already self-learning software environments, which can adjust the machine parameters to a certain extent within set limits. You should get the general understanding for the need of constant processes to increase production and product qualities. The question is, how to transfer the need of constant manufacturing processes to individualized products? Each device has its own dimensions or mass. Therefore, these data cannot be implemented within the machine software in a self-learning process. Even statistical testing methods to evaluate retrospective the process quality aren't applicable due the permanently changing part designs due to the adaptation to the individual needs. In our opinion, it is necessary to involve new testing methods to ensure constant processes for individualized 3D printing. In this case, process quality can be translated

1. The autosterile production approach is currently investigated for casting plastic manufacturing procedure due to its advantages regarding material behavior, limitations, or aging effects. Further details are presented for autosterile injection molding within the Emerging Manufacturing Technologies chapter.

to dimensional deviation between virtual data and printed device. The human body may adjust to a certain extent variations, especially in less sensitive cases like teeth aligners. For more risky patient-specific devices, it is necessary to guarantee high device quality regarding its tolerances. The manufacturer for current individual applications has done considerable efforts already. For instance, dimensions of printed sawing templates (see Section 4.2.1) are tested by laser scanning after production. This approach of testing each device is suitable for small batches of individually printed devices, but should be reconsidered for less expensive or bigger volumes due to the high testing costs.

Firstly, we have considered the process stability by regarding testing and correlation aspects. Secondly, the printing machines themselves offer room for improvement. A perfect machine does not only print a device as close as possible to the virtual set dimensions, it would also print the same device with the accurate and same dimensions every time it is printed on the same type of machine. Individual devices may fail during their application at patients, maybe due to compliances issues, just think about previously mentioned occlusal splints for bruxism therapy: During the nightly application damages are unavoidable. It would be a tremendous possibility to print the next splint on the same type of machine, but not necessarily on the actual same machine, and it is still possible to guarantee same device dimensions.

The hygienic handling offers some improvement potential, which can be summarized under the process stability aspect as well. Conventional manufacturing methods for medical devices are established to achieve a certain clean environment. To reduce hygienic challenges, many processes are based on fully automated processes to decrease the interaction between medical device and employee. Therefore, many manufacturers work with automated production and packaging machines. These approaches should be translated to the production of individualized medical devices to increase hygienic level more easily. However, it means to develop (fully) automated production cells, which includes printing itself, postprocessing steps like surface finishing and packaging. Currently, these processes are not established due to the lack of sufficient need plus a relatively small market volume. A visionary approach would be to have a fully automated 3D-printing process chain under hygienic, let's call it clean room, conditions, which allows to manufacture individualized medical devices for many different types of applications. This would help to increase occupancy rate and device quality plus decrease manufacturing costs. This aspect brings us to the final aspect of these subsections about technical challenges for manufacturing patient-specific medical devices: the creation and maintenance of a liable planning and process chain.

4.2.2.7 Liable Planning and Process Chain

Previously, the challenges regarding process stability have been introduced. However, an individual medical device production is only realizable with an all-embracing planning (including generating individual anatomic data!) and process chain. In contrast to conventional designed and manufactured devices, each printed part has to be planned virtually with appropriate software tools before manufacturing. Easily spoken, it means that the software must be able to create the individual medical device and ensure the inclusion of the necessary implied treatment. A constant manufacturing environment will be pointless, if the previous design planning is not reliable. Hence, the term "manufacturing" should be extended with the virtual device planning. It is not helpful to focus on the device development on the one hand and the manufacturing on the other hand. Production errors may appear during planning, manufacturing itself, and each postprocess. Therefore, the virtual planning environments should be considered with the same look concerning production quality.

All aspects can be summarized as followed:

Device quality depends on **each step of patient specific device creation**: accuracy of digital anatomical data, virtual planning environment, 3D-printing and post-processes including packaging.	

4.2.3 *Legal Challenges of Individual Manufactured Devices*

Though 3D printing is already in use for medical device manufacturing and some processes have been approved by regulatory bodies so far, the rising star 3D printing may cause some legal challenges for further medical device applications. Existing approvals have been granted with some stomachache, especially noticed by the U.S. FDA, due to a lack of regulatory boundaries for 3D-printing processes including the whole manufacturing chain up to the chosen materials. The FDA announced an official notice in 2014 with the following quote:

> "[...]Additive manufacturing may or may not present new questions depending on its use. However, there are technical challenges associated with the process from design to

final product that need to be properly addressed in all cases to ensure patient safety and to promote innovation in a fast-moving field. Process verification and validation are especially important when devices are produced individually or in very small batches.[...]"

FDA notice, May 19th, 2014.

This statement indicates clearly the current lack of trust and knowledge about handling 3D-printed medical devices in general and patient individualized devices in specific. Easily spoken, regulatory bodies are unsure about how to work with 3D-printed medical devices due to the same reason, why engineers faces technical challenges as described in the previous subsection. Usually, the goal behind regulatory efforts is to increase device qualities and decrease potential safety issues for individual patients. The interesting fact for 3D-printed medical devices is that not only a new medical device causes headaches concerning the approval process, but the used manufacturing approach (3D printing) is under scrutiny as well. In contrast to other long-existing manufacturing techniques, 3D-printing technologies have been invented and developed after major provisions—established by regulatory bodies worldwide. Therefore, no grandfathering of existing technologies was applicable. In addition, the general knowledge about 3D printing, including quality and risk management methods, can be considered as improvable and relatively low in comparison to long-standing and well-researched production methods. Along with the current developments within the 3D-printing world, regulatory bodies have acknowledged current lacks within their regulatory framework. Within the next years, new provisions will be published with reasonable certainty, especially due to the fact that the FDA is already publishing about the unsatisfied situation.

> Regulatory bodies will address the 3D-printing topic with further provisions with a reasonable certainty within the next years.

The general concerns and lack of knowledge about how to handle manufacturing with 3D printing apply for 3D printing of individualized plastic medical devices as well. Regarding process stability, material questions or software validation, it makes no difference if one equal part or a small batch of equal parts are manufactured. The mentioned aspects have to be addressed in similar way for regulatory issues.

Individualized medical devices may include further issues, which are not just a regulatory burden, but also legal or better-called malpractice concerns. Think about following, possible arising, questions:

- Who is liable for personalized medical devices, the prescribing physician or the manufacturing facility?
- Who performs the individualization procedure (physician, physician and technician, technician, or an automated software solution)?
- Decentralized production at the medical facility versus centralized production within a plant facility?
- Who is liable to generate the individual patient's data needed for individual devices and who is liable for mistakes in the manufacturing process (data collection, manufacturing process, etc.)?

The above mentioned questions are definitely the most obvious ones, many more are likely. Currently approved patient-specific devices, some have been introduced in this book, can be considered on uncertain grounds, if it comes to questions about malpractice situations. This is simply caused by the lack of regulatory frameworks or legal rulings, e.g., in law courts or legislations. Due to enormous difference within the legal systems, not only for the approval process, but also for prescribing individualized medical devices, malpractices laws, and so on, a worldwide comparable regulatory solution might be tough to achieve regarding the liability question.

Summarizing this chapter about legal challenges of individualized medical devices, it is most likely to have many good manufacturing practice rules for 3D-printed medical devices, which includes virtual planning environments, 3D-printing machines, materials, and postprocessing steps. More invented and applied individualized medical devices offer huge potential for new or better treatment options, not only for illnesses with high prevalence, but may also cause interesting legal questions in the future.

4.3 Individual versus Mass Production of Medical Devices

Many plastic medical devices have been produced in large quantities with the major aim to reduce manufacturing costs per part consequently. The term *mass production* has been used regularly to describe the manufacturing approach. Prior to the mass productions period, most medical devices have been made manually in small batches or only have been manufactured on behalf of physicians' desires, often made with metals or glassware. The development of modern plastic materials in combination with constant manufacturing progress has led to an enormous usage within medical devices. Major reasons are the relatively cheap manufacturing, high degree of design freedom, availability of materials with strong resistance toward sterilization, disinfection or body fluids, and satisfying biocompatibility. Mass production technologies seem unlikely to generate patient-specific medical devices, however. These manufacturing techniques have been developed for high throughput, which is definitely the gold standard for the production of most plastic medical devices. On the other hand, we have described it regularly, patient-specific medical devices may have certain advantages, surely not for every application, but likely for specific or so far unthinkable treatment options. Another opportunity is replacement of currently manually performed production with patient-specific 3D printing.

The logic behind the presented patient-specific devices can be understood easily and why they should be developed in the described way. Especially, patient-specific devices, which have no cheaper mass production counterpart so far, are not subject to discussion, weather individual, or mass production of these medical devices are suitable. However, there are many more approaches of individualized medical devices thinkable, but do have already a practicable mass-produced solution. Some existing devices or even new ones may offer certain room for improvement, if (partial) individualization is applied. We are discussing a relatively abstract topic, due to the lack of sufficient real-world examples. To understand our thinking about this topic a little bit better, we try to bring up a solely fictional example. Surgical devices can be relatively made simpler, e.g., scalpels, or be made highly complex, e.g., stapler for minimal invasive surgeries. Especially, the complex devices are under scrutiny regarding ergonomic (for the surgeon) and patient-specific issues. Addressable ergonomic topics are handling comfort or necessary mechanical forces for application. Surgeons, as patients, have logically different physical attributes. Patient-specific topics might be extraordinarily anatomical situations. Mass-produced plastic medical devices hardly can address both general topics in an appropriate way, as these usually are best possible solution for average cases (alike readymade clothing). Patients and operators are able to work with such devices for sure, but it may be helpful to increase patients' outcomes or operators' performances, if some for longer periods or highly specific situations used devices are individually adaptable.

The general question behind the current subsection is: Under which circumstances it might be useful introducing individual alterations of mass production medical devices. The focus lays on existing restriction of individualization due to manufacturing and process limitations, including regulatory questions, and possible unification approaches to combine 3D printing ("individual manufacturing") with mass production ("uniform manufacturing"). Just to make sure: It won't be a feasible approach for most plastic medical devices, but for some specific situations, which are currently addressed by standard products, individual alterations may result in better patients' treatments by better medical professionals' performances.

4.3.1 Standard Mass Production Technologies

The popularity of plastic manufacturing techniques can be explained by the vast variety of existing materials with broad ranges of properties (e.g., mechanical, optical, resistance) and the ability of producing highly complex medical devices fully automated, under clean room conditions and with low cost per part in comparison to other technologies and materials. For processing polymeric materials, many manufacturing approaches have been developed. Thermoplastic materials can be considered the standard type, which is processed for medical devices. Sure, other types like silicones or elastomers are utilized for many applications, but most parts are made with thermoplastics. Most (semi) finished products are manufactured with primary shaping technologies like injection molding or extrusion. As you may have learned so far, many adaptions of these technologies regarding functionality integration, multicomponent, surface coating, and so on are available and applied regularly. An overview of major plastic manufacturing technologies for medical device manufacturing is shown in the upcoming Table 4.2. To gain deeper understanding of typical mass production technologies, as summarized, we want to refer to standard literature about plastic manufacturing technologies and the upcoming chapters about emerging manufacturing technologies for plastic medical devices, which includes in our opinion interesting trends or opportunities for future device and manufacturing improvements.

Standard mass production technologies for plastic medical devices are **injection molding** and **extrusion** systems including all thinkable **descendant technologies**.

Table 4.2 Selection of the Major Plastic Manufacturing Technologies for Medical Devices

	Mass Production Capability	**Design to Production Complexity**	**Device Design Variability**	**Functionality Integration**	**Process Automation Effort and Process Speed**	**Clean Room Capability**
Injection molding	+++	++	+++	++	+++	+++
Multicomponent injection molding	+++	+	++	+++	++	++
Extrusion conventional	+++	++	+	+	++	+
Blow extrusion	+++	+	o	+	++	+
Thermoforming	++	+++	o	o	++	++

The choice of accurate production approaches depends among others on the device design, the integration of additional functionality, process ability of selected materials, and production volume.

+++, best; ++; +; o, worst.

The utilization of these manufacturing technologies may be reasoned by bringing the cost per part to the lowest level possible (in such cases every tenth of a second shorter production cycle lead to severe cost advantages) or by the fact that a product must be produced in a certain way to achieve the desired mechanical properties in combination with optical issues or any other thinkable option. Often forgotten, not only the cost factor is important, but also the mentioned fact, that some parts are only producible in the desired design and characteristics, if primary shaping technologies are used. In these cases, the major reason is not the high-volume output, but just to get the desired device manufactured. Surely, it is the aim of 3D-printing machine entrepreneurs to achieve comparable manufacturing conditions, which is doubtable, however, due to different molecular structures, crystallinity, or just available materials.

Mass production technologies can be surely used for small batch productions, but this approach won't be feasible due to major cost issues. Manufacturing costs depend on the overall complexity of the shape forming tools, automation, postprocessing, and resulting necessary operating resources (e.g., power supply). Postprocessing summarizes factors like surface treatments, packaging, or sterilization. Each factor can be translated into accountable costs, which can be lowered per part by simply producing more parts within a condition. Each economist and hopefully most engineers have the understanding about cost incurrence factors within establishing a manufacturing line and during its operation.

> Standard mass production technologies for plastic medical devices are not only used due to cost advantages in comparison to other technologies, but also due to feasibility issues: Some techniques imply unique device properties.

4.3.2 Restriction of Individualization and Mass Production

The naming of this subsection implies the existence of actual physical boundaries between individualized products and mass production. We use the word restriction in the sense of technical and economic challenges for individualized high-volume products. In our opinion, individualization of mass products makes no sense for plastic medical devices, which are only used short times or do not have any treatment impact on a patient. This limitation of possible devices can be considered a logical restriction based on economical, ergonomic, and treatment factors. You are probably confused right now about the meaning. It might be easier to explain with the upcoming two examples:

- Individually adapted surgical instrument for minimal invasive surgery: Most devices are single use and have to meet for a certain application. It might be feasible to have patient-specific instruments to address special cases or highly complex anatomical situations, but caused by the complexity of most devices it is not likely to achieve economical acceptable manufacturing costs for a whole 3D-printed device. Here, economical, ergonomic, and treatment factors have to be addressed for possible individualization approaches.
- Individually adapted 3-way-valves for drug application: Ergonomic issues might imply reasonable facts, why 3-way-valves should have for medical professional adapted designs. However, due to ergonomic issues, such devices are high volume and low cost, and treatment facts, ergonomic adapted devices won't have any impact on the patient's treatment due to the short time of manual handling, it is absolutely unlikely ensuring a positive business case for such devices.

Due to the complexity, it is not easily definable under which circumstances a partial individualization of high-volume products may be feasible. It is surely a question of lack of sufficient data, knowledge about possibilities, and depends on future, probably highly interesting, research efforts to understand this manufacturing approach more. A general evaluation method has not been developed or used so far. It is our aim to incite the reader's imagination to think about the existing restriction and the evolving challenges by asking the following, not directly answerable, questions.

- Under which economic, ergonomic, and medical treatment circumstances the partial individualization of mass production products seem feasible? How can these aspects be evaluated a priori of a development effort?
- How can an individually manufactured part be integrated into the basic, mass-produced, component?
- How can material combination, mechanical, sterility, or biocompatibility issues be addressed? Is it possible to evaluate the individual and standard part by its own?

- Individualization means the availability of user or patient data. How would a corresponding workflow of data generation, virtual planning, 3D printing, postprocessing, and integration in the standard part look alike?
- Is it feasible to combine single-use standard products with reusable individually manufactured parts, for instance, in case of ergonomic handholds for surgeons?
- How can a feasible quality and risk management be reached for centralized production of standard components and decentralized 3D printing of individual parts, which might be necessary due to manufacturing and logistic reasons?

Hopefully many more questions have not been mentioned in the listening, and you have gained some understanding of the issue or have developed additional questions as well. Besides more general hurdles, partly individualization of mass-produced plastic medical devices offers interesting matters like combinability of injection-molded basic part with 3D-printed individual part. Thinkable options might be to print the individualization part directly on the standard component or having some sort of integrated combination concept, which can be a fusion process or mechanical bonding process.

The previously established questions cannot be answered easily without any research or development work. Especially, economic or medical treatment circumstances and the establishment of acceptable and approvable decision-making and workflow processes are tough fields to consider. Besides these more process and liability orientated questions, issues about manufacturing approaches can be discussed as part of this book about emerging technologies for plastic medical devices. Therefore, the upcoming subsection should be considered as think tank about possible technological approaches for unification of mass-produced standard components with user- or patient-specific manufactured special components, which have to be fitted together for the actual application or treatment.

4.3.3 Unification of Individualization and Mass Production

This chapter is about possible technological approaches to combine mass and individually produced parts of medical devices for overall user- or patient-specific (partly) plastic medical devices. Possible unification approaches for mass and individually 3D-printed medical device parts can be simplified as some sort of fusion or combination process or let's call it as *personalized add-ons on standard products* to stay in the wording of the digitalized world. Plastic materials tend to be relatively tricky in regard of fusion. It depends on the basic material plus the added material and, not to forget about, the fusion technology itself. However, tricky does not mean that it is not possible. Different fusion approaches have been used for plastic devices for years. In regard of the individualization of mass products or a cheaper and faster production of individual devices with standard produced cores, following approaches might be feasible:

- 3D printing an individualized component directly on a mass-produced standard or basic component,
- welding together a mass-produced basic component with a 3D printing individual component,
- using bonded joint to combine individual and basic component, or
- working with mechanical bonding approaches, like plug connectors, to fixate both components.

Experienced plastic device engineers may recognize a simple pattern behind our suggestion: using existing fusion approaches for plastic devices, from multicomponent injection molding to laser welding, and translating them into unification approaches for individual and mass-produced components for patient-specific medical devices. In this chapter, it is not our aim to address the previously established questions about meaningfulness, economic, and further issues about individualized plastic medical device, but to show possible technical approaches of combining mass-produced standard components with individually printed parts to address individualization advantages with the advantages of standard manufacturing technologies and mass production. The following described approaches can be considered as fictional idea and are not assessable with engineering and business standards so far due to the lack of sufficient research, development, and general experience.

4.3.3.1 Printing Individualization on Mass-Produced Basic Component

This manufacturing idea is based on the multicomponent approach, which is widely used within injection molding. A basic component is (partly) overmolded with a second component within to injection steps. Thermoplastic–thermoplastic or thermoplastic–silicone is often used.

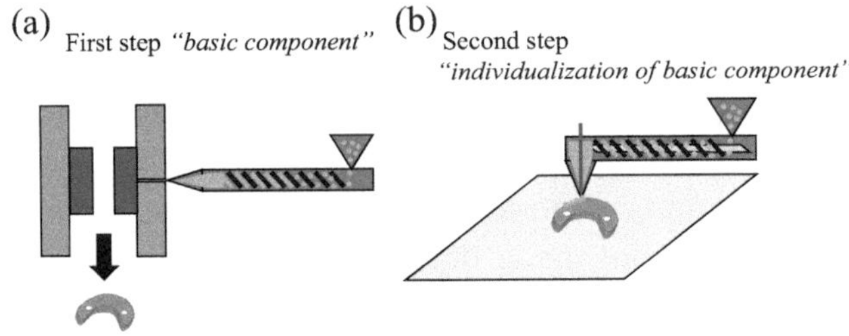

Figure 4.17 Printing individual component directly on mass-produced basic component: (a) First, a standard component is mass produced, e.g., with injection molding, including the mass production advantages like production speed and costs per part. (b) Second, standard component is individualized based on patent's anatomical data with direct three-dimensional printing on standard component. It combines the advantages of faster and cheaper production of standard mass production technologies with individualization aspects for patient's treatment.

The actual bonding depends on the chosen material combination, processing parameters, and design of the device. Actual bonding of new material combinations cannot be simply predicted and has to be evaluated with actual experimental setups. Transferred to our approach of individualizing standard components, the mass-produced basic component may be "overmolded" to a certain extent with a second component by using a 3D-printing machine and material. An explanation graphic is shown in Figure 4.17.

Major open questions are the compatibility of conventional-produced basic component materials with 3D-printed counterparts. The basic components would need some kinds of landmarks or fixation options within a 3D-printing machine to ensure a correction positioning prior to the individual optimization.

This approach offers following advantages and disadvantages, besides probably many more:

- Advantages:
  - no additional bonding material (e.g., glue) necessary,
  - the bonding process is integrated within 3D-printing step (less manufacturing steps),
  - no additional mechanical bonding necessary (however, often additional used within conventional multicomponent techniques to strengthen the bonding; typical example is using undercuts).

- Disadvantages:
  - issue of problematic hygienic conditions in 3D-printing machines (an additionally cleaned 3D-printed component cannot be used, the printing process itself has to meet the hygienic requirements),
  - rare experience about the bonding behavior,
  - 3D-printing machines using polymeric powder or resin basins are not suitable (basic component cannot be integrated in those basins, so far!),
  - time-consuming bonding process (faster printing technology might be more feasible, but might offer worse integrated bonding characteristics).

4.3.3.2 Welding of Individualized and Standard Component

Welding is a widely used technology to bond thermoplastic components together. Several welding approaches are available, like laser, rotation, or friction welding, but all are based on the same principle: inserting heat energy to induce local melting (therefore, thermoplastic behavior is necessary!) and implying a bonding process. Welding is often used for relatively simple geometries and bonding areas, which can already be interpreted as a disadvantage of the bonding technology. In Figure 4.18, a possible transfer approach of the welding technology is described for the individualization of standard products.

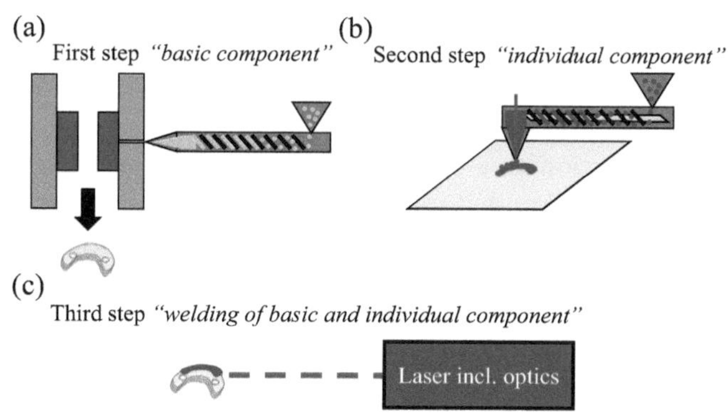

Figure 4.18 Separate manufacturing of basic and individual component: (a) The basic component is manufactured by a conventional mass production technology. (b) The individual component is manufactured by a three-dimensional printing machine based on individual anatomical data and a virtual device planning. (c) Both components are fused with a bonding technology, in this case with plastic welding like laser welding.

This approach offers following advantages and disadvantages, besides probably many more:

- Advantages:
  - no additional bonding material (e.g., glue) necessary,
  - no restriction of basin-based 3D-printing technologies,
  - no additional mechanical bonding necessary,
  - welding technologies are widely used under clean room conditions and therefore no hygienic concerns regarding the bonding process.

- Disadvantages:
  - additional processing step is necessary,
  - welding works with thermoplastic plastics only (exemptions might be possible) and therefore limits the range of possible 3D-printing approaches,
  - welding procedures have limitations regarding possible geometries and bonding areas,
  - rare experience with bonding behavior between printed and conventionally manufactured thermoplastic components.

4.3.3.3 Bonded Joint between Individualized and Standard Component

Bonded joint technology works with glues adapted to perform well with plastic materials. Its bonding behavior depends among others on the used materials, the surface structure and the geometrical design. In regard of a possible utilization as a technology for unification of individual and standard components, bonded joint technology implies in general similar advantages and disadvantages as the welding technology. However, the chemical structure and its possible effects on biological and mechanical issues for medical devices are under scrutiny, regularly.

4.3.3.4 Mechanical Bonding of Individualized and Standard Component

Mechanical bonding can be considered the longest existing technology to bond two separate components together without primary shaping. Pins, screws, clips, rivets, dovetail joints, and many more invented techniques

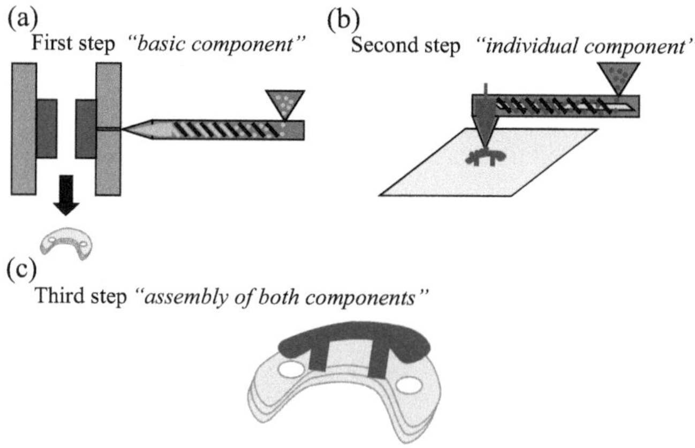

Figure 4.19 Integration of mechanical bonding for assembling individual with standard component: Mechanical bonding can be realized with frictional connections or form closure. A corresponding mechanical bonding part, e.g., pins, has to be integrated standardly within the individual component to fit it into the standard component.

are still regularly used within medical devices (not only focused on plastic parts). Mechanical bonding may be an interesting approach for integrating an individual component onto a standard component, especially if it is designed in an easy to-assemble and to-use way. Especially, clipping seems to be a good way to combine both parts. Designs can be highly sophisticated, e.g., easy to assemble with integrated locking functionality to disable dissembling. The individualization of standard medical devices might be practiced as described in Figure 4.19 by simply assembling a conventionally manufactured component and an individual component.

This approach offers following advantages and disadvantages, besides probably many more:

- Advantages:
  - no additional bonding material (e.g., glue) necessary,
  - no general restriction regarding manufacturing technologies and materials,
  - assembling with no-specific technologies possible, e.g., manual assembling prior to application possible,
  - minor concerns regarding hygienic situation.

- Disadvantages:
  - additional processing step is necessary,
  - integration of additional mechanical bonding functionality necessary, which may lead to more elaborate device designs,
  - no adhesive bond between both components, which may lead to earlier component failure.

5 Emerging Manufacturing Technologies

OUTLINE

Emerging Trends in Medical Plastic Engineering and Manufacturing
http://dx.doi.org/10.1016/B978-0-323-37023-3.00005-1

The previous chapters were focused on the demanding field of regulatory affairs with upcoming restrictions and did provide an outlook of future design challenges for plastic medical devices. Beginning with the generative manufacturing chapter, we have shifted our focus from the design to the actual manufacturing of plastic medical devices, which will be our main focus of attention within the upcoming chapter.

The topic of manufacturing of plastic medical devices summarizes development potentials for the production environment itself plus implementation of additional procedures like surface treatment, antibacterial processing, or anticounterfeiting technologies. In contrast to small-batch or individual-manufactured medical devices, most plastic medical devices are fitted for high-volume markets, produced by high-throughput manufacturing technologies. As, however, generative manufacturing technologies already play a vital role, that may be expected to significantly expand over the next years, these are covered by an own chapter. Now, we are looking into presumably emerging manufacturing technologies, which can be implemented within the so-called classic technologies for polymer processing, like injection molding, extrusion, thermoforming plus possible fusion processes.

Mentioned many times, the world of medical device engineers and manufacturers can be considered as relatively conservative regarding the introduction of new technological trends, as this might be close to state of the art in other more progressive engineering and manufacturing fields. Therefore, it is always worth having a look into approaches to plastic applications of other well-established fields of technology, such as consumer electronics or automotive. The big picture here is technology transfer. Some are definitely implantable within medical devices, if regulatory issues are adaptable or more generally spoken: safety issues have to be addressed adequately. Interesting developments are seen within the fields of sensors, which are regularly used within smartphones, but are not yet accepted within plastic medical devices at comparable extent. We have identified major emerging manufacturing technologies based on the general analysis of other engineering subjects by evaluating their potential for medical device application. It is necessary to adopt these general technological ideas into the medical device world to meet its specific requirements, such as sterilization ability or the often-mentioned biocompatibility.

Generally spoken, it sounds like, that future manufacturing trends for medical devices are easily predictable by observing major engineering fields. The medical device industry might be not the major player in developing groundbreaking new manufacturing technologies, but also it is not running after every trend due to issues of legal liability as well as high barriers to entry for new competitors. The manufacturing of plastic medical devices involves aspects of hygienic manufacturing, risk, and quality management plus further biological concerns. These branches must be driven by inner motives of the medical engineering community. Surely, clean room applications play a crucial role in other fields, especially the semiconductor industry, but without focusing on the major issue of sterility, which can be translated to the absence of living or devitalized microorganisms (as explained in Section 2.3.3). And if required, it can get a considerate engineering challenge for plastic medical devices. During product development processes, there are many demands and wishes for a product, but hygienic points are always the key aspect. If you develop a brand new biocompatible sensor technology integrated in plastic implants, these sensor will have no success at all without having an acceptable sterilization procedure available. Sterilization does not mean simply the process itself. It requires clean manufacturing conditions, which is applied usually by clean room production or at least some sort of cleaning processes. Emerging manufacturing technologies are underlying tougher restriction than in most other fields: beginning with the mentioned hygienic conditions, followed by highest quality and lowest risk reasonably possible, as these are demanded by international standards and regulations (like International Organization for Standardization, ISO 13485 or 21 CFR 820, see Section 2.3) to be considered without including financial considerations. Surely, everybody, who sees no financial aspects within medical device manufacturing, can be called a dreamer, but in contrast to most other technological fields, financial aspects must play a minor role during quality and risk evaluations.

Based on our experiences and current developments, we have chosen in our opinion emerging manufacturing technologies from within and beyond the medical device world and evaluated these within the specific requirement context for the convergence of plastic and medical engineering. Beginning with the unique point of sterility and its technological counterpart, the sterilization, new sterilization approaches are discussed and followed by the ultimate approach for sterile products: manufacturing sterile without any subsequent sterilization procedure. This would lead to enormous possibilities for new technologies to be introduced into the plastic medical device world. Of course, the assumption of having biocompatibility guaranteed, had been done before. However, it shows how a simply seeming sterilization procedure is actually the bottleneck for emerging technologies within plastic medical devices. Nevertheless, there are many upcoming manufacturing technologies, which might pass this hurdle and may lead to exciting new plastic medical devices with more integrated functionality. The discussed hot topics are antimicrobial device design as response to antibiotic-resistant bacteria, nanomaterials with focus on their antimicrobial potential, miniaturization for less-invasive plastic devices followed by combined and fully integrated and automated assembled devices. This leads us to the sensor integration approaches, which will be a major trend not even from a technological view, but also a more wide emerging trend of sensor integration in the daily life of future human beings to catch growing diseases as soon as possible. Health-related wearables are the catchy phrase for the upcoming opportunities. These more general trends are based on the emerging manufacturing technologies and are presented in Chapter 6. The current chapter will end with anti-counterfeiting technologies for medical devices. Anticounterfeiting will not directly improve any therapy, but will be more and more important to avoid the usage of fake medical devices, especially for the more delightful and therefore expensive representatives, improving the benefit for patients indirectly. It may sound surprising, but it is already a major problem within the heavily regulated and legally controlled pharmaceutical industry. Highly priced pharmaceuticals, like many for cancer treatment, face severe counterfeiting already, even in industrialized first world countries as EU and the US. It would be absolutely unlikely, if such illegal activities did not occur with medical devices as well. Therefore, it is worth having a deeper look into existing and upcoming technologies. Some of them seem likely to be relatively easily integrated within existing plastic devices, especially solely optical-based approaches.

5.1 Emerging Sterilization Methods

In many different applications, medical devices have to be sterile (Table 5.1). The polymeric medical device industry largely can be divided into single and reuse applications. Sterility is a hygienic standard, whereas its understanding had been developed for decades in the twentieth century. Some introducing words are necessary to understand the need of sterility and its problems within the medical device industry.

Nowadays, sterility is defined as a contamination probability of 1–1,000,000. The definition can be expressed as following: only one surviving germ is allowed on one million manufactured sterile devices. Bacteria, funguses, and other microorganisms are not easily detectable with existing technologies. A method for direct counting of organisms unit would be amazing to detect augmentable germs on medical device surfaces. There are no suitable inline systems available to monitor sterilization procedures on surfaces. Future developments might be interesting,

Table 5.1 Mainly Used Sterilization Approaches for Single-Use and Reusable Plastic Medical Devices

Sterilization Method	Sterilization Type	Issues with Plastic Materials
γ-Radiation	Radiation	• Inducing severe aging effects in many materials • Complex processing effort • Logistical costs
Ethylene-oxide	Chemical	• Inducing aging effects in some materials • Complex processing effort • Long process duration • Geometric restrictions
Heat-steam	Heat	• Processing temperature above operating temperature for many plastics • Inducing aging effects in some materials • Geometric restrictions

Besides the availability of more methods, γ-radiation and ethylene oxide can be considered the state of the art and primarily applied technologies for industrial-based sterilization efforts for plastic medical devices (especially single-use). Heat-steam with up to 134 °C is mainly used within medical facilities to reprocess reusable plastic medical devices.

however, the state of the art to validate sterilization methods is an indirect approach by measuring sterilization kinetics with so-called test germs, which are considered a worst case contamination. For example, the bacterium *Geobacillus stearothermophilus* is used to validate heat-based sterilization procedures. A sterilization kinetic is determined by measuring the duration to inactivate 90% of a given amount of germs. The duration is known as the D-value (decimal reduction time value). Sterilization methods are usually grouped in heat, radiation, or chemical systems.

Each procedure is common that a lethal dose necessary to inactivate the worst case germs is applied. Unfortunately, each treatment includes certain disadvantages regarding the use of plastics. Typical problems are a lack of temperature resistance, optical changes, or decreasing mechanical properties. Additionally, geometrical characteristics may exclude gaseous techniques, because it cannot be assured the necessary lethal doses of gas accessing difficult to reach areas (e.g., gastight-sealed voids).

It is easily imaginable, that there is no easy way to define which sterilization procedure is suitable or even best fit for the designed medical plastic device. Industrial standard is to use existing material–sterilization combinations based on own experiences. The introduction of new materials needs to be addressed with a certain amount of testing worst case scenarios to ensure the intended use and duration. The gold standard of the production of sterile single use is to manufacture and package under clean room conditions (usually ISO 6–8) and to add a subsequent sterilization like γ-radiation or ethylene oxide. Single-use medical plastic devices are manufactured with several machine techniques, like injection molding or extrusion, which are commonly used within the plastic industry to create plastic products. To understand the state of the art, the injection molding process is used, which is the standard manufacturing method for syringes, connectors, or diabetes pens. Typically, the injection molding machine can be enclosed entirely with a clean room or only the clamping unit with the mold is attached to a clean room for further processing as seen in Figure 5.1.

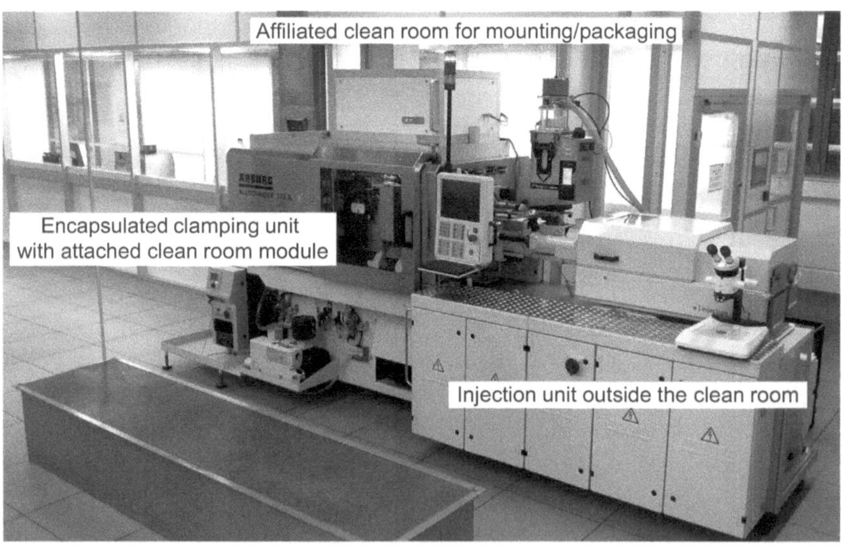

Figure 5.1 Injection molding within an International Organization for Standardization 6/good manufacturing practice-C clean room: the clamping unit with the injection mold is encapsulated and connected with the clean room to ensure hygienic manufacturing conditions. *Courtesy: Horst Scholz GmbH & Co. KG.*

However, there exist only recommendations or standards which clean room regarding hygienic standards have to be used. In contrast to the pharmaceutical industry, it is not regulated by law within the European Union, so far.

5.1.1 Material Issues with State-of-the-Art Sterilization Methods

Application of any sterilization methods implies always some conflict regarding the necessary sterilization kinetics to ensure actual sterility as defined and aging effect within plastic materials. Standard sterilization methods have been developed mainly for metal-, ceramic-, and glassware-based medical devices, especially for reuse applications. These materials generally show marginal influence by standard sterilization techniques like γ-beam, ethylene oxide, or heat-steam. Meantime, plastic materials always are affected, although at different extent, and so even polyetheretherketone (PEEK), known for its remarkable endurance, can be altered by applying to many heat-steam sterilization cycles.

5.1.2 Environmental Issues with State-of-the-Art Sterilization Methods

A vast majority of plastic medical devices, which are applied sterile, are sterilized by γ-radiation or ethylene-oxide, especially almost all single-use devices. Both technologies are highly compliant with industrial packaged goods. Simply spoken: palettes full of card boxes loaded with packaged medical devices can be sterilized at once without any necessary repackaging. Both methods can be considered state of the art. It can be summarized that γ-radiation may be preferred due to its faster and less-restrictive sterilization procedure regarding the actual geometry and shape of the device, however, it may cause more aging damage to the chemical structure of the plastics. Therefore, ethylene oxide, which is highly toxic by the way, is often applied for more critical devices. Ethylene oxide is under scrutiny to cause cancer, which is addressed by long-term airing times to decrease the ethylene oxide concentration on a sterilized good to the lowest level possible. As you can imagine, a radiation-based and a highly carcinogenic approach imply some significant problems. Environmental issues are often not the major thought when discussing advantages and disadvantages of sterilization procedures, but they are already within a general focus and will gain more relevance. As standard source of radiation, radioactive cobalt-60 isotopes are used to generate γ-radiation within specific sterilization plants. Nuclear power is already under scrutiny in many industrialized countries, particularly after the Fukushima incident. Some countries have stopped their plans to implement nuclear power and some have started to terminate such plants. So, it is just a question of time, when the first demands will be spoken out to terminate γ-radiation plants as well. A highly environmental toxic chemical substance like ethylene oxide is probably not the best alternative either, besides simple technical problems, which already exist and some are mentioned above.

5.1.3 Emerging Technologies for Medical Device Sterilization

Thankfully, parallel to medical device industry many other life sciences have to deal with sterilization issues. Besides the pharmaceutical industry, the food sector is working with interesting approaches, which may be in use for some medical device application already, but may also have some impact futurewise for a broader application. The most important aspects of plastic medical devices can be broken down to just two points: large-scale industrial style with lowest cost and time consumption possible and minimum impact on material selection or polymer aging. Research groups have investigated many different possible sterilization procedures for many years. And every single group advocates its approach the most that is for sure. To be honest, at the beginning, sterilization procedure includes always some disadvantages due to the simple fact that there is a certain amount of energy necessary to destroy living germs, even those, which are specialized on harsh living conditions. On the other hand, a sterilization procedure should be as fast and reliable as possible and has no impact on plastic materials as well. Interesting emerging technologies for medical device sterilization might be:

- Plasma beam sterilization
- Hydrogen peroxide
- X-ray beam sterilization
- Electron-beam sterilization (as shown in Figure 5.2).

But all these sterilization procedures have still one major disadvantage in common, which is independent of the approach itself: it is always an additional manufacturing step, the sterilization, necessary prior distribution of sterile and packaged plastic medical devices. Additionally, it is not possible to integrate these approaches simply within a plastic manufacturing line due

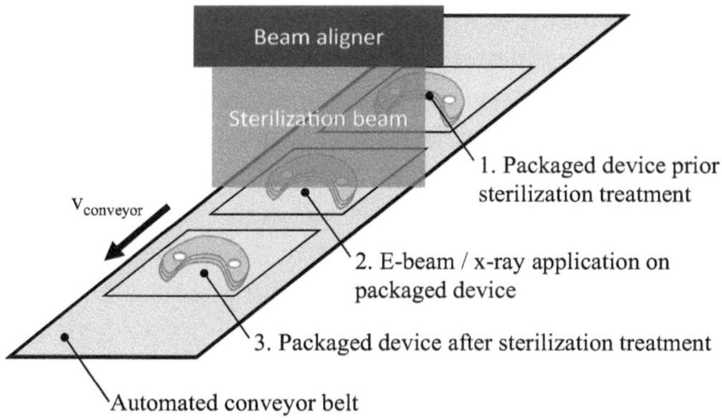

Figure 5.2 Beam sterilization equipment are built similar to γ-radiation plants. A sterilization beam is focused on packaged devices, which are driven through the beam by an automated conveyor belt. It depends on the packaging, the devices, and the actual amount, how many devices can be sterilized at once in one package. An X-ray/electron beam used for sterilization is less energetic than γ-radiation and therefore it is expected to cause less aging than γ-radiation would be.

to safety reason, sterilization time, and simply the cost for a sterilization unit, which is often many times more expensive than a plastic processing machine. Interestingly, the pharmaceutical industry utilizes an approach already for decades, which avoids having a subsequent sterilization, and that is called aseptic production. Transferred to plastic manufacturing, this could be translated into an autosterile manufacturing and packaging approach.

5.2 Autosterile Manufacturing and Packaging

A subsequent sterilization may imply increased manufacturing costs of up to 10% for logistics and for the procedure itself. Sterilization methods like the mainly used γ-radiation or ethylene oxide application hardly can be implemented meaningful in an automated inline-manufacturing process. Reasons are the required space, sterilization duration, or additional safety policies. γ-Radiation is generated within cobalt-60 source, a highly dangerous isotope, which needs to be handled with additional protective barriers to avoid potential harm to employees. In addition, the sources must be kept in a high-security area, due to potential terrorist action, and generate radioactive waste, issues which have to be mentioned within these times. Even the use of ethylene oxide gases implies enormous health hazards to the operator and has to be addressed by strict safety regulations.

The achieved hygienic standards are absolutely blessing, but due to the necessary inactivation kinetics also a huge liability for the plastic industry. Plastics include probably a wider spectrum of geometrical, mechanical, or optical qualities than any other materials. However, the necessary sterilization procedure limits the possible use of plastics within the medical device industry dramatically and don't forget about the significant costs.

The pharmaceutical industry has already a solution to avoid subsequent sterilization: **aseptic production**. Active ingredients are often absolutely not sterilizable due to their chemical nature. The major legislators (the US and European market) determined regulations how to manufacture under aseptic conditions, which are known as good manufacturing practice, EU (EU-GMP) or current good manufacturing practice, USA within the pharmaceutical industry. Exemplary, the European GMP implies certain requirements concerning air and surface contamination within the cleanest areas (often referred to GMP-A) and the surrounding spaces (GMP-B, -C, or -D), as well the behavior of the employees. Quality and risk management measures have to be taken into account to verify the production process. Sterile packaging systems have to be implemented, which are indispensable for the transportation of sterile goods out of the cleanest zone. Packaging units can be shipped through a sterilization unit to the GMP-A zone or multilayer-packaging, which are sterilized before, are used. There are already useful regulations, guidelines, and standards, which can help to establish an autosterile manufacturing approach for single-use medical devices (see Table 5.2).

The question is now, why not to benefit from the knowledge of the sterile production of drugs within the plastic device industry? In Figure 5.3, we have transferred the GMP standards for aseptic production to an injection molding process scheme, how it seems reasonable to establish an autosterile injection molding procedure. The GMP approaches with room in room technologies are utilized. However, there are some open questions, which have been addressed to a certain level by current research. On the one hand, sterility for the inserted ingredients (here: polymeric melt plus packaging) and the product touching surfaces have to be guaranteed. On the other hand, the manufacturing costs are essential for the industry and the usability of the system must remain for the employees. For example, think about implementing a new material within the injection molding process. Every technician knows, you need to perform some (up to 50) cycles to establish a well-running system with stable process, before the system can run automatically. This has to be addressed by enabling starting procedures. Or think about the change of an injection mold, which bears the risk of destroying the hygienic (or sterile) conditions within the clean room. How is it possible to avoid the contamination of other production lanes?

Table 5.2 Selection of Hygienic Regulations and Standards within the Pharmaceutical and Medical Device Industry, Which Can Be Helpful to Achieve the Goal of an Autosterile Polymer Processing Process

Codification	Type	Special Feature
2009/C 163/01 and 02—Publication of titles and references of harmonized standards under the Directives (90/385/EEC and 93/42/EEC)	Regulation	Overview about the harmonized standards and therefore acknowledged as state of the art within the EU
Good manufacturing practice guidelines for medicinal products for human and veterinary use (especially: annex 1—manufacture of sterile medicinal products)	Guideline	Required by law within the EU
Guidance for industry: sterile drug products produced by aseptic processing—current good manufacturing practice (cGMP)	Guideline	Required by law within the US, based on cGMP as codified in 21 CFR parts 210 and 211
EN ISO 13408—aseptic processing of health-care products	Standard	Defines necessary requirements for an aseptic/autosterile manufacturing
EN 556—Sterilization of medical devices—requirements for medical devices to be designated “sterile”	Standard	Especially 556-2: Requirements for aseptically processed medical devices
EN ISO 11138—Sterilization of health-care products—biological indicators	Standard	Validation method by applying biological indicator
EN ISO 14937—Sterilization of health-care products—general requirements for characterization of a sterilizing agent and the development, validation and routine control of a sterilization process for medical devices	Standard	General requirements for sterilization processes for medical devices

ISO, International Organization for Standardization.

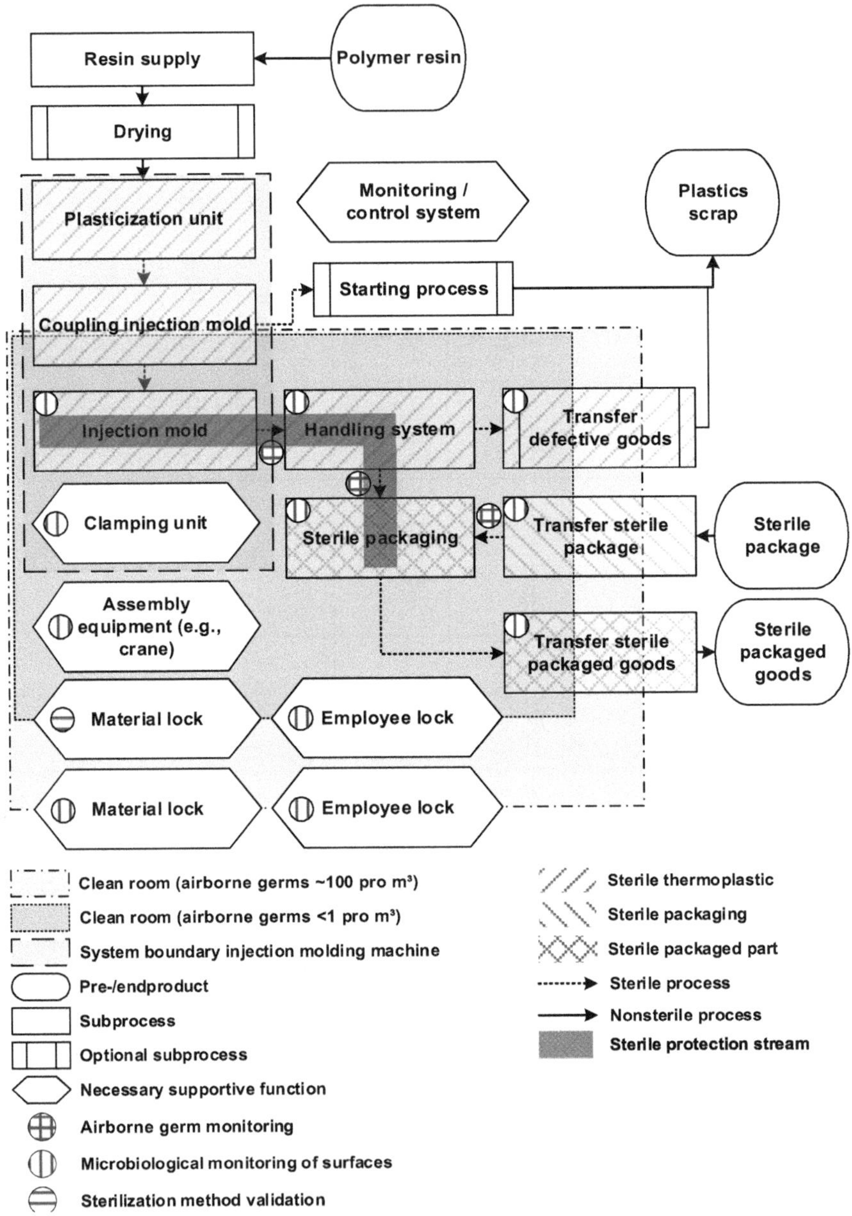

Figure 5.3 Possible autosterile manufacturing procedure of medical single-use products: the proposal is based on the good manufacturing practice guidelines for the aseptic drug production.

It is not our aim to determine, how an autosterile manufacturing process has to look like in detail, because different approaches seem suitable. Overall the major task would be to establish a plausible (cost-based) benchmark regarding possible potential for development by eliminating the disadvantages of subsequent sterilization and the needed technical equipment for an autosterile manufacturing unit. In Table 5.3, we have summarized the amazing potential of an autosterile manufacturing technique within the plastic manufacturing world for medical devices.

The potential of an autosterile injection molding is outstanding, especially as it is actually quite clear how it is realizable, as the pharmaceutical industry clearly shows. However, probably the most important step is to establish an acceptable method to validate the autosterile manufacturing process and to convince the conservative medical device industry about the described positive effects. It is inescapable to declare conformity with applicable standards. No approving organization (e.g., accredited notified body within the European Union) will accept an autosterile polymer manufacturing process without meeting general acknowledged standards. The development and proof of accuracy of new validation methods is cost intensive and exposed to the risk of being not accepted. Fortunately, the ISO has already defined the necessary standard for aseptic production in general: ISO 13408—aseptic processing of health-care products. In addition, it exists already one certified and comparable manufacturing technique within the pharmaceutical industry for filled medical drugs container, which is known as the **blow-fill-and-seal-technology**. This technology is highly comparable to an injection molding process for plastic bottles (stretch blow molding). First, polymer melt is extruded in the mold. Second, the shape is formed by applying sterile gaseous pressure within the mold. Third, the liquid and sterile drug (sterilized by filtration for example) is injected by the so-called filling needles. Finally, the container is sealed. The whole process works within an isolator, which avoids human interaction consequently. Transferred to standard manufacturing techniques like injection molding, it means to ensure absolutely sterile ingredients besides the overall sterile hygienic manufacturing conditions. Corresponding to thermoplastic injection molding or extrusion techniques, it can be translated to ensure sterile melt before entering the mold plus sterile packaging afterward (and of course any insert). A quite common used assumption is that the melt is always sterile due to the applied temperature and dwell period within the plasticization unit. First of all, a presumption is not proved for a necessary system validation and second, which temperature and dwell period can be set as minimum level? Current research approaches have shown interesting results at the Institute of Medical and Polymer Engineering at the Technische Universität München: sterilization

Table 5.3 Overview of Likely Effects and Development Potential of Medical Devices by Introducing an Autosterile Plastic Production Technique

	Effect	**Development Potential for Medical Devices**
Plastic material	• Increased raw material availability • Increased likelihood of new material development for medical devices	• Material selection based on nonsterilization-related requirements • Faster introduction of new materials within medical devices
Medical device design	• No consideration of sterilization effects on new design functionalities • No consideration of sterilization procedure compliant design	• Decreased testing efforts for new medical plastic devices • Easier transfer of plastic design knowledge to the medical device industry (especially for nonrelated device engineers)
Medical device manufacturing	• Increased manufacturing standards concerning hygienic conditions within the production process • Likelihood of adapted or renewed manufacturing equipment	• Ultrahygienic handling of manufactured medical devices (→ interesting for DNA-free production)
Material transfer and logistics	• No additional sterilization process necessary • Shorter production to customer time • Easier adaption of production in-line with demand	• Decreasing production periods • Decreasing production costs regarding logistics • Increased production variability

testing with *G. stearothermophilus* spores recommends a minimum dwell period of about 5 min at 200 °C melt temperature to ensure sterile polymer melt by all means. If you have some knowledge about injection molding processes, then you can imagine that these conditions are definitely within the typical process parameter range. Simplified spelled, it is only necessary to implement an acceptable method to provide GMP-A level clean room conditions and sterile packaging plus introducing acknowledged validation methods. Of course, there are still some unanswered questions (e.g., how to obtain GMP-A level within an injection molding clamping unit), but the future generation of medical manufacturing engineers is hopefully capable to solve upcoming hurdles.

5.3 Antimicrobial Device Design

Any medical device, regardless if intended for sterile application or not, is manufactured at clean conditions in order to minimize contaminations with dirt or microorganism. Beyond aesthetic considerations (who would trust a soiled device?), this comes from biological requirements as even devitalized germs may induce an immune response via endotoxins (see Section 2.3.2). This aspect explains sophisticated techniques such as clean room manufacturing or sterilization utilized for medical device manufacturing. Anyhow, any medical device will be exposed to living microorganism during application. These so will find a breeding ground and start reproduction, finally **creating a biofilm**, if not hampered adequately. This is a widespread problem known with many medical devices, especially those with prolonged application. **Urinary catheters** will see the formation of a biofilm that will migrate along the tubular structure and eventually entering the body, presumably causing an infection. Comparable but in result much worse problems may occur with long-term implants. Even if surgery is performed at ideal clean conditions, a minimal number (maybe just on single) of bacteria may be attached to the implant, which then will start reproduction. Thereby, the human body sometimes is unable to defeat these intruders as the immune system either generally is not capable of doing so (immune suppression, elderly or sick people) or does not gain appropriate access to the site of infection (insufficient vascularization, complex implant design). Anyhow, the result frequently is an **implant infection** that, if reached a sufficiently advanced stage, needs revision surgery to replace the implant and treat the infection. Even health-care systems in highly developed countries see a considerate number of such cases, most frequently for load-bearing orthopedic (hip and knee) or dental implants.

These induce additional costs, tie up resources, and generate in best-case inconvenience, in worst case severe health issues for the patient. This problem is superimposed by an emerging number of bacteria that developed an **antimicrobial resistance (AMR)**, making them unsusceptible to many or even all antimicrobial agents. Because of excessive and inappropriate application, these bacteria performed a genetic mutation making them resistant to the effect of one or more antimicrobial agents that were once effective. This term is not to be confused with the closely related term of **antibiotic resistance**, which refers to bacteria immune to the effect of antibiotics. Anyhow, the early identification of all these infections is crucial for appropriate treatment and many interesting approaches to do so based on lab-on chip devices (Section 6.2) or in vitro diagnostics (Section 6.3).

Anyhow, infections that occur during (or are caused by) a medical treatment commonly are labeled as nosocomial or hospital-acquired infection. To emphasize the fact that these infections can be correlated with the entire health-care system (not only hospitals), the appropriate name should read **Healthcare-associated infection** (HAI). Thereby, AMR infections play a superior role as the usually best performing antibiotics and antimicrobial agents frequently are applied without effect. In result, HAIs are an emerging problem for the health-care systems on global base, affecting third world as well as first world countries in comparable extent. Within the European Union, approximately 4.1 million patients do acquire an HAI per year, and the number of deaths occurring as a direct consequence of these infections is estimated to be at least 37,000. The World Health Organization (WHO) does estimate that at any given time, 7 in developed and 10 in developing countries will acquire at least 1 HAI. Thereby, about 20–30% of these infections are considered as being preventable by appropriate actions, such as intensive hygiene, comprehensive control, and new technologies to prevent infections. Antimicrobial design for medical devices can contribute to the attempts to fight HAIs. Thereby, many approaches are available, and while some are still subject to current research, others already found serial application. Anyhow, as antimicrobial devices are predicted to see a significant emerging application, first regulations dealing with them currently are developed, such as a draft guidance issued by the FDA. The following chapter will give you an overview upon basic scientific principles and their possible applications.

5.3.1 Antimicrobial Surfaces

Like any other living organism, germs are dependent on the presence of water. While many bacterial and fungal spores may survive extended periods of extreme drought, none of them is able to reproduce itself in the absence of water. In consequence, a hydrophobic surface may hamper the growth of germs and so strong nonpolar polymers show an inherent microbiological effect. By micro- and nano-structuring of the surface, even polar polymers may exhibit hydrophobic properties, an effect commonly known as lotus effect. The functional principle is a double structure, as displayed in Figure 5.4, which minimizes the surface of contact to a water droplet. That way, the resulting adhesion forces are reduced and that so superseded by the surface tension and water is repelled. Put simply, the surface structure, although rather rough than smooth on microscopic scale, does minimize the grip for a water droplet that will fall off. Further, many bacteria need a surface to be attached on for surviving. This may be a macroscopic surface like a medical device or a microscopic particle. This is why bacteria in the air are not airborne but rather are attached to a floating particle[1] or floating in a micro-droplet of liquid. Repelling both, particles and liquids, exhibits an antimicrobial effect by physical mode of action. Specific types of such structuring do exhibit a lotus effect like action toward bacteria that consequently will not find appropriate grip to the surface. A big advantage of this approach is the fact that it does base on the morphology of the processed polymer only. This does significantly facilitate testing for biological safety and approval of a device.

5.3.2 Antimicrobial Monomers

While surface modification features a passive antimicrobial effect, polymers may be tailored to actively devitalize germs by following one of three basic approaches. The simplest one is to **polymerize antimicrobial monomers**.

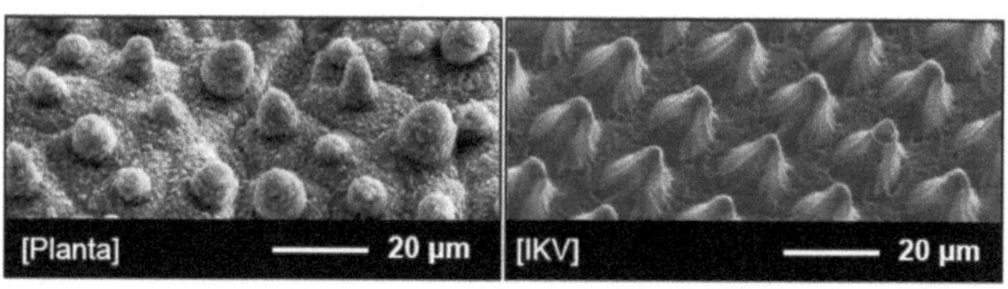

Figure 5.4 SEM pictures of the surfaces of a plant leaf and a polymer film. Both exhibit a microstructure that significantly does increase hydrophobicity. Additionally, those bacteria that require attachment to a surface for survival will not find adequate "grip." Both effects may hamper the reproduction of germs and thus create an antimicrobial surface. *Image in courtesy of IKV, RWTH Aachen.*

---

1. This is why the air within clean room usually exhibits very low numbers of cfu, as airborne particles are missing. Anyhow, this may not be transferred to the surfaces of the clean room that need disinfection on regular basis to be free of bacteria.

Depending on the monomer used and the length of macromolecules, these plastics will kill bacteria in contact to them by slowly releasing single monomers. Most of these polymers are less suitable as material for medical devices from an engineering point of view, but may be interesting candidates for antimicrobial polymer coatings. For the other, antimicrobial monomers may be integrated into the basic polymer backbone chain during synthesis, forming a **copolymer**. Finally, antimicrobial monomers such as phenol groups, ammonium salts, or antibiotics may be anchored to an existing polymer via **covalent bonding**. Anyhow, regardless the approach utilized, as these are illustrated in Figure 5.5, it is important to remember that doing so significantly may alter the mechanical properties of the polymer. The idea of antimicrobial polymers still is comparatively new, and thus still topic of current research with only very few industrial application for medical devices yet. Anyhow, the opportunities are very promising and so the development of these materials is worth tracking. Currently some devices are subject to research that serve as antimicrobial wound dressing.

5.3.3 Antimicrobial Compounds

Well established is the approach to add antimicrobial agents to an existing polymer by forming a compound. Put simply: you mix a disinfectant agent into the polymer, creating an antimicrobial modified polymer.

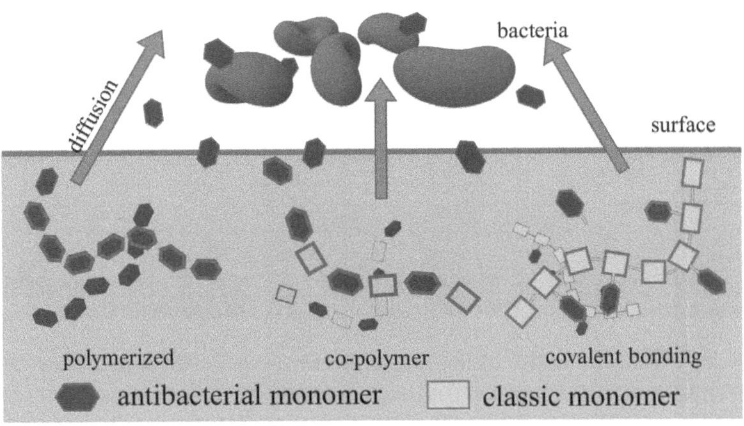

Figure 5.5 Utilizing antimicrobial active monomers may follow three basic principles. The antimicrobial agent may be directly polymerized, combined with a classic monomer forming a copolymer or anchored to the backbone chain of an existing engineering plastic by covalent bonding. In all approaches, single antimicrobial monomers will slowly be released and diffuse to the surface of the device, devitalizing the germs present.

These agents either may base on metallic ions, ceramic particles, or antimicrobial chemicals, such as established disinfectants or antibiotics. Anyhow, adding any compound to a polymer may significantly alter its mechanical properties. Further, the antimicrobial effect frequently does depend on eluting the antimicrobial agent. If so, the effect will decrease asymptotically and furthermore either show a strong effect over a long period or vice versa.

It is known for long time that many metals, e.g., zinc, silver, or gold hamper the growth of bacteria. The metal is added to the polymer as **finely dispersed particles** by classical techniques of compounding. Thereby, the mechanical properties of most polymers are altered only insignificantly, making it an interesting approach from an engineering point of view. During application, the particles will disperse ions that will find the way to the device surface by diffusion. As most bacterial cell walls are negatively charged, the positively charged metallic ions easily make contact and unfold their antimicrobial effect. Most commonly, **colloidal silver** is utilized. When grinding pure silver to a particle size smaller than about 100 nm, it will turn into a sticky (*kolla*=Greek for *glue-like*) paste of brownish color. As alternative to its pure form, compounds or nanospheres containing silver may be used too, as illustrated in Figure 5.6. Colloidal silver or its

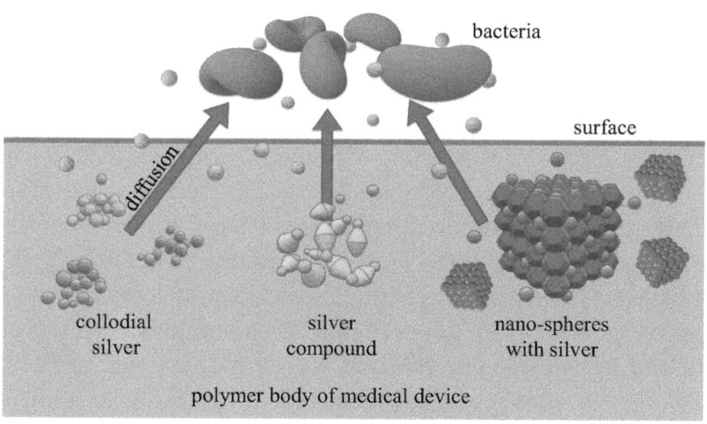

Figure 5.6 For antimicrobial modifications of polymers, silver may be added in three basic modifications: as extremely fine grinded (then labeled colloidal), as chemical compound containing silver, or as nanospheres containing the metal. Anyhow, silver ions will make their way to the device surface by diffusion, then making contact to present bacteria that will be devitalized. Nevertheless, the excessive use of silver may induce allergies or turn skin and mucosal tissue into a blue or bluish-gray color, a condition called argyria. As alternative, other metals like zinc, nickel, or gold may be utilized too, whereas all critical aspects mentioned for silver will remain valid.

derivates easily may be added to any polymer, giving it an antimicrobial activity, and so beyond medical devices, many products are commercially available basing on this technology. These comprise antimicrobial modified clothing for sporting that release less odor when sweating. Metabolic degradation products originating from bacteria cause the unpleasant smell of sweat. On the other hand, objects of daily use those frequently are touched by different people, such as doorknobs, handholds, or work surfaces in health-care environments are modified that way. Anyhow, although generally considered as biological inert in low concentration, there are emerging concerns about impacts on health and environment related to the excessive utilization of colloidal silver. Long-term exposure to silver may cause irritations of the skin and the ions accumulate within the body. This can cause a condition known as argyria (from Greek argyros = silver) that in worst case may result in locally limited or generalized blue or bluish-gray coloring of the mucosal tissue and skin. Although this requires the intake of considerate amounts of silver, the plentiful applications of silver ions must be seen critically. The FDA issued a consumer advisory dealing with dietary supplements containing silver, explaining that inappropriate consumption of these may cause permanent discoloration of skin and mucous membranes. Via sewages and clearing sludge, the silver ions will find way into the ecosystem so will find their way into our food chain. The far-reaching consequences are not predictable yet. Currently colloidal gold or other metals (e.g., zinc or nickel) are advertised as superior alternative, but all critical aspects mentioned for silver will remain valid.

Beyond those compounds acting disinfecting via the diffusion of antimicrobial agents, finely dispersed particles that induce **photocatalytic reactions** when exposed to ultraviolet light may be used as well. When activated by light exceeding a defined energy (minimum wavelength), these will serve as catalyst for manifold chemical reactions, whereas those affecting water and oxygen are from greater interest, as both always are present (air humidity and moisture). The reaction will reduce oxygen molecules (O_2) to superoxide (O_2^-) and oxidize water molecules (H_2O) to hydroxyl radicals (OH^-). However, do not get afraid. The precise reaction is complex but shall not be subject of this book. Anyhow, both ions belong to a group of molecules known as **reactive oxygen species** (ROS) that are known to exhibit considerate antimicrobial effect. As catalytic agent usually serve ceramics, whereas **titanium dioxide** (TiO_2) currently is the gold standard. It features a brilliant white color and does exhibit a superior biocompatibility, which is why it has a wide range of applications, including paint, sun blocker, coloring of food and consumer goods (e.g., toothpaste, laundry detergent), and many more. Further, it is utilized for manifold medical devices, such as dental of orthopedic implants. It is worth mentioning that TiO_2 frequently is labeled as gold standard for long-term implants. For antimicrobial modification of polymers, it is added as finely dispersed particles by compounding, as illustrated in Figure 5.7, or as coating.

The antimicrobial effect may be **enhanced by adding silver** ions to the titanium dioxide. This not only promotes the formation of ROS, but also does add the antimicrobial effect of silver ions. As TiO_2 serves as catalyst, its disinfecting action will remain perpetually, differing from metal ions that are consumed, and thus exhibit a decreasing effect with sagging concentration. Anyhow, the fact that antimicrobial action does depend on activation by ultraviolet radiation comes along with some disadvantages. Meaningful applications require the device being exposed to daylight or a source of ultraviolet light, making it not suitable for devices penetrating the human body (e.g., implants, catheters). Further, ultraviolet light as well as ROS induce aging processes within the polymer, changing it in color (yellowing), and frequently making it brittle. Further, only TiO_2 particles that are present (or close to) the surface will feature an antimicrobial effect. Thus, when added by compounding, the majority of particles are found inside the material and will have no effect. In consequence, the ideal application is coatings for devices that easily may be exposed to strong ultraviolet light on regular base. Broad applications are paintings and coatings for working surfaces and walls in doctor's offices and operation theaters. Nevertheless, antimicrobial modification for classical medical devices is comparatively new and many new ideas may be expected.

Material suppliers realized the trend and so even global players of polymer synthesis launched entire product lines of **antimicrobial modified resins** as part of their medical grade portfolio. These sometimes

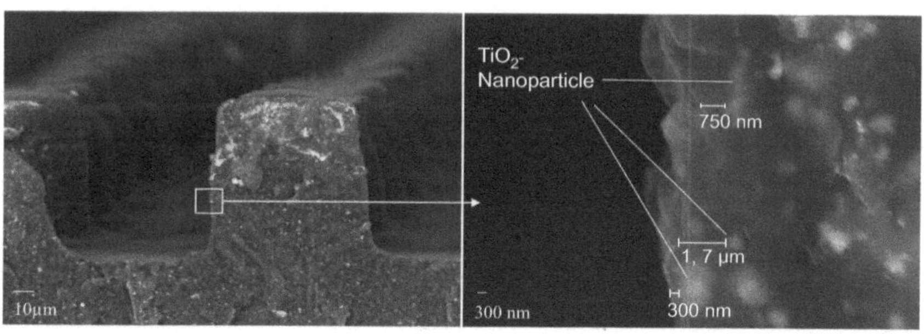

Figure 5.7 Polymer with added titanium dioxide nanoparticles. When exposed to ultraviolet light, these induce a photocatalytic effect that generates reactive oxygen species that show an antimicrobial effect. This approach is ideal for surface coatings. *Image courtesy Teresa Huppmann, Technische Universität München.*

are intensely advertised for applications in medical devices, whereas the precise agent utilized frequently is disclosed. Anyhow, pretty much all of them either base on the techniques presented in this section, or slightly adapt and/or combine these.

5.3.4 Antimicrobial Coatings

Utilizing antimicrobial coatings offers several advantages. These may be applied to readily developed or existing medical devices with negligible influence on its functionality. Currently there are many technologies for plastic coating of surfaces applied for medical devices and many more about to be developed (Section 5.6). Many of those coatings may combine antimicrobial effect with additional functionalities. A prominent example is a coating with antimicrobial parylene. **Parylene** is the trade name for a group of polymers that were developed for **chemical vapor deposition**, designed to create moisture or dielectric barriers or to create an antifriction layer. This aspect is from greater interest for devices that benefit from reduced friction, such as tubes or needles that penetrate the human skin. Less rubbing during application will reduce the trauma and so accelerate wound healing after treatment. Moreover, some parylenes exhibit a considerable antimicrobial effect, reducing the number of bacteria present on the surface (cfu, see Section 2.3.3) by one magnitude (Figure 5.8). This is an interesting aspect for devices such as a central venous catheter, a tube

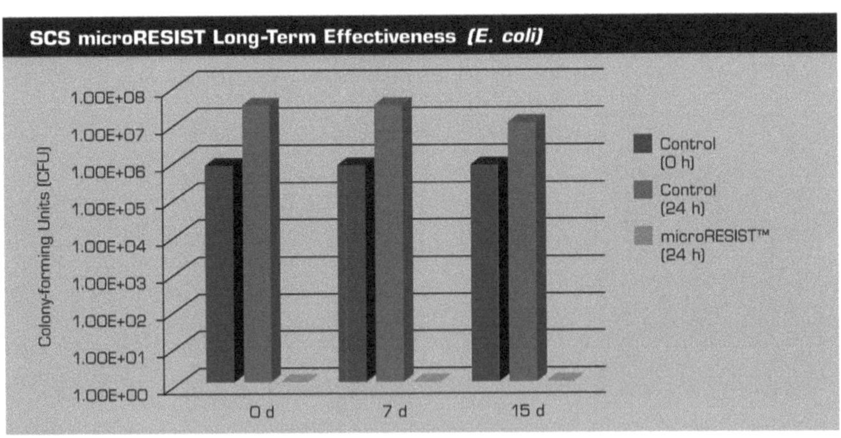

Figure 5.8 Long-term antimicrobial effect of a coating with parylene. These coatings may be used for additional features, such as moisture barriers or antifriction layers, making them interesting for many medical devices. *Image courtesy of Special Coating Systems.*

placed into a central vein close to heart in order to get access to the central blood circulation. As the tube usually features a comparable large diameter, application induces a considerable soft tissue trauma, and due to its location close to the heart, migration of a biofilm along its tube must be prevented in any case. Coating of a central venous catheter with parylene enables to reduce the trauma induced by application and the risk of infection during utilization simultaneously.

Other interesting approaches base on surfaces modified with silicone oil. Most silicone oils exhibit an excellent biocompatibility and are used for a wide range of life science products, such as lubricants, massage oil, ointments, cosmetics, filling for aesthetic implants, and antiflatulent drug. When applied in moderate amount to the human body, it is bioinert and thus not harmful, even within the blood circulation.[2] Currently silicone oil is used as lubricant for venous catheters with larger diameter and sealing for vascular locks. In consequence, comprehensive knowledge upon its risks and benefits of application for catheters is established. A novel application was developed at Harvard University, called liquid-infused silicone as a biofouling-free medical material. A catheter made from polydimethylsiloxane, a specific type of silicone, is infused with liquid silicone. The result is a stable, very slippery surface that exhibits exceptionally low bacterial adhesion and in result helps to prevent the formation of a biofilm. Moreover, the antimicrobial action is combined with the lubricating effect of the silicone oil, making it very interesting for catheters that induce less soft tissue trauma during application. Thereby, the antimicrobial effect shows at least an order of magnitude reduction of biofilm formation, as displayed in Figure 5.9.

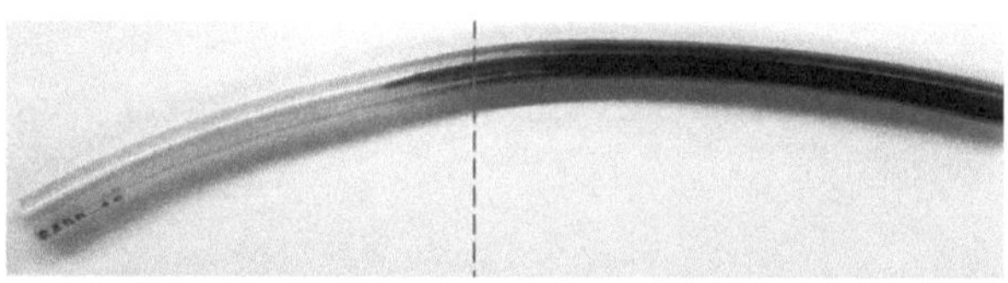

Figure 5.9 Catheters produced from silicone may be manufactured that way that a slippery surface containing uncured silicone oil is created. That way, germs and bacteria will find no grip on the surface that therefore exhibits an antimicrobial effect. *Figure Courtesy of Noah MacCallum and Joanna Aizenberg, Harvard University.*

2. Bigger amounts of silicone oil are administered to the body may induce severe health issues, which is why leaking or rupturing of silicone oil-filled breast implants usually leads to severe medical conditions.

This approach still is within its early stage of development. However, it gives a good example that creating innovative medical devices frequently does base on the transfer of existing technologies from related fields or the combination of known features for novel applications. Residue of uncured silicone oil frequently is regarded as a problem, as the resulting slippery surface is not suitable for further processing (e.g., printing). In this particular case, this seeming disadvantage was turned into a benefit as it does implement a novel functionality.

5.3.5 Ideal Approach

Of course there cannot be anything like an ideal approach for antimicrobial modification of polymers or medical devices. Any modification intended to reduce the creation of biofilms or to devitalize germs does rely on effects that show adverse impact on human living tissue as well. Put simply, antimicrobial modification is an antagonist to biocompatibility, resulting in an endless discussion about the combination about both features. However, following the appropriate approach will generate an antimicrobial effect where the benefits will outweigh the cutback on biocompatibility, or even increase biointegration. A prominent example is material used to build bone structure of the jaw. After removal of a dent, the implantation of screws is not possible due to a lack in bony structure. In this case, a biomaterial, consisting of hydroxylapatite (mineral phase of the skeleton), growth factors, and surface disinfectant (less than 1%) is used to induce formation of bone. Thereby, the disinfectant not only shows an antimicrobial effect but also even enhances the formation of bone structure, although generally considered from minor biocompatibility. This shows you that combining two aspects that were expected to compound in adverse effects suddenly exhibit great opportunities for medical device design.

5.4 Nanomaterials for Medical Devices

Nanotechnology and nanomaterials are catchwords you probably frequently encounter in many aspects of daily living. Generally, both are associated with innovations and emerging technologies and many imagine these to spark a technological leap like the invention of steam engine or digital electronics. However, mankind has been utilizing nanomaterials as early as premodern times, but without realizing about doing so. Dyed glasses (~fourth century) or sabers made from Damascus steel (thirteenth–fourteenth century) contain materials and structures that base on nanotechnology from a technical point of view. However, well-founded scientific approach to the topic of nanotechnology started in the mid-nineteenth century, but it took another 100 years until the first groundbreaking innovation related to nanotechnology, namely, the semiconductor transistor (1947). Hardly any other invention boosted the development of computer technology in comparable extent, and in consequence IT still is the dominant application for nanotechnology. However, many more discoveries broadened the knowledge upon this designated field, with the detection of fullerenes (1985) and carbon nanotubes (CNTs) (1991) probably among the most important ones for material sciences. Nevertheless, except from computer technology, it was not until the millennium that industrial products basing on nanomaterials became commercially available in a significant extent. The application of nanomaterials for medical devices comes in various forms, but currently does focus on using these either to modify existing raw materials for or coating of products. It is worth mentioning that nanoparticles can be generated as a result of the wear and tear of medical devices, even if the medical device did not originally contain nanomaterials. The following list will provide you an overview upon first established applications.

5.4.1 Antimicrobial Modification of Medical Devices

Using nanotechnology, materials and surfaces may be modified to exhibit an antimicrobial effect. The most common approach is to utilize colloidal silver or finely dispersed titanium dioxide as additives to raw materials. This enables to implement the desired antimicrobial effect in close to any polymer-based medical devices, such as examination gloves, wall paintings for surgery rooms, or wound dressings (see Section 5.4). Anyhow, the mode of action does not require, but rather is enhanced when using nano- instead of microparticles, as doing so significantly does increase the active surface of the particles. Alternatively, nanotechnology may be utilized to create a defined surface structure within the submicrometer range that is repelling almost any other material, giving the surface self-cleaning properties. This action is commonly known as **lotus effect**, and is well suited for antimicrobial modification of a surface (see Figure 5.4). Moreover, doing so enables to simultaneously implement other features, as these surface structures may serve as counterfeit protection (see Section 5.7) or optimization of gliding properties at the same time.

5.4.2 Surface Modification

Nanomaterials enable to produce low-friction surfaces that exhibit an exceptional wear resistance. This is from greater interest for medical devices used for pricking or cutting, such as a surgical blade or needle. The trauma induced during penetration significantly correlates with the friction between device and tissue. A needle modified for lower friction will cause less pain while piercing and a scalpel or suture material is more convenient in application for the surgeon. Moreover, a smooth and low-friction surface is from great benefit for devices making contact with the stream of blood, as this will lead to a significant lower tendency to induce coagulation. So many venous or arterial grafts and coronary stents are coated with an ultrathin layer of nanomaterials.

5.4.3 Materials for Dentistry

The dental industry has many applications for nanomaterials, a fact that easily may be explained. When restoring teeth, it is of high importance to work at high precision, as any deviation to the ideal shape of the chewing surface of more than ~10 μm will give the patient a strange feeling or even lead to occlusal problems (bad bite). Consequently, any powder-based material for reconstruction or filling should feature a grain size significantly smaller, which makes nanomaterials well suited. Moreover, dental fillings must exhibit a considerate life span while being exposed to harsh mechanical and chemical conditions. Nanomaterials allow to cope these aspects by enabling to develop materials with improved strength and wear resistance. Hence, common dental applications for nanomaterials are as reinforcement of polymer-based materials for filling or reconstruction or as nano-ceramics.

5.4.4 Reinforcement of Medical Devices

Increasing the stiffness of an implant is from greater interest especially for orthopedic implants. Frequently these are fixed to the bone using a polymer-based adhesive known as **bone cement**. In order to minimize the trauma induced during implantation, the amount of adhesive utilized should be reduced to the max. This requires a bone cement with high strength whereas a reinforcement with CNTs is from greater interest. Moreover, the rapidly increasing miniaturization of medical devices (see Section 5.5) does trigger the demand for high-performance materials that exhibit high mechanical strength. Within a miniscule device, even a seemingly small force applied may induce significant stress and strain. Thereby, established approaches for reinforcement, such as carbon or glass fibers (typically 10–100 μm in diameter) are not applicable, as these frequently are far too big in dimensions. CNTs enable to reinforce even polymer structures with sizes of just a few microns, enabling to create miniaturized medical devices with exceptional mechanical strength. Currently, CNTs reinforced catheters for coronary intervention and stent delivery are under development.

5.4.5 Enhanced Biointegration

The reaction of the surrounding biological system toward a medical device generally is influenced by its material and surface presented toward the body (see Section 2.2). Especially for load-bearing orthopedic implants, a positive interaction is from great importance to achieve fast healing and a long-term stable flow of forces between skeletal system and implant. Nanotechnology enables to produce coatings that attract cells of the respective target tissue. For orthopedic implants, a promising approach is coating with hydroxyapatite (HA).[3] Plasma-based techniques for coating are well established (e.g., for hip or knee replacement implants), but nanotechnology enables to do so in a characteristic that features enhanced biointegration. HA shows a high tendency to attract bone-forming cells (osteoblasts) and as naturally occurring material within the human body features an excellent biocompatibility. Hence, nano sized HA also does find application as major component for biomaterials, utilized for reconstruction of defects or deficiencies of osseous structures, as this may be required within the jaw bone prior placing a dental implant.

Anyhow, most of these applications rather improve existing medical devices than offering groundbreaking new applications. Approaches basing on nanomaterials that are very likely to enable innovative therapies commonly are summed up as **injectable medical devices**. This term is not to be confused with pharmaceuticals administered by injection. By definition of many competent authorities, which is used within this book too, a pharmaceutical drug features a chemical mode of action, while a medical device does exhibit a physical mode of action. Anyhow, this categorization becomes more and more blurred due to emerging trends in medical engineering (see Section 2.7).

---

3. Hydroxylapatite (or hydroxyapatite) is the main component of bone mineral, the inorganic component of bone.

Among the first injectable medical devices are some that are intended for local tumor therapy. Nanoscaled iron oxide or gold particles are biochemically modified (chemical bonding of bioactive molecules) in a way that these accumulate within the degenerated cells, making them so susceptible to externally applied electromagnetic fields or radiation. This allows a locally limited heat input, restricted to the spatial expansion of the tumor. An established approach to do so is called **boron neutron capture therapy**, which does base on the observation that boron-10 nuclei exhibit a large cross section for thermal neutrons of defined energy, while these show a very low interaction with other elements. Primary step is to accumulate boron-10-containing nanoparticles within the tumor cells. If now the patient is exposed to radiation of thermal neutrons, these primarily will interact with the boron, creating alpha particles which in turn immediately interact with the tumor cells. Although still under development, this is a very promising approach for radiation-based local tumor therapy. Although technically seen not basing on nanotechnology, another approach is worth mentioning. **Selective internal radiation therapy** does base on radioactive polymer or glass spheres with 20–60 μm in diameter that are injected into the artery supplying the tumor. When traveling along with the stream of blood, the spheres eventually will physically block the vessels, as these taper down to a diameter of 4–10 μm. This induces two effects: the tumor cells are cut off from blood supply, and the sphere is affixed in a position ideally for the desired local delivery of radiation.

These approaches, as well as many more, commonly are summed under the label nano medicine. Although this term faces many different definitions, it is commonly accepted that it does comprise any approach for healing basing on physical manipulations on molecular scale. Consequently, an ongoing miniaturization of medical devices, as presented in Section 5.5, sooner or later will lead to nanoscale devices. Although this might sound very futuristic to you, first ideas doing so do exist with initial samples being available, as illustrated in Figure 5.10. A CNT does serve as rack for a nanoscaled device that can be equipped with additional components, as these are required for the desired therapy. These may include components for drug delivery, sensors, nanoparticles susceptible to physical forces (e.g., magnetic fields or radiation), or biochemical molecules that interact in specific metabolic processes via a lock and key principle. Developments like these will fuel the convergence of the nanotechnology-related efforts of many scientific, such as medicine, biology, physics, (bio-) chemistry, and engineering toward the field of nano medicine.

Anyhow, while the benefits of nanomaterials for medical devices still are discussed and investigated, there are considerate concerns about their safety,

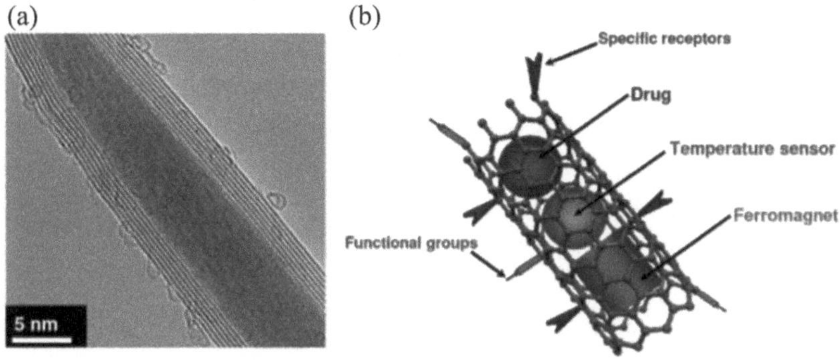

Figure 5.10 Example of a nanoscale injectable medical device, (a) as SEM image and (b) as illustration. A carbon nanotube (left side SEM image) does serve as rack that, depending on the desired therapy, may be equipped with different components such as drug delivery, sensors, nanoparticles susceptible physical forces, or bioactive molecules. *Image courtesy of Mark Hermann Rümmeli of IFW Dresden and the Journal of Materials Chemistry B.*

especially in the long term. These issues frequently are triggered by the lessons learned from **asbestos**, a naturally occurring silicate-based nanomaterial, which was utilized by mankind as early as the year 300 BC as reinforcement for pottery. Due to its outstanding heat resistance, its primary application in the industrial era was (and still is) as fire-resistant materials for insulation and fire protection. Although first concerns upon its health-damaging effects were raised as early as the end of the nineteenth century, it encountered emerging application in housing construction with peak application in many developed countries in the second half of the twentieth century. As the impact on public health became visible with significant delay, some scientists expect the peak of asbestos-induced disease still to come. In consequence, there are considerate concerns that comparable problems may result from widespread application of nanomaterials, primarily for life science products. First investigations indicated that incorporated nanoparticles show a tendency to accumulate within human cells, whereas the impact on health is not fully understood yet and thus not predictable. In consequence, many competent authorities acknowledge the beneficial potential of nanomaterials for medical devices while meantime expressing considerate concerns upon the long-term safety. In consequence, this topic is addressed by the FDA guideline to ISO 10993 (see Section 2.4.1), the revision of ISO 10993 (see Section 2.4.2), and a new project of the Technical Committee of ISO 10993, basing on a technical report issued as "Guidance on nanomaterials." Especially the Scientific Committee on Emerging and Newly

Identified Health Risks (SCENIHR) as part of the scientific branch of the European Commission does express considerate concerns upon the health risks possibly induced by nanomaterials as part of medical devices. A document issued by SCENIHR in early 2015, strongly recommends a phased approach to nanomaterials. Whenever you think about utilizing nanomaterials for a medical device, you should consider these regulations and documents and weigh the advantages and disadvantages as this involves the significant risk of not adequately addressing a risk with long-term effect or consequences.

5.5 Miniaturization of Medical Devices

Without doubt, miniaturization is one of the technological trends that had and still has major impact on all aspects of our daily living. Thereby, it is anything but easy to give a general definition for this term as most areas of our life in general (and technology in particular) usually have a very differing understanding about this term. However, the largest common denominator for miniaturization is that due to the technological evolution any existing machine, system, or apparatus is getting smaller in its general dimensions over time while meantime featuring more. The most prominent example for this trend can be found in microelectronics, where Moore's Law[4] still describes the ongoing trend toward miniaturization. Moreover, the evolution of all production technologies shows a trend toward miniaturization. You now may ask: aren't there some technological fields that rather focus on enlargement, like aviation or shipbuilding, where the products are getting larger and larger over time. First of all, manufacturing of the transportation giants only is feasible as a result of miniaturization that enables the technologies required (e.g., computing). Further, miniaturization not necessarily involves the entire product to become smaller but rather that it does exhibit an increasing amount of miniaturized components or substructures. In this meaning, a macroscopic product such as a foil that does exhibit a microstructure intended to repel dirt, commonly known as lotus effect (see Section 5.7), may be assigned as a product of miniaturization as well.

It is not surprising that miniaturization had major impact on the world of medical devices as well. Only the emerging computing power of modern

4. "Moore's law" is the finding that the number of transistors in an integrated circuit has doubled approximately every 2 years since the early 1970s. Although a saturation was postulated several time, the trend still continues.

microelectronics allows the construction of sophisticated machinery like those for magnetic resonance imaging and it was only microelectronics that enabled to treat people with devices such as an implantable pacemaker or a cochlea implant. Moreover, it was the general trend toward miniaturization that significantly fueled the medical fields of microsurgery and interventional cardiology. Both disciplines are in essential need for micro tools, manipulators, and devices, a need addressed by medical device manufacturers. Like in most cases, technological advancement of medical devices rather bases on technology transfer than on development or basic research (see TRIZ, Section 3.2.5). By utilizing established methods for micro manufacturing, medical device companies are capable to offer more elaborate micro medical devices, what in consequence broadens the applications of microsurgery and in return does increase the demand for appropriate devices. An aspect frequently encountered within polymer engineering is the impressions (you even may call it prejudices) that plastic is suited for rather coarsely shaped products, manufactured at large quantities. Even many experienced engineers are not aware about how far miniaturization within polymer processing has gone so far. Hence, in a first step, we will show you some examples for medical devices (or components for them) at the edge of polymer processing, and then in a second step show what development for miniaturization of plastic medical devices is to be expected.

Within the general field of techniques for minimal invasive therapies, especially **interventional therapies** as these frequently are applied in cardiology, neurology, and radiology, essentially require catheters. These tubular structures are used to access locations deep within the human body (e.g., heart or brain) via a peripheral penetration of a blood vessel and subsequently following the path of the arterial or venous system. The tubes required as precursor for these catheters should be as small as possible while capable of handling considerable mechanical loads. Moreover, frequently multilumen tubes are desired as these allow separated paths of access for different tools, fluids, fiber optics, or to administer drugs. Another application of microtubes in medical devices is in **oxygenators** or for **dialysis**. In both applications, the stream of blood is diverted through an external medical device in order to allow an exchange of gasses or liquids, while keeping the blood entirely enclosed. As the rate of exchange is proportional to the surface available for diffusion, the blood is passed through a large number of parallel aligned microtubes that are surrounded by an appropriate processing media. A good analogy from traditional engineering for this approach can be a heat exchanger where a large number of parallel aligned tubes allow the transfer, for example, from traditional engineering thermal energy between two media without mixing them. As you can imagine, reprocessing of these devices is close to infeasible (see Section 6.1) which is why these usually are produced as singe-use devices. The considerate need for these tubes is addressed by elaborate techniques for **extrusion** (see Section 3.1.4) that enable to produce tubes with an outer diameter of less than a millimeter that still exhibit several different lumens. Thereby, the resulting wall thickness may be as low as 25 µm (see Figure 5.11). The precise designs feasible (diameters, number of lumen, wall thicknesses) are highly dependent on the material utilized and the technical capabilities of the producing company. In consequence, it is not possible to give a general statement on the current technical boundaries. However, the market of micro extrusion does exhibit a considerate evolution that is worth tracking when deigning medical devices for interventional therapies.

Over the recent years, traditional **injection molding** also did exhibit a considerate development when looking at miniaturization. Thereby you should remember that within this context, miniaturization not necessarily involves a microscopic part to be produced but also may be a macroscopic part that does exhibit micro sized elements. However, modern techniques of injection molding enable to produce parts with shot weights

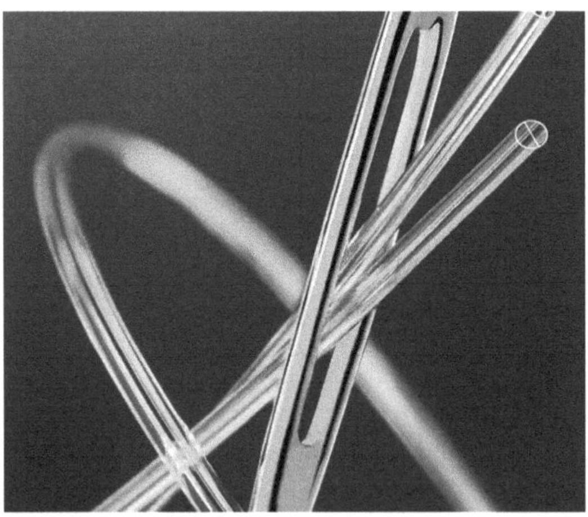

Figure 5.11 Example of a multilumen microtubing, as these are utilized as precursor for many devices, such as catheters for interventional therapies, dialysis, or oxygenators. The technical design limits (e.g., diameters, amount of separate lumen, wall thickness) are influenced by the plastic material used and the capabilities of the producing company. The two-lumen microtube displayed is utilized as diagnostic micro dialysis catheter. *Image courtesy of RAUMEDIC AG.*

lower than 1 g and structures smaller than 10 μm are feasible. This pushes plastic processing close to precision manufacturing of metal. Once more, the technical limits are influenced by the plastic material used as well as by the capabilities of the tool maker and the processing company. Injection molding is of greater interest for the manufacturing of complex designed components in large quantities. Although costs for an injection mold significantly may increase when getting into micro production, the running costs for an injection machine are largely independent from the design produced. Thereby, current technical capabilities of microinjection molding allow to easily implement defined **surface structures** on implants that allow to improve the response of surrounding tissue. This response is as a result to the material as well as to the surface structure presented, as explained in Section 2.2. Figure 5.12 does display an SEM image of a micro surface texture that is designed to attract soft tissue cells in order to improve the bonding between an implant and the tissue.

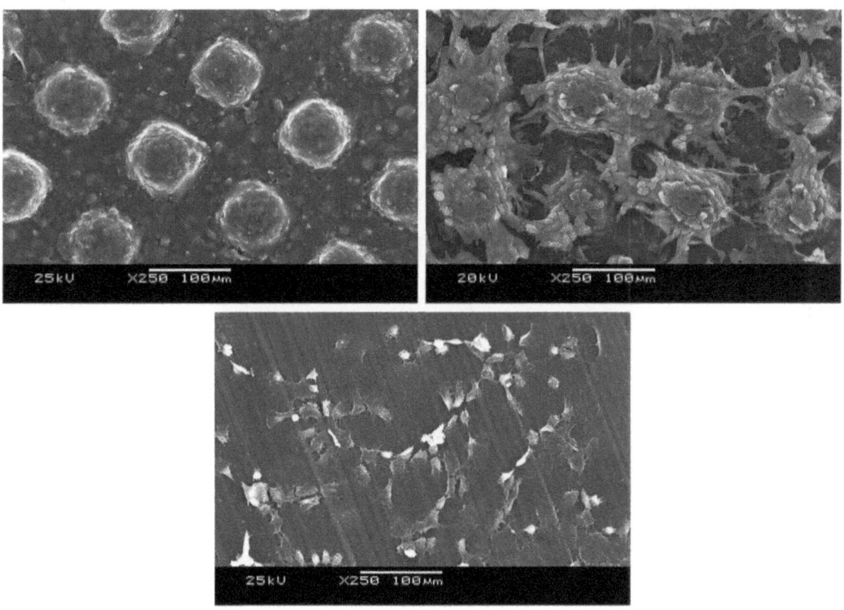

Figure 5.12 Micro surface structures intended to improve the biological reaction of the surrounding tissue. The microstructure (left image) consists of knobs, 50 μm in diameter and about the same distance. Cell culture (middle image) shows this structure to be highly attractive for soft tissue cells that appear (proliferation rate and morphology). The same material, identically processed into a flat surface (right image) shows to be less attractive to the very same cells.

The structure consists of knobs with 50 μm in diameter and the same distance in between. Investigations basing on cell culture show that the same material, identically processed into a flat surface shows to be less attractive for the cells.

Another interesting application for injection molding is the manufacturing of miniaturized tools and implants for microsurgery. In order to reduce the trauma induced during the surgery, the amount of tissue affected should be minimized. Nowadays, even elaborate surgical therapies like coronary bypass surgery at the beating heart may be performed minimal invasive via endoscopes. This generates a strong demand for appropriate micro tools and implants. A medical field with long tradition in such micro implants is middle ear surgery, where defective auditory ossicles[5] frequently need to be partially or entirely replaced. Thereby an appropriate implant must fit to the narrowed anatomical conditions and the delicate structure of the middle ear. While established implants exhibit a rather simple rod-shaped structure, novel approaches try to implement additional features like the ability to automatically adapt in length or to damp excessive sound levels. This necessarily involves a more complex geometry without a significant increase in implant weight, as it must be able to oscillate at frequencies within the spectrum of human hearing. Microinjection molding allows to manufacture a middle ear implant that does exhibit complex kinematic comparable to the native auditory ossicles, while still fitting within the cavity of the middle ear and not excessing a mass of 20 mg. The implant displayed in Figure 5.13 is manufactured from PEEK and the integral hinges (flattened structures) exhibit a wall thickness of less than 100 μm.

Combining products from micro extrusion and microinjection molding allows to manufacture complex miniaturized active implants such as minimally applicable heart support systems. Many acute heart diseases, such as heart attack or failure, result in an insufficient pump performance, although the heart muscle is working close to or even over its capabilities. Meantime the heart would desperately require a release from mechanical load in order to regenerate. A meaningful solution to this condition can be a miniaturized blood pump. Current systems at the edge of technology are capable of replacing the entire workload of the heart while still exhibiting dimensions that are well suited for interventional cardiology (see Figure 5.14). It is worth mentioning that

5. The auditory ossicles are a structure of three tiny bones, commonly known as malleus, incus, and stapes, located within the cavity of the middle ear, that play a crucial role for the perception of sound. They are by far the smallest bones within the human body.

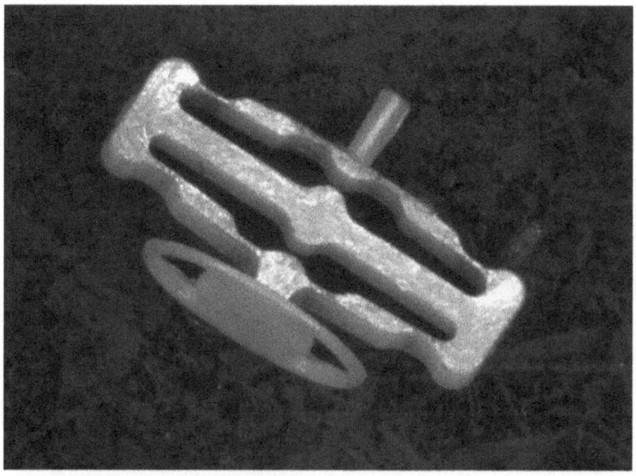

Figure 5.13 A novel middle ear implant, manufactured by injection molding. Established implants exhibit a rather simple rod-shaped design that does not allow to automatically adapt the length of the implant or to damp excessive sound levels. The implants displayed solves these disadvantages by featuring a kinematic comparable to the native auditory ossicles, while still fitting into the middle ear cavity and not exceeding a mass of 20 mg. *Image in courtesy of Scholz-HTIK.*

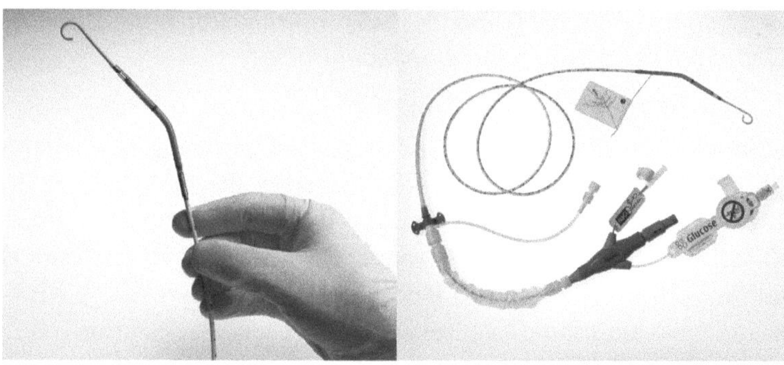

Figure 5.14 Display of a heart support system at the current edge of technology. The system is capable of replacing the workload of the heart, giving it time to recover, while still featuring dimensions that are suitable for interventional cardiology (the pump displayed is 4 mm in diameter). *Images courtesy of Abiomed Inc.*

reprocessing (see Section 6.1) of such a device is close to infeasible which is why these are intended for single use only.

The trend toward even smaller micro tools and implants that meantime exhibit additional integrated features will continue. As a good example for this, development may serve the idea for a bioresorbable electronic stent

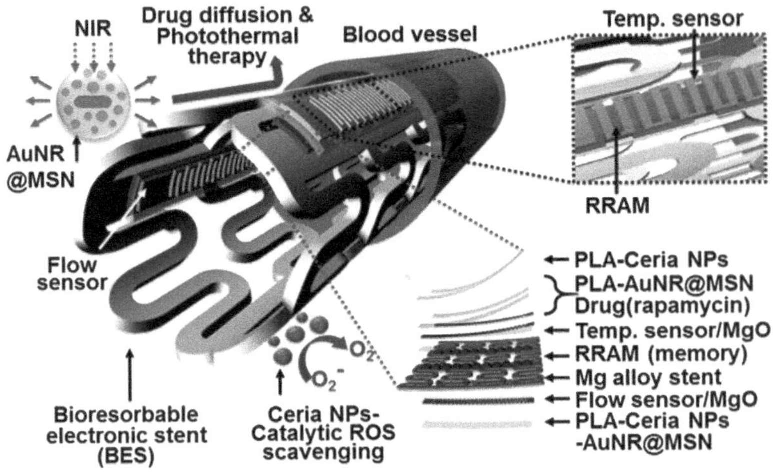

Figure 5.15 Illustration of a bioresorbable electronic stent (BES). Established stents, as these are utilized to treat constrictions of a blood vessel (stenosis), face an emerging trend to bioresorbable implants that frequently base on polymers. When considering the opportunities of miniaturization, it is the logical next step to integrate additional feature, such as sensors, drug delivery, or micro actuators into such a bioresorbable stent. ROS, reactive oxygen species. *Reprinted with permission from Donghee Son et al. Copyright 2015 American Chemical Society.*

(BES). Stents are well-established devices used to treat a constriction (stenosis) of a blood vessel (Figure 5.15). Currently the trend is going toward bioresorbable stents that frequently base on biodegradable polymers (see Section 6.5.1). When reflecting the advantages of bioresorbable stents and the opportunities of miniaturization a BES is the logical next step. A BES would allow to integrate additional features such as sensors (see Section 5.6.2), drug delivery (see Section 6.6), and micro actuators. This device already is very close to the idea of a miniaturized submarine that treats life-threatening conditions, a vision already presented in some science fiction movies.

The world of medical devices has already seen many miniaturized devices that were thought to be impossible no long time ago. These enable to ease the patient's condition minimally invasive and so to increase the therapeutic outcome while reducing the costs for treatment. And the trend toward miniaturization may be expected to continue, whereas especially shape-memory polymers significantly contribute to these developments (see Section 6.5.2). But when getting smaller and smaller, the dimensions of such a micro tool, implant, or device are getting closer and closer to the magnitude of molecules. The manipulation of molecules or even a single atom commonly is labeled nanotechnology. Interestingly, nanotechnology (see Section 5.4) does exhibit developments that yield toward the manipulations of objects rather big in size within the nano world, developments that are expressed as devices for nano medicine. You might call this an upscaling of nanotechnology. As miniaturization and nanotechnology approach to each other, future trends accordingly will see a merger of both disciplines.

5.6 Fully Integrated and Automated Device Manufacturing

Many medical devices are composed of different components or materials. This necessarily involves additional steps for assembly those, like within any other discipline of engineering, do increase production costs and the risk of faulty products. However, approaches to avoid additional processes for mounting are from particular importance for medical devices. Any step of assembly bears the risk of adding bioburden to the product that may cause harm to the patient, even if the device is sterilized prior application (see Section 2.3.2). This is why manually performed assembly should be replaced by automated processes as far as possible. Moreover, although assembling a medical device does allow to utilize more simple designed components, it comes along with significant disadvantages. For example, frequent bonding is utilized to join different components. For this, a predominant role play UV curing adhesives with many glues suitable for medical applications are available on the market. A prominent example is hypodermic needles, where a hollow needle (metal) is joined with a Luer-Lock[6] connector (plastic). However, these mass produced SUDs are cost sensitive and creating the adhesive sealing a challenging process. Now and again, the bonding does fail in field causing sometimes fatal consequences, as the fluidic system may leak without noticing it. Less dramatic, but still as severe event, are small adhesive particles that may become detached by the bypassing fluid. Once injected into the body, these may provoke a fever, whereas its precise cause frequently remains unknown to the treating medical professional. However, many medical devices or components of these are produced by injection molding. This technology offers great opportunities to avoid most of these problems mentioned by means of fully integrated device manufacturing. There are many examples from manufacturing of consumer goods or toys that show the great cost-saving potential.

---

6. Luer-Lock is the worldwide established standard system of small-scale fluid fittings, which are used to create leak-free connections between different medical devices, named for its inventor Hermann Wülfing Luer.

Moreover, doing so usually does increase the automation of assembly and may replace some or even all subsequent steps of assembly. These advantages are even more relevant when thinking about approaches to autosterile manufacturing, as these are explained in Section 5.2. The ideal would be a fully integrated and automated manufacturing by means of autosterile manufacturing. Put simply, manufacturing an equipment that, fed with the relevant raw materials and components, does produce sterile and ready-to-sell medical devices. And coming back to the example of the hypodermic needle: why not replacing adhesive-based bonding by an automated assembly during manufacturing? This may sound futuristic to you, but it partially is established in the medical device world, and it already is state of the art in other industries. The next chapter will give you some examples of fully manufacturing processes that are suitable for medical device manufacturing and show their enormous potential by the example of emerging approaches to treat diabetes.

5.6.1 Mechanical Assembly

Mechanical assembly during manufacturing of plastic components is anything but new. There is an impressive number of technologies for **multicomponent injection molding**, that all stand for the approach of assembly during manufacturing. A good example is tooth brushes, which nowadays feature a rigid handle with soft grips attached to it. It is unknown to many people that an ordinary tooth brush (see Figure 5.16) is considered

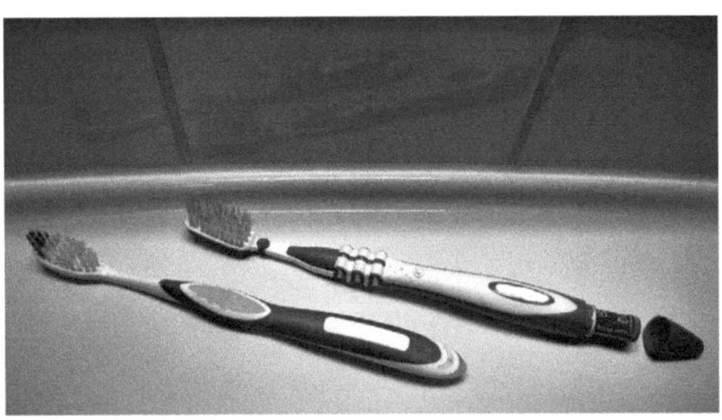

Figure 5.16 Tooth brushes commonly are produced by multicomponent injection molding, whereas a rigid component for the handle is combined with soft materials for the grips. Some competent authorities consider ordinary tooth brushes as medical device. The one displayed on the right is an electric tooth brush (battery case opened) intended for complete disposal when outworn. Thus it may be seen as example for established single-use electronic medical devices.

a medical device by some competent authorities, making them an unexpected still well-suiting example. The established standard process of manufacturing tooth brushes is based on multicomponent injection molding utilizing thermoplastic elastomer systems (see Section 6.4) and does result in a ready-to-pack product. But multicomponent injection molding is not only suitable for rigid bonding. For moveable, still inseparable connections (form-locking), one may make use of the shrinking of the polymer part during cooling, a process known as **assembly injection molding**. In a first step, the component featuring the female part of the joint is manufactured. Next, the component with the male part is produced, whereas the void of the female joint serves as partial mold for the male. The latter will shrink during cooling and thus create a joint space that allows movement. Frequently, two materials featuring different processing temperatures are utilized to avoid a tight connection. Nevertheless, by selecting appropriate process parameters, even the very same material may be processed that way. This technology is well established for the production of plastic toy figures with moveable legs and arms. The very same principle may be used as well to manufacture a ready assembled lead or translation screw, and first attempts are taken to manufacture ready assembled gearboxes and transmissions that way. This would enable to utilize these mechanisms for cost-sensitive SUDs, which require manufacturing costs that do not allow to integrate these in traditional ways.

Both approaches presented are not limited to the application of plastic materials. Any material processible by injection molding may be utilized, whereas this most frequently does imply to find a material exhibiting a melting temperature within the range of those of plastic materials. Accordingly, there are some metals available that may be integrated within a process of multicomponent or assembly injection molding, which may serve as electric conductor or wiring integrated during manufacturing. Combined with inlay molding, a technology presented in the next chapter, this exemplary allows to manufacture a product such as a battery-powered bedside lamp fully automated and ready-to-use by means of fully integrated and automated injection molding.

Although a consumer product, the bedside lamp indicates the enormous potential of fully integrated and automated medical device manufacturing. And why not imagine a single-use lamp as medical device? For full anesthesia during an operation, the patient usually gets a flexible plastic tube placed in his trachea (windpipe) in order to maintain an open airway. As axillary for this process known as (tracheal) intubation, the performing medical professional usually utilizes a device called laryngoscope. Among other things, its primary function is to lift the tongue and to provide light in the patient's throat. As state of the art, a laryngoscope is a reusable medical device that does require reprocessing prior its next application (see Section 6.1). Besides the costs and manpower required for doing so, this in particular is a strain for the electric components (wiring, source of light), that would be meaningless when using a single-use laryngoscope. So, why not imagine a (partially) single-use laryngoscope, produced by means of autosterile and fully automated manufacturing? As mentioned within the first chapter of this book, medical engineering is probably more subjected to technology transfer than any other technological discipline. And looking at the manufacturing approaches utilized in other industries, combined with your knowledge as (bio) medical engineer, creates an almost endless source for novel medical devices.

5.6.2 Automated Sensor Integration

The ongoing miniaturization (see Section 5.5), combined with the advances in manufacturing of microelectronics nowadays enable to produce sensors at costs that allow to their integration into single-use devices. So within this chapter we want to focus on an aspect that you could call **single-use sensors or electronics**, an approach that comes along with some distinctive advantages. In fact, single-use medical devices are already commercially available, as illustrated in Figure 5.16. However, prior reuse of a medical device, any biological remains sticking to it must be removed thoroughly (see Section 6.1) in order to avoid cross-infection or faulty measurement. The task of reprocessing is rather complicated when performed at delicate or tubular structures or even more at rough or uneven surfaces. Most of these problem cases are combined in measurement equipment that features microfluidic components (see Section 6.2) that in many cases hardly may be reprocessed in a way appropriate for reuse. Single use seems to be the only meaningful solution to this problem. A prominent example for this is the meter-strips used for the measurement of blood sugar level, as displayed in Figure 5.18. A blood droplet is sucked into a microfluidic system by capillary forces and eventually finds access to a reaction chamber where distinct chemicals are present. Although many different biochemical reactions are utilized to quantify the amount of glucose present in the given blood sample, close to all systems eventually utilize an electrical sensor which is why those test meter-strips feature two electrical contacts. As you may imagine, removing all remains of blood after measuring is close to impossible. Moreover, reprocessing would require restocking of the chemicals, which is why meter-strips virtually exist as single use only. As meter-strips are utilized on global base (see Section 5.6.3), you see that integration of sensors as well as single-use sensors are well established. However, the meter-strips are rather simple in design and usually feature sensors of moderate complexity. The tricky part is to be found in the biochemical reaction, which is why these systems commonly are classified as In Vitro Diagnostics (see Section 6.3).

Larger or more complex sensor systems may be integrated during manufacturing using the technology of **inlay molding**. For this, the component desired for integration is placed within the mold prior injection. After demolding, the component is firmly joined with the plastic part. Thereby, the process of inlay molding allows the part to be partially (e.g., the LED in Figure 5.17) or fully within the plastic part. Moreover, even wiring and bonding may be performed during manufacturing. While sensor electronics usually exhibit a printed circuit board, these elements may be replaced by structures directly attached to the surface or even integrated within the part or component. A closer look to consumer electronics shows a remarkable integration of functions on minimal space. Just think about a state-of-the-art smartphone, that, beyond the electronics for wireless communication (GSM, LTE, WIFI) usually exhibits an impressive amount of sensors, e.g., intended to measure global position (GPS), acceleration (linear and rotatory, in three dimensions), magnetic fields (compass), and many more. You might wonder about the relevance of medical devices? Well, there is a general lack of sensors in medical devices, especially those intended for single use.

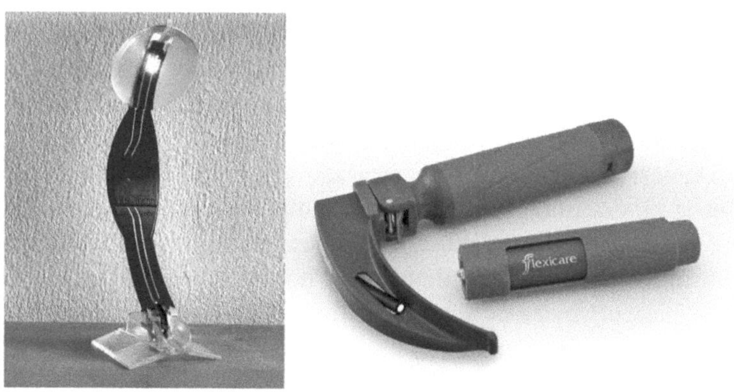

Figure 5.17 On the left, bedside lamp produced by fully automated multi-component injection molding, as it is produced ready-to-use in one single production step. The very same technology could be used to produce single-use laryngoscope, as displayed on the right. *Image on the right, courtesy of Flexicare Medical Limited.*

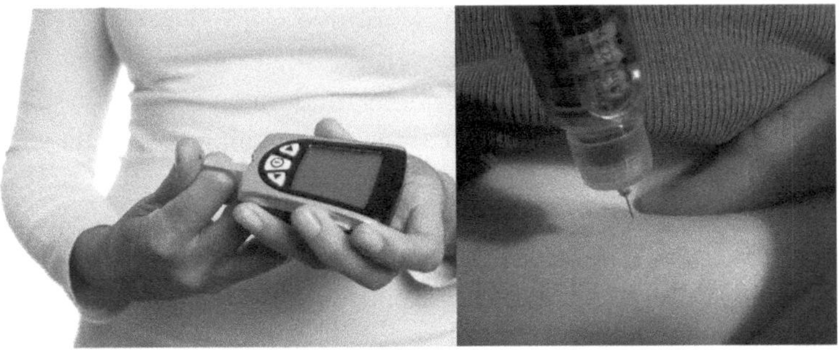

Figure 5.18 Left side: State-of-the-art measurement of the blood sugar level by performing a finger prick to harvest a droplet of blood that subsequently is analyzed by a glucometer. From this analysis, the appropriate amount of insulin is derived and administered as subdermal injection by an insulin pen (displayed on the right) or partially automated by an insulin pump (not displayed). This entire, rather unpleasant procedure must be performed several times a day, a major reason for incompliance to diabetes therapy. *Image on the right, courtesy of Danielle Laun.*

Of course, there are manifold medical devices that feature elaborate measurement equipment. Just think about the equipment for electrocardiography and ultrasound examination or implantable pacemakers. However, these are not subject to the proclaimed lack of sensors. The call for more sensors rather shall concern the countless number of single-use devices and implants that seldom feature any kind of sensors, which does result in an enormous, yet largely unused potential to improve the efficacy of therapies. Accurate information about the patient's state of health is crucial for deciding upon the next steps for therapy. Currently, acquiring this information usually is performed in a step completely independent from the actions following it. Getting back once more to the example of measuring the level of blood sugar: in a first step a finger prick is performed in order to harvest a droplet of blood. In the next step, this sample is analyzed with a glucose meter. Why not imagine a miniscule lancet that does perform the measurement in the short time while puncturing the skin? During most therapies, most patients make contact for different durations to a great number of single-use devices, such as tubes, needles, catheters, and many more. And as explained in Section 2.2, this contact always will induce a foreign body reaction. As consequence, this necessarily occurring contact should result in a maximized benefit for the patient, e.g., by implementing sensors into these devices. Ideally, a catheter used for intravenous administration of liquids (a drip) should exhibit sensors to measure the current blood pressure. Or why not implementing a temperature sensor into a plaster or brace, allowing conveniently determining the blood heat? This would allow to save the time required for treatment and could ease a problem that is fundamental to most processes of measuring as these are performed during medical treatment: **measurement** usually does spot the state of the human body **at a distinct moment only**. However, the human body as biological system is highly dynamic. Blood pressure may change within seconds and body temperature within minutes. Moreover, most quantities of the human body to be measured are highly influenced by the reaction of the patient. Think about a patient who is scared by the doctor's examination. This anxiety will result in the release of adrenaline, what in return will result is an increased blood pressure and thus the value determined will not represent the "normal" state. It is well known that appropriate data upon the biological system of the human body do require repeatedly performed measurements. Just think about fever chart, the depiction of many temperature measurements performed over time, intended to gain information upon the temporal evolvement of the body temperature. Ideally, any medical **measurement** should be performed **over an extended period**. And integrating the required sensors into a single-use device that is applied anyway, does represent the ideal solution for doing so. Transferring this idea to implants allows to imagine many more opportunities. Load-bearing implants could be equipped with sensors to measure the mechanical load and movement. This would allow an improved observation of their postoperative biointegration. And why not finding more uses for the very same sensor? An emerging problem within our society is the overaging population, whereas beyond those caused by medical treatment, significant costs are related to care and nursing. A meaningful solution to this problem is any approach that does enable the elderly people to live at home as long as possible. Thereby, frequent medical alarm systems, e.g., ported as necklace or bracelet, are utilized to call for help in case of emergency. Frequently an elderly person makes use of these systems after stumbling and subsequently falling, resting on the ground, unable to ease his situation himself. What if the person is unable to press the alarm button? These problems are addressed by an approach called **ambient-assisted living** (AAL). And sensors integrated into implants ideally could be integrated into systems for AAL, as these allow to detect potential hazardous conditions that may not be tracked by conventional external sensor systems. Partially this already is done. An implantable cardioverter-defibrillator does sensor the electrical activity of the heart and in case it is required, automatically perform defibrillation. However, AAL could be significantly improved by integrating these mechatronic systems into an extended network for monitoring. A load-bearing implant featuring a shock sensor combined with an artificial heart-valve could help to detect if the patient did collapse after defibrillation and is in urgent need of help. You see, these developments are closely related to parallel development within our society. More and more people are wearing devices that track their physiological condition (see Section 6.7), e.g., during sports. Meanwhile, we integrate more and more sensors into our home, in order to adapt heating and air conditioning to our personal needs or even to monitor the content of our fridge. These developments will result in an all-embracing network that significantly will improve our daily living. And medical devices will become an integral part of this network. In result, the precise boundaries between medical devices and consumer products will get more and more blurred. In fact, we are already deep inside this process of merger, as explained in Chapter 7. Nevertheless, as promised in the beginning of the chapter, we now will focus on the impact of sensor integration into medical devices on the treatment of diabetes.

5.6.3 Continuous Glucose Monitoring

Integration of sensors into medical devices does enable, among others, innovative approaches to treat **diabetes**. As consequence of overaging population combined by an unhealthy lifestyle (e.g., malnutrition, lack of exercise, obesity), the amount of people suffering from diabetes within the industrialized countries have reached considerate numbers that are expected to rise even more within the upcoming decades. The WHO estimated a worldwide number of 30 million people suffered from diabetes in 1985 that will increase to 300 million by 2025. This induces a significant financial burden to the health-care systems, induced by direct costs that are required for treatment of diabetes and indirect costs, e.g., those caused by secondary complications, loss of productivity, and many more. Hence, it stands for a good reason that the diabetes drug and device market, although exhibiting a remarkable size already, is expected to grow even further. To give you an idea, the U.S. National Diabetes Statistics Report for 2014 estimated the total diabetes-related costs to be $245 billion.

To get closer to emerging trends in the diabetes medical device market, it is helpful to make a short excursion into the **blood sugar regulation**. The concentration of sugar, the main source of energy for human cells, is kept at constant level by a complex biological system that involves many setting parameters, as a level to low will cause coma (and eventually death) while a level to high will cause considerate harm to the blood vessels increasing the risk for diabetes-induced blindness, diabetic feet, cardiovascular diseases, and many more. The hormones, insulin and glucagon, both are synthesized within the pancreas, play a vital role within the regulation and act as antagonists. Insulin is released in case of high blood sugar and enables the uptake of sugar by the cells and simultaneously stimulates its storage as glycogen (polymerized glucose) within the human liver. Glucagon is realized in case of low blood sugar and triggers the breakdown of a glycogen, what in turn does raise the level of blood sugar. Similar to all types of diabetes is that the amount of insulin and glucagon required is not covered adequately due to a lack or total loss of its production.

Easing the harm from diabetes requires the patient to actively participate in this regulation by closely monitoring his blood sugar level (see Figure 5.19). This is commonly done via a **finger prick**: with a blood lancet, a fingertip is punctured in order to harvest a small droplet of blood that is analyzed by a glucometer (see Figure 5.18), a method basing on In Vitro Diagnostics (see Section 6.3). This rather unpleasant method should be repeated several times a day, especially every time prior food intake, and in consequence is one of the primary reasons for the patient's incompliance to diabetes therapy. Approaches to allow more convenient methods to measure the blood level will be discussed later in this chapter. The lack of glucagon may be managed rather easy: a low level of blood sugar

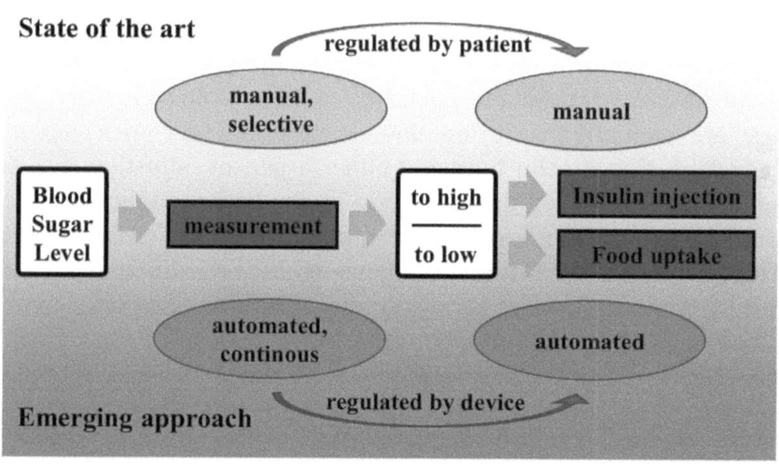

Figure 5.19 Schematic illustration of the way of diabetes treatment according to the state of art and as it could be done by an emerging approach by means of an artificial pancreas. The current approach represents an open-looped control that requires action of the patient several times a day. Emerging approaches utilize a closed loop that automatically and continuously measures the level of blood and delivers the appropriate amount of insulin. This significantly will improve the quality of life for a diabetic, equipped with an artificial pancreas.

will be noticed immediately by a feeling of weakness and intense hunger and is corrected the consumption of food rich in sugar and hence always should be carried along by diabetics. Managing the lack of insulin is more difficult, as an acute increase in blood sugar level hardly is sensible. In consequence, regulating the appropriate amount of insulin requires to closely monitor the blood sugar level (finger prick) and correspondingly administering insulin via subdermal injection. This usually is done with an insulin pen, a medical device designed for multiple subdermal injections (see Figure 5.18). Alternatively, an insulin pump can be used, an electric-driven device that continuously releases insulin via a tube that is placed subdermal and may stay in place for several days to weeks. In most cases, the constant administering of insulin is beneficial for the treatment of diabetes and many patients enjoy the reduced number pricking. However, in both cases require the manual determination of the blood sugar level by doing a finger prick and regulation of the dosage of insulin.

And exactly this comes along with several disadvantages. First of all, doing so is a selective measurement while the blood sugar level ideally should be tracked continuously. Additionally, many diabetics are anything but happy to perform this rather unpleasant procedure several times a day. In fact, the effectivity of current diabetes treatments is primarily influenced by the patient's compliance that requires active participation. From an engineering point of view, the active participation of the patient covers two major aspects. These are repetitive, rather simple to perform actions as these are manually measuring blood sugar (via finger prick) and manually administering insulin by using either a pen or adjusting the setting of the insulin pump. And the regulation by the patient, which in this case deriding the appropriate dosage of insulin required, derived from the blood sugar level determined. Although this task must be learned and intensely trained by diabetics, it does follow known algorithms and once more is a repetitive task, as illustrated in Figure 5.19.

Consequently, current developments for medical devices for diabetes therapy follow two main aspects. The first one is to replace the established finger prick by a more convenient method. Ideally this technology does allow an **automated and continuous measurement** of blood level for a period of several months up to dates. Current approaches utilize either a subdermal placed sensor, making direct contact to the blood, or perform measurement transdermal (without penetration of the skin) using laser-based systems. Continuously tracking the blood sugar level allows to significantly better cure diabetes and bypasses the aspect of noncompliant patients that are not willing to perform a finger prick as frequently as it ideally should be done. Moreover, those systems are ideal to automatically store the measurements, whereas long-term data form great interest for the treating physician. The other main aspect of current interest does focus on the **automated administration of insulin**, an approach you may call **artificial pancreas**. Although established insulin pumps allow a continuous dosage, these still must be manually programmed basing on the data that are derived from the equally manual performed measurement of blood sugar, as illustrated in Figure 5.19.

Therefore, the logical step should be to close the loop from an automated measurement to an automated administration of insulin. From an engineering point of view, this would mean to transfer the control system from open-looped to closed-looped, be automatically and continuously adapting the delivery rate of insulin to the blood sugar level measured. This combination of medical devices could be labeled as artificial pancreas, as it almost entirely may replace the functionality of the original biological system—at least for a period of several days, and that is an enormous period for any diabetic, that is used to focus on his disorder several times a day. In fact, the very first system that features a closed loop for automated and continuous control of the blood sugar level came to market in 2015, as displayed in Figure 5.20.

It is obvious that the primary goal of this development is to improve the diabetes therapy, and therefore it may be called **primary benefit of therapy**. But the secondary goal is to improve the quality of life for people treated with the system. Needless to say that those systems are experienced as significantly more convenient by many patients as less action is required. And exactly this fact does help to improve the compliance of the

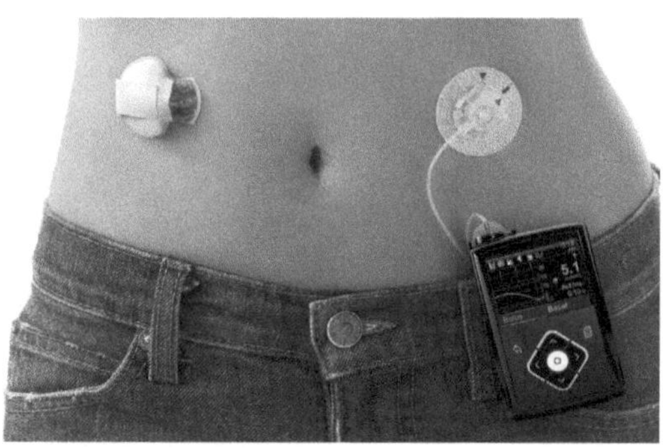

Figure 5.20 System for automated control of the blood sugar level, consisting of a sensor for continuous measurement (left) and fully automated delivery via an insulin pump (right). This system already may be labeled as artificial pancreas as the system may run several days without any action, compared to traditional methods (see Figure 5.19) that need attendance several times a day. *Image courtesy of Medtronic.*

patient, a fact you may call **secondary benefit of therapy**. The augmented acceptance to the therapy will improve its outcome directly, by optimized regulation of the biological system, as well as indirectly, by giving the patient a good feeling. Many people suffering from a chronic disease are engaged in their treatment on daily basis. Consequently many of them state that they dream about not having to think about their condition, even if it was for just a couple of days or even just hours. The artificial pancreas presented is a considerable step toward this for diabetics. As mentioned in the previous chapter, any medical device should feature sensors intended to gain additional information. Following this call, currently contact lenses are developed that feature sensors to measure the blood sugar (see Figure 5.21). As the cornea of the eye is alimented only by the tear fluid, it contains glucose in a concentration directly proportional to the level of blood sugar. Integrated into a system of an artificial pancreas, this contact lens even more would increase the convenience for a diabetic. And this probably is just the first step toward an entire network of sensor-equipped medical devices that are not only intended to treat a disease but meantime as well to maintain our health. And this further will blur the distinction of medical devices, consumer electronics, and consumer products.

5.7 Anticounterfeiting for Medical Devices

Due to the fast progressing globalization, product piracy is an emerging problem for the entire manufacturing industry. Usually the risk of plagiarism correlates with the product price and thus not only manufacturers of

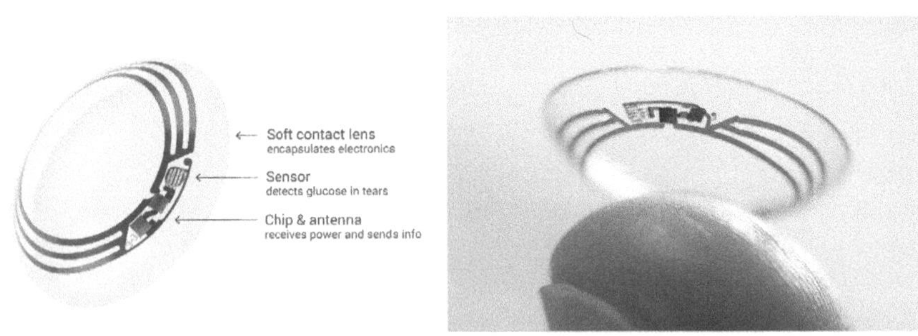

Figure 5.21 As the cornea of the eye is alimented only by the tear fluid, it contains glucose in a concentration directly proportional to the level of blood sugar. Current research does focus on the integration of continuous blood sugar measurement into contact lenses. This would allow a very convenient way for continuous blood sugar measurement. *Images courtesy of Google.*

trademark products are affected, but also small companies that sell valuable goods. So manifold technologies were developed to prevent or at least significantly complicate counterfeiting. We all have seen many of these: just think of banknotes that feature elaborate microprints and holograms to prevent falsification, or software that requires a serial key for activation prior use. While counterfeiting conventional consumer goods usually will result in annoyed consumers and a loss in business, falsified products from life sciences may lead to severe risks for health or even death. Unfortunately, these products increasingly are subject to criminal activities, as the possible benefits are rather high while the consumer awareness still is comparatively low. Just think about the considerate trade of pharmaceuticals via the Internet, which does focus on prescription or not marketable drugs. Many buyers rely on the effectiveness of these drugs due to the packaging and labeling they are accustomed to without really questioning its quality. On the other hand, can you imagine a surgeon checking the authenticity of a medical device during an operation? Presumably most medical professionals will not, as although knowing about counterfeit medical devices, they usually will consider this a rather distant problem. Triggered by these facts, the global health market faces a rapid growing number of false medical devices and pharmaceuticals, an issue addressed by competent authorities via the creation of special task forces, e.g., the *International Medical Products Anti-Counterfeiting Taskforce* (IMPACT) that was established by the WHO. The fight against piracy and counterfeiting of life science products requires a strong collaboration between governmental bodies and industry on global scale. The contribution from the medical device industry must be at least appropriate technologies that prevent the counterfeit of their products. The motivation therefore should not only be the protection against economic damage or legal safeguarding, as failure of a forged medical device always will fall back on the assumed manufacturer. **Counterfeit protection for medical devices is crucial** to protect the health of patients. Anyhow, preventing the falsification of medical devices involves some boundary conditions that are different to those for consumer goods. The following chapter will present established and emerging technologies for counterfeit protection while considering their suitability to safeguard medical devices. Thereby, it is important to remember that not only a product but also counterfeit protection itself may be subjected to falsification. Therefore, any measure taken for protection should be so complicated to reproduce, that any attempt to do so appears to be not worth the effort. At the end of this section, you will find further general considerations with a short overview upon pros, cons, and their respective specifics.

5.7.1 Security Printing and Holograms

Both technologies are well established with broad applications. Close to all banknotes and identity documents issued by states and countries are protected by different types of security prints and holograms. Just take your wallet and have a look. **Security printing** comprises many techniques at the edge of printing technology, such as microprint (minuscule block letters), watermark, guilloché (ornamental arrangement of fine lines), special inks or intaglio (raised or textured print work), and many more (as illustrated in Figure 5.22). Moreover, by combining elaborate printing technologies and special inks, objects can be created that change color when either conditions of observations are changed or the object is warmed, e.g., by pressing ones finger on it (Figure 5.23). Both techniques allow to easily check on originality for any

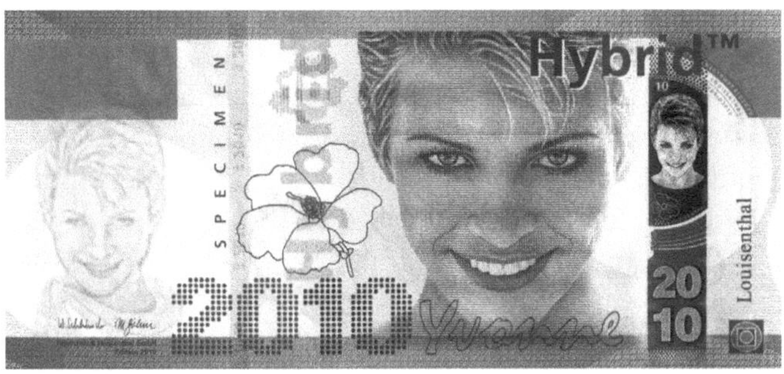

Figure 5.22 Sample of a banknote, featuring state-of-the-art security printing. Manufacturing features such as microprint (minuscule block letters), watermark, guilloché (ornamental arrangement of fine lines), color-changing objects, special inks, or intaglio require elaborate machinery and specially trained employees, giving a high barrier for counterfeiting. *Security printings and image in courtesy of Giesecke and Devrient GmbH.*

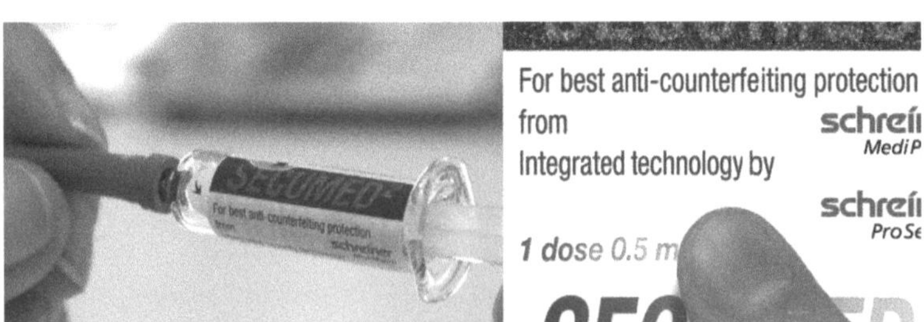

Figure 5.23 By combining elaborate printing technologies and special inks, objects that change color when either conditions of observations are changed (left image) or the object is warmed, e.g., by pressing ones finger on it (right). Both techniques allow to easily check on originality for any layperson. *Images courtesy of Schreiner Group GmbH & Co. KG.*

layperson. Counterfeit protection by security printing does result from the high-end machinery, well-educated personnel, and restricted precursors that are crucial for production. Even untrained layperson will easily detect plagiarism, a fact from great advantage for objects that change hands many times, making banknotes the ideal application for these technologies. However, a growing number of medical devices and pharmaceuticals are equipped with security printing on the packaging. This enables easily checking on plagiarism by every single person involved during the distribution, from custom officers over retailers to end customer. Anyhow, security printing is less advantageous for marking the medical device itself.

Holograms may be produced by many different means of manufacturing, whereas currently electron-beam lithography is probably the one most frequently utilized. Reproduction requires a master hologram as well as expensive, specialized, and technologically advanced equipment and so these usually are sold as labels or stickers, making them a standard bought-in part. In its most common version, a hologram does show an artwork consisting of two or three layers that in sum create a static three-dimensional image with characteristic color pattern, like it can be found on close to any credit card. Compared to micro printing, electro-beam lithography allows creating structures significantly smaller and complex, which enables to manufacture holograms that are more delicate, and by combining several layers more sophisticated effects can be generated. As these frequently are combined, four of these will be presented more detailed. Each requires the development of complex algorithms to create optical elements that shape scattered radiation patterns. Computing the nano-structures is a complicated mathematical task, giving them a very high level of protection. A **dot matrix** is a hologram that consists of arrays (dots) of down to 10 μm whereas each dot consists of smaller optical units and thus creates its own unique scattered radiation pattern. Put simply, a dot matrix is a hologram created by superimposing manifold micro holograms. This does result in an eye-catching colorful appearance that changes when conditions of observations are changed. This easily allows distinguishing these from conventional holograms that show a rather static image. More elaborate algorithms to compute the structure and alignment of these arrays allow implementing more features. Although technically still a dot matrix, these commonly are known by different names. **Covert Laser Readable** images are invisible to the naked eye, but suddenly appear when illuminated with laser light of defined wavelength. Most of these images are designed for readability with class-2 laser pointers (620–780 nm) that are easier to access. **True color holograms** are an attractive feature and are easy to verify even by uninstructed layperson. Even without further explication, everyone will become suspicious if the holographic image of an everyday object or a brand sign appears in unfamiliar or strange colors. Anyhow, the widest distributed features are **kinetic images** or **kinegram**® as the trademark name of the inventing company. Although technically seen a real hologram, these images seldom give a real three-dimensional impression. The feature is rather a two-dimensional artwork that moves when conditions of observations are being changed. Turning or tilting the hologram in any direction allows studying this movement or detecting details only visible at distinct positions, as illustrated in Figure 5.24.

However, while attaching a label to the packaging is rather easy, direct marking on a medical device involves some issues. Many medical devices require high hygienic conditions or need to be sterilized prior application. However, any additional handling of a manufactured device, such as attaching a hologram label, increases the risk of contamination and requires additional processing. Further, the adhesive of the label may influence the polymer it is attached to and so alter its mechanical properties. Moreover, this interaction may produce leachables (see Section 2.1) with possible negative influence on biocompatibility and biological safety. Most holograms are not suitable for common techniques of sterilization and thus not suitable for sterile devices. All these aspects mentioned must be properly addressed by risk management and biological testing, significantly increasing time and effort to do so. An interesting technique to avoid these problems is to **embed holographic effects** into the product during the manufacturing. A nano-structure, comparable to those utilized for printing, is engraved into the surface of the device and so creates the hologram. This easily can be integrated into serial production like injection molding or hot stamping and bypasses the regulatory and biological aspects mentioned for holograms attached as label, as no material or

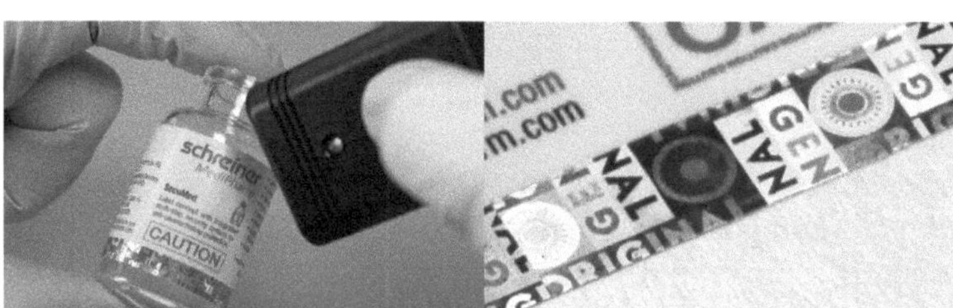

Figure 5.24 Holograms produced by electron-beam lithography allow implementing many features additional to a three-dimensional effect. The left image does display a label intended to prove originality of a pharmaceutical. The right image shows in detail how complex and delicate holograms may be designed. *Images courtesy of Schreiner Group GmbH & Co. KG.*

compound is added. This makes it a very interesting approach for high-volume disposables, such as syringes, as these are driven by cost-reduction where an expensive system for counterfeit protection is not economical. If placed advantageously, the hologram is easy to spot during application and allows an ultimate check upon originality prior to use. Figure 5.25 illustrates a specially treated injection mold for a single-use syringe and the resulting product bearing the embedded hologram.

5.7.2 Surface Structuring

As explained, the integration of a hologram can be done by appropriate surface structuring. However, counterfeit protection may be achieved as well by such a surface structuring that does not produce a hologram but

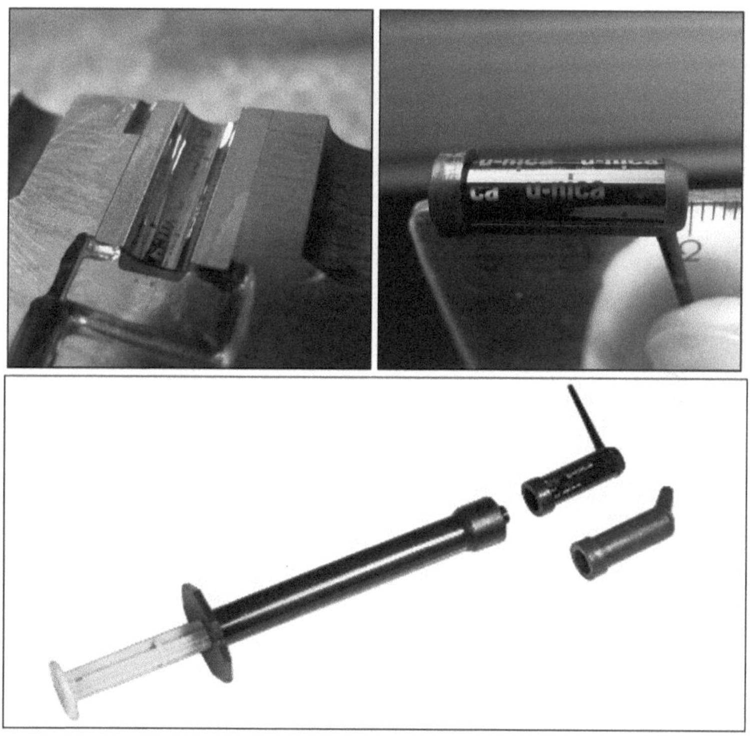

Figure 5.25 Injection mold for a single-use syringe that imparts an embedded hologram directly onto the product during production. As no materials or compounds are added, this approach bypasses many regulatory and biological aspects. It is an interesting technology for high-volume single-use devices and allows an easy ultimate check of originality prior to application. *Pictures of the intraGRAM® system courtesy of U-NICA Solutions AG.*

still is very difficult to copy. Thereby, it would be ideal to have access to a portfolio of patterns that features manifold unique designs while still being easy to access at low costs. An interesting approach to such a portfolio does base on diatoms, which are a major group of algae, and are among the most common types of phytoplankton. Diatoms are usually between 0.1 and 1 mm in size and it is expected that over 100,000 different species do exist. As supporting structure they posses a skeleton that does base on silicon dioxide (or silica) and that is unique to every single species (Figure 5.26). Following the death of a diatom, its ornate silica shell remains as mineral material, still exhibiting its unique nanoscaled structure, as displayed in Figure 5.26. These shells may be either added to a polymer by means of compounding or utilized as agent to produce an imprint into the surface of the plastic pat during injection molding. In order to copy this tagging, it is necessary to know which species was utilized, as well as getting access to its shells. While it is rather easy to find a species with a shell structure never used before, the other way round, finding the appropriate species to a given structure is just alike finding the needle in the haystack. Moreover, silica is a mineral with known high biocompatibility. Consequently diatom shells are within the focus of nanotechnology in general, as well as emerging approaches for nano medicine (see Section 5.4) and drug delivery systems (see Section 6.6).

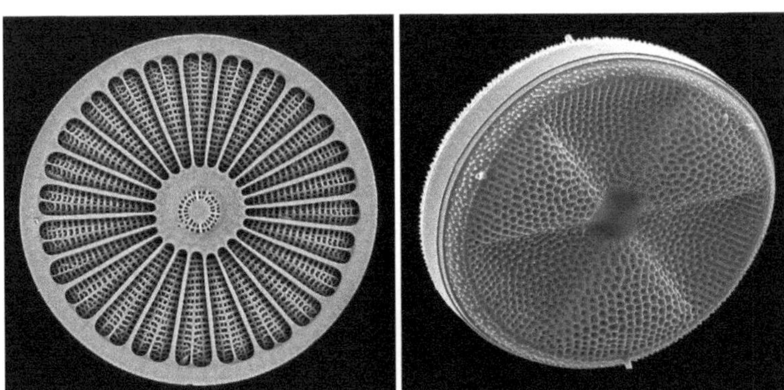

Figure 5.26 SEM picture of Diatoms. These are algae with sizes of 0.1–1 mm that feature supporting structure basing on silicon dioxide (or silica) as shell. It is expected that over 100,000 different species do exist, whereas each does exhibit a unique structure for its ornamented shell. While diatom shells are already within the focus of nanotechnology, these also may serve as unique pattern for counterfeit protection of medical devices. *Images courtesy of Dr Lars Friedrichs, Alfred Wegener Institute, Helmholtz Centre for Polar and Marine Research.*

5.7.3 Radio-Frequency Identification

The technology of radio-frequency identification (RFID) allows wireless transfer of data and found wide application for identifying and tracking of objects. The automobile industry uses this technology to control the flow of goods and as near-field communication or it allows customers to use their smartphone as credit card or electronic wallet. RFID is an integral part of any biometric passport and has emerging use as microchip implant for the identification of animals. Mandatory legal requirements to do so either exist (e.g., Israel, New Zealand, or Ireland) or are in preparation (e.g., England, Germany). Although counterfeit protection is not within the primary scope of RFID, protecting medical devices is feasible. Moreover, this allows providing each product with individual information, making it interesting for the implementation of a unique device identifier (see Section 2.4.5) or as approach to prevent reprocessing of medical devices (see Section 6.1). Still, both applications might be subjected to the regulations of 21 CFR 11 (see Section 2.3.9) if intended for marketing in the US.

Until now, RFID has found broad applications in the health-care industry as well, primarily to online track the flow of supplies as well as to locate personnel and patients within the building, although this may impose issues concerning personal privacy. If already attached to a medical device or a package of pharmaceuticals, it is easy to expand its functionality toward counterfeit protection. The most convenient way to do so is to provide the RFID chip of each medical device, an individual unique license number. As the code is invisible for the naked eye, an additional equipment for decoding is required, that easily may be attached to existing medical devices that run with a desktop computer that additionally is used to verify the code ideally performed online. However, there are some concerns that the electromagnetic radiation necessary for wireless transfer of information may interfere with other electronic medical devices. This may falsify the measurement signals of devices for electrocardiography and so impose health risks. Attaching an RFID chip directly to a medical device features boundary conditions comparable to those for hologram label. It requires additional steps of processing and the combination of plastic device and adhesive for attaching induces complex regulatory aspects. Most commercially available chips will be destroyed by established techniques for sterilization, making RFID unsuitable for direct labeling of medical devices. Most of the problems can be solved by integrating the chip within the medical device. While this easily can be done for complex devices that require assembly, simple ones require more elaborate techniques to do so. An interesting approach is to integrate a chip into injection-molded products already during manufacturing. The integration of solid object is a well-established technique and has wide applications as insert-molding. Chips are available that easily endure the heat and pressure during injection molding. As the RFID chip is entirely concealed by plastic material, the regulatory and biological issues induced by attaching it via an adhesive are bypassed.

5.7.4 Invisible Tagging

Novel approaches utilize techniques to tag a material or product that is not visible by the naked eye, but are detectable with minimal or moderate effort. But why hiding a counterfeit protection? Any known approach to prevent product piracy will trigger efforts to bypass copy protection. A prominent example is illegal programs designed to generate a license key, required to activate a software purchased. So hiding such a feature improves protection, as any attempts to reproduce it requires knowledge about its existence. Anyhow, in case a check upon falsification is desired, the tagging should be easy to decode.

An interesting approach bases on the application of **micro color codes**. These are microscopic particles, 5–45 μm in size, that consist of typically 4–11 layers in different coloring. Current technologies allow about one dozen different hues for each layer, that additionally may be magnetized or exhibit luminescence if exposed to infrared- or ultraviolet light. By additionally varying the thickness and arrangement of each layer, several billion unique codes are feasible. The micro color batch appears to be a white powder to the naked eye and easily may be dusted on surfaces, added to liquids or compounded into polymers. Many established systems utilize melamine–alkyd polymers that exhibit a long-term thermal stability of 200 °C and are resistant to most organic solvents, thinners, acids, and bases. While marking with a micro color code is invisible for the naked eye, the code easily may be discovered with a normal light microscope, and to learn decoding requires only a minimal briefing (Figure 5.27). This allows even laypersons checking on counterfeiting at almost any place. First investigations indicate that melamine–alkyd polymers-based codes are nonhazardous for application in primary or secondary packaging of food or pharmaceuticals. Moreover, as produced with modern printing technologies, these are available at moderate costs. While compounding a micro color batch into the polymer for a medical device probably is critical in terms of regulatory affairs, marking the packaging is well conceivable and gives an interesting approach to prevent counterfeiting.

Instead of polymers, ceramic may be utilized for invisible tracking as well, giving it a heat resistance of up to 2000 °C. This allows to add

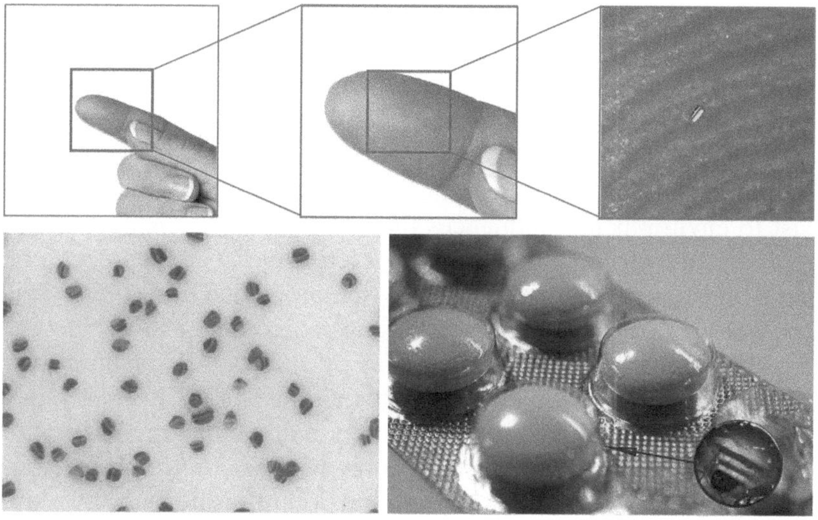

Figure 5.27 Examples of polymer-based micro color codes. While these are invisible for the naked eye, the code easily may be read with a microscope. Some systems were tested and found compliant for application in food and pharmaceutical packaging. *Lower left picture in courtesy of Stealth Mark®, upper row and lower right in courtesy of 3S Simons Security Systems GmbH.*

such systems as compounds to the raw materials, making it an interesting approach for manufacturers of raw materials. Invisible tagging just as well may utilize a unique combination of molecules or elements. This approach, commonly known as **molecular tagging** is even more complicated to counterfeit, but usually requires more elaborate equipment for checking on originality. However, when thinking of a unique code, basing on molecular base, it is easy to get an association with the unique genetic code, every single organism does bear within its DNA.

5.7.5 Artificial DNA

The genetic code of every living organism is encoded in deoxyribonucleic acid (DNA). Although always consisting of the identical basic compounds, it is unique to every individual due to differing sequence of arrangement. This way DNA profiling is a well-established forensic technology to identify individuals. Modern methods of biotechnology allow comparing DNA to existing samples in short time and at moderate costs. By providing an object, a comparable "genetic code," therefore, is an interesting approach for counterfeit protection.

From a chemical view, **artificial DNA** does not differ from its real counterpart, as it consists of the identical compounds. However, it does not contain the information required to create a living organism. It simply serves as a series of unique combinations of A (adenine), C (cytosine), G (guanine), and T (thymine), as illustrated in Figure 5.28. For protection of an object, a short-chain of artificial DNA synthesized, making it more robust to environmental influences than human DNA. This genetic code is reproduced and subsequently used for tagging. This approach comes along with many advantages for counterfeit protection of medical devices. As it is part of the human body, it has no toxic effect and is biocompatible without restrictions. Adherence of nonviable DNA is plain sailing for most medical devices, and uncritical for those used for gene analysis, due to the artificial nature that does not accord to any living organism. It easily may be applied as gel, grease, or spray whereas UV luminescent may be added to facilitate detection. Reproduction of artificial DNA requires either knowledge about the precise code (arrangement of amino acids) or an existing sample. Anyhow, both approaches require complex machinery

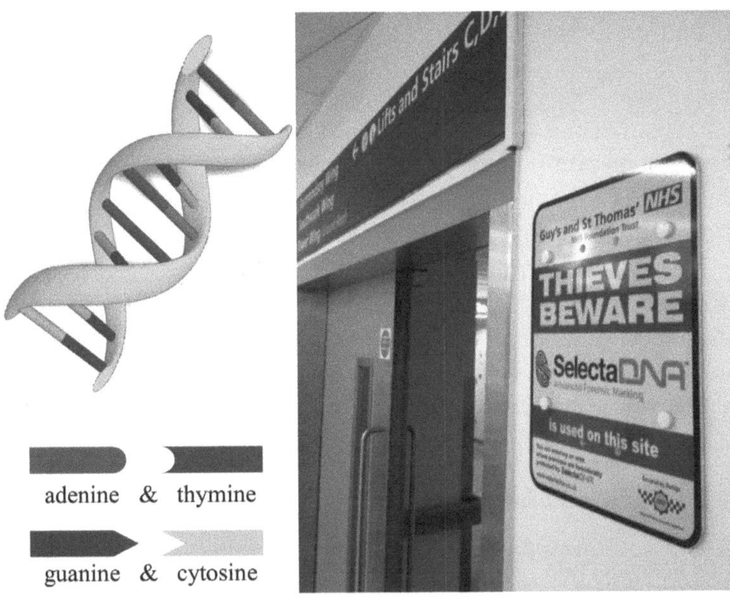

Figure 5.28 The DNA of every single living organism is unique, although consisting of an arrangement of two basic pairs of amino acids. An artificially created DNA sequence does not contain the information relevant for the creation of life, but is suitable to provide any object or group of them with a unique encoded number. *Images on the right courtesy of SelectaDNA™.*

and thorough knowledge about genetics, presenting a considerate hurdle. For checking upon originality, a sample is taken and analyzed by means of DNA profiling. In consequence, this approach is less suitable for products that frequently need control of counterfeit.

Beyond counterfeit protection, artificial DNA is successfully used as theft protection. This tagging may be applied to many objects easy and at moderate costs, while removal is rather difficult as even miniscule remains are sufficient for DNA profiling. Many railway and telecommunication companies in Europe use this method to protect their infrastructure, as copper is an object of increasing interest for metal thefts. But also many companies operating hospitals, such as the Ealing Hospital NHS Trust as part of the British Public Health System, started to use it as general protection against theft of valuable goods (see Figure 5.28).

5.7.6 General Considerations

Selecting the appropriate technology for counterfeit protection sometimes is anything but easy, as several aspects should be considered. First of all, it is important to bear in mind, that any approach to counterfeit is anything but impossible to copy. It rather is a question of time, money, and knowledge upon the protection to find ways to falsify it. Just think about banknotes that are over subject to falsification at almost the same since their first application, although the efforts of protection consistently are extended. Within this race between those, seeking to protect their established market shares and good reputation, and those, trying to illegally benefit both, it is crucial to have an appropriate advantage in time and technology.

An **apparent visible** security label comes along with many advantages. It does create confidence among the end user and allows to perform a final check on authenticity prior application. However, if such an apparent visible label is falsified in a sufficient quality, this advantage is reversed. A solution might be to increase its complexity in order to improve the protective effect. But in turn, this frequently does induce significant cost increase and may complicate checking on authenticity or, as you may say, decoding. Moreover, if decoding does require any special equipment or training, it is very difficult to implement multiple checkpoints during the global travel of goods. Anyhow, a security label as complex to copy as possible that still may be screened even by an untrained layperson frequently is the ideal for medical devices. That way, the applying end consumer, regardless if patient or medical professional, may perform a final check on authenticity prior application.

When utilizing **invisible tagging**, it requires knowledge upon its existence and composition for counterfeiting. This may give a time advantage for protecting products, as it presumably will take longer until first falsification will appear. And even if these appear, the style of invisible tagging could be altered, once more giving time until the product pirates get aware of this fact. Still, if checking on authenticity should take place rather frequently, decoding an invisible tagging ideally should not require elaborate equipment. Systems, such as micro color codes or molecular tagging, appear to be ideal e.g., for the protection of raw materials, such as plastic resin, or medical devices in big boxes for shipping.

Counterfeit protection technologies could be seen as part of an even bigger picture. It is the whole picture of ensuring the correct application of a medical device according to the intended use. Counterfeit protection helps to provide the correct medical device for the actual intended use. This may be seen with the establishing of UDI numbers (see Section 2.4.5). A combination of counterfeit protection technologies, which is accompanied by UDI numbers, and technologies, which may prevent reprocessing of intended single-use devices (see Section 6.1), may be helpful to ensure the correct medical device for future patients even in a dark world of counterfeit or intentional misuse. This might be triggered by the pressure to cut costs. However, this should be prevented by technologies as far as possible, simply for the patient's sake.

6 Emerging Trends

OUTLINE

There is no exception, every branch, industrial field or business model, is hunting the next emerging trends, sometimes even though there is no actual need for it. This effect can be transferred to the plastic and medical device world as well. Some phenomena may occur just due to the fact they are trendy currently. In regard to plastic medical devices, the major trends are not driven by the public opinion. These public-driven appearances are usually part of some sort of campaign based on ideology. Typical topics are bisphenol-A free materials, polyvinylchloride free devices, or plastic materials in general as harmful to the environment. Interestingly, most of these public-driven trends are following some sort of cycle: becoming public and disappearing regularly without major changes. That should not be interpreted as a general negation of public-driven trends within plastic medical devices. There are surely some trends not coming from the plastic device industry, which should have, like reduction of waste. But, most

Emerging Trends in Medical Plastic Engineering and Manufacturing
http://dx.doi.org/10.1016/B978-0-323-37023-3.00006-3

emerging trends for future plastic medical devices are generated within research groups, industrial R & D departments, and during application. Just to make it clear, not every nice looking idea will be an actual trend. Based on our experience in the plastic medical device world in specific and the whole engineering world in general, we have chosen some interesting approaches, which have already left the point of an idea and are investigated heavily, but also show some potential to be implemented actually. The trends are mainly driven by general aspects of higher integration level of technologies, but also between engineers, medical professionals, and patients. This can be seen in the emerging trend of preventing the reprocessing of medical devices, simple due to the fact of safety or also economic reasons, but as well in topics like lap-on-a-chip devices, in vitro diagnostics (IVDs), or drug-delivery devices. Besides, more material-based trends like biopolymers, we are getting into the aspect of health-related wearables, which might be a relatively small field currently, but might be a major tool to increase the general health of societies in the future. This is based on the understanding of catching deriving illnesses as soon as possible and increasing the interaction level between patients, medical professionals, and also engineers more. Nevertheless, these are topics, where nobody can leave the medical plastics technologies out of the game. In comparison to metals or ceramics, the costs are acceptable and, the more technological point of view, fully integrated manufacturing processes are and will be available. Think about the topics of sensor integration within clothes; without plastic technologies these ideas would be unlikely to be realizable.

6.1 Preventing Reprocessing of Medical Devices

While counterfeiting medical devices is illegal, reprocessing is in accordance to general laws and regulations. However, both usually are not in the interest of medical device manufacturers and solutions to fight product piracy may be suitable to prevent reprocessing as well, thus generating synergies for simultaneous actions against these two aspects. Therefore, the approaches presented in this chapter are closely linked to the previous chapter and vice versa.

6.1.1 Reusable Medical Devices

The reuse of medical devices is very common. Elaborate devices such as surgical instruments are expensive in purchase and thus typically utilized revealingly, therefore, commonly known as reusable. This does require a step of reprocessing after each use, essential to thoroughly remove biological remains sticking to it, such as blood, proteins, body liquids, pyrogens, and of course germs. While purifying a simple shaped device, such as a surgical blade or retractor, may be executed rather simply, cleaning a complex built device like an endoscope with its long tubular structures is rather challenging. Where needed, the device will be sterilized and packaged, making it available sterile for the next application. Any step of reprocessing and sterilization must be validated (see Section 2.3.8) and is heavily regulated by the respective competent authorities. This poses significant financial and personal burdens to hospitals, doctors, or dental practices that intensively utilize reusable. Industry does address this issue by designing single-use devices (SUDs) that are intended to bypass a reuse, thus eliminating any risk of deficient in-house reprocessing. Modern technologies of mass production like injection molding enable to produce high volumes at comparatively low costs, which allow selling prices undercutting the costs for reprocessing. Today technological advances allow designing more elaborate SUDs and so even video endoscopes that are partial or entirely single-use are available in the markets.

In the early 1990s, during the peak of bovine spongiform encephalopathy (BSE), the animal disease affecting primarily cattle, and thus commonly known as mad cow disease, the practice risk of reusables was discussed intensely. At that specific time, the precise method of infection was unknown, and there were doubts if established processes for cleaning and reprocessing are sufficient to prevent infection. As Great Britain was seriously affected by BSE, this problem leads to dramatic decision. Many hospitals completely stopped reprocessing and started to utilize SUDs only. This generated a considerable business and fueled the development of devices that, although complex in design, were intended for single use.

6.1.2 Reprocessing of SUDs

Some companies make business with reprocessing of medical devices that were initially designed and produced by the original manufacturer for single use only. Even high-risk devices like intracardiac (inside the heart) catheters that are intended for disposal after application, may be collected, reprocessed, and sold again. Thereby, the original manufacturer has no legal options to take influence on this business. Although this may sound close to fraudulent, this approach is approved by many competent authorities, including the FDA[1], and thus completely legal in many places. Still, reprocessing is subject to vigorous discussions, with supporters highlighting possible cost savings and environmental issues, while opponents emphasize health risks caused by possible device failure or faulty reprocessing. Moreover, reprocessing an SUD may lead to complicate legal entities. If such a device does malfunction during application, who is responsible: the original manufacturer or the company that performed reprocessing? While the US does market exhibit precise regulations for reprocessing of SUDs, Europe still has country-specific regulations for this aspect. This shortfall is addressed by the planned amendment to the EU Medical Device Directive (see 2.4.4), as it will increase the responsibility for companies that perform reprocessing. Considering this and other current developments in many regulatory entities, it is well expectable that reprocessing will remain an established element to the medical device world.

6.1.3 Preventing SUD Reprocessing

Although some medical device companies do business with reprocessing of SUDs, the majority distance themselves from this practice. This may be triggered by loss of business, the risk of legal issues, or simply the business model. The most common approach to avoid reprocessing is the device **selling-price**. Modern technologies of mass production enable to produce at unit costs so low, that reprocessing is no longer competitive, but this will not work for more complex and thus in consequence more expensive devices. However, reprocessing may be hampered or prevented by means of device design or packing.

Complex electronic medical devices, such as ultrasonic scanners or laser systems for cosmetic treatments, frequently come along with an additional protective SUD. It is intended to safeguard fragile machinery parts (sensors or lenses), to facilitate cleaning (no direct contact from patient to machinery) and to easily provide appropriate hygienic conditions (single use only). Simple designed versions are protective caps (like those for a pen), e.g., a cover mounted on the sensor of a clinical thermometer, before used on the patient. Others are more complex in design and challenging in manufacturing. As prominent example may serve transparent caps, as these are used during laser treatment of the eye to ease ametropia. The covers are mounted on the laser first and subsequently used to adhere the eyeball, necessary to secure and flatten it during the treatment. To assure

1. Although it would be legally possible, up to date (2015) no company was seeking FDA approval for a reprocessed Class III SUD (e.g., an intracardiac catheter).

appropriate results, these devices are subjected to very high requirements in terms of optical quality and dimensional stability, although intended for single use only. Falsifications of minor optical quality are hard to detect without elaborate optical measurement equipment, but may lead to disastrous results of treatment. An emerging approach to prevent counterfeit is to provide every medical device with a **license** just alike you know it from computer software. The number is printed on the packaging or the device as plain text (readable to the human) or as normal or matrix barcode (readable to machine), requiring an adequate scanner. The license enables to unlock the device system online and the desired treatment can be performed. It seems reasonable to combine a license printed on the device with the UDI—number (see Section 2.4.5) that will be mandatory in near future. A matrix code could combine all information required and easily may be integrated into almost any enterprise resource system. But you should consider that by doing so, the label will be subjected to 21 CFR part 11 (see Section 2.3.9). Additionally an approach based on licenses allows new business models. The expensive machinery for medical treatment may be sold at cost, and profit is generated through selling the auxiliary device.

Other approaches to complicate reprocessing usually remain secret, and there are good reasons to do so. As mentioned, close to all relevant authorities generally allow or even promote reprocessing, as this is an appropriate measure to reduce health-care costs. So when seeking approval for a new medical device, the respective company is asked to state its reasons, why the device is intended for single use only. It is a common misbelief that it is the competent authorities decision whether to classify a device as SUD or not, but in fact this must be done by the manufacturer, as only he has the relevant expertise. However, many competent authorities are aware that from an economical point of view, some companies might have a tendency to generously judge in favor of marketing a medical device as SUD. To avoid this conflict of interests, measures to prevent reprocessing may be taken by **means of device design** including process of manufacturing. And all of them should be triggered rather by attempts to reduce legal liability or to improve functionality than by ogling to prevent reprocessing of a device, which in fact easily could be reused. Those attempts e.g., may include specific materials that required special methods for cleaning or sterilization. To give an example, a plastic SUD is manufactured from a polymer that is not suitable to all commonly established methods of cleaning or sterilization (see Section 5.1). Any attempt of reprocessing must fail, as no applicable method of doing so is available. Or the device may be designed in a way that during its application an irreversible mechanism is activated. You know this from soft drink bottles, where a plastic ring breaks

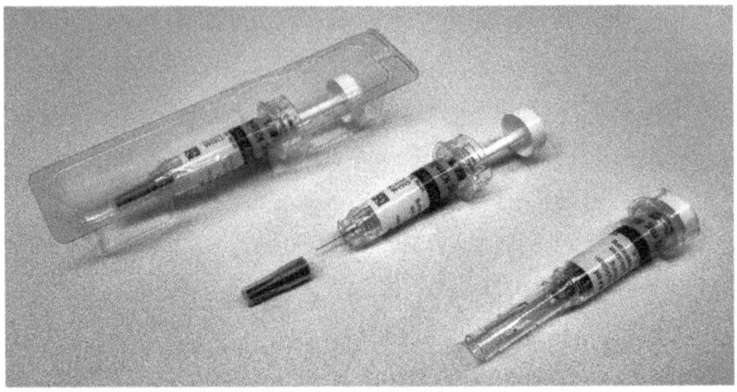

Figure 6.1 Prefilled syringe, intended for home application of subdermal injections, on the left in sterile packaging and in the middle ready to use. A mechanism does eject a protective cap covering the needle after removing it from the skin, in order to prevent needle-stick injuries. As sidekick, the same mechanism does prevent reprocessing effectively, as reversing only is possible destructive.

when opening for the first time. A good example for this approach is prefilled syringes intended for subdermal injections performed by patients at home (Figure 6.1). Many of those systems feature a mechanism that does eject a protective cap covering the needle after removing it from the skin, in order to prevent needle-stick injuries. Moreover, statutory provisions in most countries require that used medical needles must be disposed as biological hazardous waste, unless appropriate measures are taken such as the protective cap, to prevent injuries caused by the needles. Thus in fact, it is only these protection mechanisms that allow an application at home. Meantime, reprocessing of such a device usually is not possible, as the ejection of the cap only may be reversed destructive. As you see, implementing features only to prevent any reprocessing may induce issues during device approval, anyhow, when these come along as sidekick from other features, the implementation seldom will be questioned.

6.2 IVD Medical Devices

In many regards, IVD medical devices may be seen as products that utilize techniques derived from biomedical engineering, (bio)-chemistry, (molecular) biology, and pharmacology—and this unique blend often leads to some confusion. The main reason for this comes from the general understanding that biochemistry, just like pharmaceuticals, is a subset of chemistry, and thus does exhibit primarily a chemical mode of action, while a medical device is generally physical in mode of action. Any device combining both modes of action usually is considered a combination product (see Section 2.7.2), like many drug-delivery systems (see Section 6.6) or prefilled syringes (see Figure 6.1) and still is not to be confused with an IVD. A meaningful definition for IVD medical devices was developed by the GHTF (now IMDRF) that states:

> In Vitro Diagnostic (IVD) medical device means a medical device, whether used alone or in combination, intended by the manufacturer for the in-vitro examination of specimens derived from the human body **solely** or **principally** to provide information for diagnostic, monitoring or compatibility purposes.

And from this definition you may derive two aspects that are of greater importance within the context of this book. First, as intended for an in vitro examination (for the precise meaning, refer Section 2.7.3) that by definition does involve some sort of chemical reaction, the product generally does contain chemical compounds, regardless if as dried powder, pellets liquids, or comparable. This clearly separates them from classical medical devices. Second, an IVD is not intended for direct treatment of the patient, like a defibrillator, releasing electric energy (physical in nature), or a pharmaceutical, influencing the patients metabolism (chemical in nature). **IVDs** are utilized **to detect, diagnose, or monitor a disease** and its process, and subsequently determine the appropriate course of treatment, thus, indirectly influencing the patient. But this shall not mean that failure of an IVD is less dangerous than if occurring with a classical medical device or a pharmaceutical. Moreover, within our modern healthcare system IVDs play a role as important as pharmaceuticals or classical medical devices, and this already for several decades. For many applications, as some of these are explained in Sections 2.7.3 and 5.6.3, modern medicine was not imaginable without IVDs. Nevertheless, for long time IVDs were available as rather simple designed test kits or strips for equally simple formulations of questions. As a prominent example you may take the test strip utilized in combination with a glucometer for measurement of the blood sugar level, as displayed in Figure 5.18. Anyhow, the last decade has seen an impressive development in complexity of IVDs and so currently systems are available that have a considerable potential to improve the outcome of therapies while reducing the associated costs. These developments were addressed by many competent authorities that currently developed or recently issued refined regulations for IVDs (see Sections 2.4.4 and 2.7.3). The following section will give you an example of such a novel approach for IVDs that in comparable approaches currently is brought to market by several companies.

An emerging problem for the treatment of patients, especially at intensive care units, is bacteria that are resistant to many or even all available antibiotics. The aspect of **antibiotic resistance (ABR)** bacteria significantly contributes to the issue of **health-associated infections**, a problem that almost equally affects industrialized just alike third world countries (see Section 5.3). To get closer to this issue, we now will give you an example for an ABR-induced critical health condition that can be treated significantly better when using novel IVDs. A patient, postoperatively treated in an intensive care unit and kept in artificial coma for several days, suddenly develops a severe pneumonia, an event unfortunately not too infrequently. As a **standard therapy**, a specimen of sputum is harvested and sent to a microbiology laboratory in order to determine the type of bacteria and to check on possible ABR. Usually this is done basing on polymerase chain reaction (PCR), the well-established technique for analysis of gene sequences. Anyhow, in its classical way, this analysis requires a well-equipped laboratory that many medium- or small-sized hospitals cannot afford, and so analysis frequently is performed outhouse. In this case, it may take several hours or even days until the analysis result is available. Meantime, without information to find a better therapy, the patient will be treated with a broad-spectrum antibiotic, presenting a heavy burden to the organism's metabolism that even may be without effect if the patient suffers from antibiotic-resistant germs. This therapeutic blind flight could be shortened significantly, or even totally avoided, by having the opportunity to perform the PCR analysis directly at the intensive care unit as **novel therapy**. And the microbiological analysis of PCR is ideal for automation within an IVD system. Consequently, there are several such systems that currently are brought to market and either are subject to, or even were granted approval by competent authorities for the respective markets. And the benefits are considerate. The time from harvesting the biological sample (sputum in case of pneumonia) is reduced significantly down to a period of just a few hours. This in turn allows to find a more appropriate treatment that consequently helps to ameliorate its outcome while simultaneously reducing its costs. Moreover, as the systems are designed to run fully automatically, a basic training is sufficient for operation, which hence may be performed by the treating professional medics. Thereby modern systems, like the one displayed in Figure 6.2, allow to perform PCR-based analysis on manifold aspects on microbiology. For every respective question, a cartridge is available that contains the required chemicals and only the specimen for analysis must be added. Thereby the system presented exemplarily, features a color-based encoding for the analysis desired, further simplifying its application.

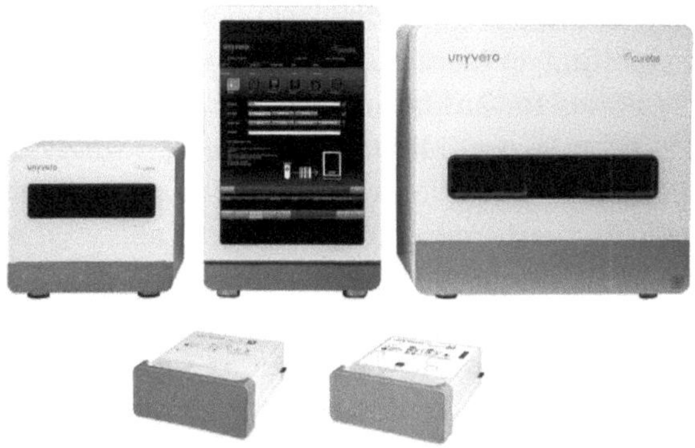

Figure 6.2 In vitro diagnostics already have a widespread application for rather simple medical tests, like those presented in Figure 2.7. Anyhow, modern systems allow to perform fully automated much more complex laboratory analysis. The system displayed enables to conduct a polymerase chain reaction analysis on a desktop, e.g., to check on the presence of specific bacteria or antibiotics resistance, on site of an intensive care unit, instead of analyzing the sample in a microbiology laboratory. This does save time and costs, while increasing the outcome of treatment. The system presented does consist of an electronic device as user interface and evaluation unit (reusable), combined with a single-use cartridge containing the chemicals required for the respective analysis, and used for one single analysis. The color of the cartridge does encode the specific type of analysis and that way allows to easily select the desired system. *Image courtesy of Curetis AG.*

The example of **fully automated PCR desktop-analysis** does depict the most likely development of IVD systems. More and more complex microbiological analyses will be transferred into IVDs that are easier to operate at the same time. Thereby the systems presumably will always consist of a console, containing the user interface and electronics for operating and thus representing a reusable, combined with a test kit or cartridge, encasing the chemicals and fluidic components, intended for single use only. Especially for the single-use portion, techniques for mass production such as injection molding are of greater interest, which is why it may be expected that companies making business with biotechnology and IVDs will gain importance as customers for plastic converters. Anyhow, it clearly should be said that the actual complexity of these systems is to be found in the formulation of the biochemical reaction and the production of the required compounds. In comparison, the plastic and automation components required remain simpler in design. Nevertheless, as consequence to the general trend of miniaturization (see Section 5.5), the IVD systems may be expected to get smaller while exhibiting an increased amount of functionalities. In parallel, the trend clearly points toward an increasing content of electronics within the disposable part, an aspect already presented as **single-use electronics** within the Section 5.6.2. However, when thinking about a miniaturized laboratory, automatically performing a biochemical analysis, still featuring a considerate amount of electronics and sensors, but that still is intended for single use only, you are very close to a discipline of engineering known as **lab-on-a-chip** (LOC) devices. Anyhow, from a scientific point of view, the differences of IVDs and LOC devices is subtle, and so both presumably will see a merger within the next years.

6.3 LOC Devices

The overarching goal of LOC devices is to integrate one or more laboratory functions into a chip only a few square centimeters or even millimeters in size. From a medical device point of view, these laboratory functions are IVD analyses (see Section 6.2), and thus LOCs can be considered as a miniaturized version of IVDs. However, within the medical device world and especially among medical professionals, there still are some misunderstandings, as the roots of LOCs trace back in very different scientific fields. Their modern times origin probably may be traced back to the development of integrated circuits in general and inject printers in particular, as these devices required technologies for micro- and nanomanufacturing and the ability to handle extremely small volumes of liquids respectively, which in turn evolved into a discipline called **microfluidics**. LOC devices are closely linked to, and sometimes overlap with, microfluidics, which describes primarily the physics, the manipulation, and study of minute amounts of fluids. However, although LOC does refer to the miniaturization of the laboratory functionality to chip size, this not necessarily involves the utilization of microfluidics, although this is done frequently. Basing on the technical origin of LOCs, they make a subset of **microelectromechanical systems** and, to underline their all-embracing approach, sometimes are referred to as **micro total analysis systems (μTAS)**.

As mentioned, LOC devices may be seen as miniaturized IVDs and in consequence are not really new. Among others, some of their specific advantages contributed to their widespread application, while funnily many operators are not really aware of technically seen utilizing an LOC device, as you soon will see by a prominent example. The probably most striking advantage is their relatively low manufacturing price. The last decades have seen exploding possibilities in micro manufacturing technologies (such as microinjection), including molding and plating, wet and dry etching, and electro discharge machining. A very heavy impact of these developments may be seen in the rapid miniaturization of integrated circuits that lead to a considerate increase in commuting power. All these allow to produce **complex micro- or nanofluidic systems** that exhibit integrated electronics and sensors (see Section 5.6.2) at prices that are reasonable for application as SUDs. Moreover, utilizing microfluidics comes along with more advantages. The required chemical compounds often are rather high in price. Especially if the chemical reaction does base on an antigen–antibody reaction, the crucially required compounds, produced by biotechnology companies, exhibit prices easily exceeding those of precious metals. Microfluidics require only **minimal amounts of** these **chemicals**, and thus may balance their purchasing price. Moreover, for analysis only a **sample minimal in volume** is required. This is from great benefit for analyses where the sample is challenging to harvest or the amount collected correlates with the pain induced to the patient. A good example for this is the test strip, combined with a glucometer, utilized to determine the blood sugar level (see Section 5.6.3 and Figure 5.18). These strips feature a microfluidic system intended to transport the blood sample by means of capillary forces (no actuator required). As a minimal amount of blood is sufficient, a smaller lancet may be used to harvest the sample, which in turn leads to less pain when performing the finger prick (see Figure 5.18). The test strip does perform an in vitro analysis on minimal space, virtually making the entire system an LOC device.

Nevertheless, it is not to be expected that in future all IVDs will be replaced by LOC devices for several reasons. First, many IVDs do and will not require any electronics, like those displayed in Figure 2.7. And for many that exhibit complex electronic systems like the one presented in Figure 6.2, miniaturization on LOC level is not beneficiary as this maybe even would hinder the application. Within the surrounding of an intensive care unit, an IVD the size of a SIM-card or small coin is anything than workable. LOCs rather are likely to conquer those areas of application where conventional IVDs fail due to their dimensions, required infrastructure (such as distribution networks, possibilities for refrigeration, operator training) and price, as this may be found for application in field. Hence, currently many LOC devices are developed or even already applied for the **detection of diseases in third world countries**. These underdeveloped regions frequently face a rudimentary health-care system combined with a lack of funding, while simultaneously impacted by plagues such as malaria, hepatitis, AIDS, or Ebola. A meaningful approach to handle these problems is LOC devices intended to diagnose these diseases. As mentioned in Sections 5.6.3 and 6.7, an enormous positive impact on these developments comes from our smartphone era. With these electronic devices, that already found widespread distribution even in underdeveloped countries, elaborate and largely standardized computing platforms are available almost anywhere and anytime. Consequently, many LOC devices for third world countries utilize smartphones as user interface and evaluation unit. The benefit for public health in underdeveloped countries is obvious. Moreover, these developments are very likely to positively turn back on first world countries. As mentioned, the functionality of IVDs and LOC devices primarily does rely on the chemical reaction and its respective compounds. Consequently, these devices may be modified at moderate effort to detect diseases that affect the public health in industrialized countries. But why should this be done by low-cost LOC devices instead of examination by a professional medic? Actually, it should not be done instead but rather in addition to the established health-care systems. Low-cost LOC systems allow to expand the coverage of preventive medical checkups significantly without exploding costs, giving additional benefits. Some diseases are associated with a social stigma, such as drug abuse, colorectal cancer, hepatitis, or AIDS. Although knowing better, the affected people avoid examination by a professional surgeon, although any delay in treatment significantly does reduce the chance for curing. Easy and anonymous to access LOC devices allow to **check on social stigmatized diseases** and thus may contribute to better and faster treatment of diseases of an affluent society. This may sound futuristic to you. Actually street side-mounted self-vending machines already may be found that sell IVD or LOC test kits respectively intended for a self-check on drug abuse or colorectal cancer, as displayed in Figure 6.3.

An other emerging technology for LOC devices, more closely related to the manufacturing of medical devices, is systems intended to check products on the presence of bacteria or remains of them. As explained in Sections 2.3.2 and 2.3.3, many medical devices must be analyzed for pyrogens sticking to the device. The established approach does base harvested from the Atlantic horseshoe crab, an endangered sea dweller. Currently test methods are developed, such as the **monocyte activation test**, that allow to perform tests on pyrogens without impact on biodiversity, and as state of the art, these are likely to be integrated into LOC devices. This would allow to perform this type of quality control closer to the production line and more frequently at moderate additional costs.

The development of more refined technologies for micro manufacturing of LOC devices presumably will further fuel these developments. As example may serve approaches to **print entire LOC systems** with inkjet technology, as displayed in Figure 6.4. This approach allows to

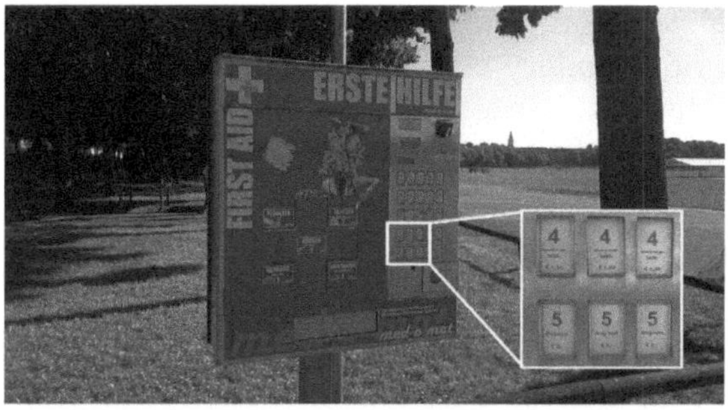

Figure 6.3 Low-cost lab-on-a-chip devices presumably will gain importance for diagnosis of check on social stigmatized diseases, such as on drug abuse or colorectal cancer. Public accessible self-vending machines, like the one displayed, enable to perform an anonymous self-check on these diseases and thus contribute to the public health by expanding the coverage of preventive medical checks. The machine is located at the entrance to the world famous Oktoberfest (beer festival) in Munich, Bavaria. *Image courtesy of Hans Peter Enis.*

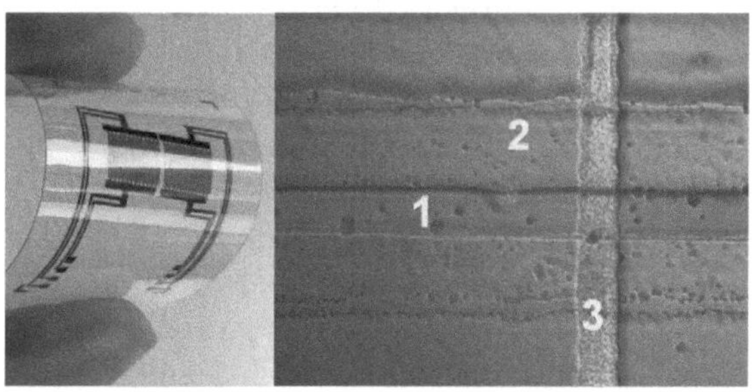

Figure 6.4 Novel technologies enable to produce lab-on-a-chip (LOC) devices, like the one displayed on the left, by printing basing on inkjet technology. Thereby, entire circuits may be manufactured that way within one single manufacturing process, as displayed in detail on the left. On a foil serving as carrier, a conducting wire (1) is covered by an insulation (2) whereas both eventually are crossed by another conducting wire (3), all manufactured by printing. Approaches like this allow to produce small batches or even individualized LOCs still at reasonable prices. *Images courtesy of Prof. Dr Bernhard Wolf, Heinz Nixdorf-Lehrstuhl für Medizinische Elektronik der TU München.*

produce small batches or even individualized designs for LOCs still at moderate costs. From a technological point of view, this development is highly comparable to the emerging field of generative manufacturing technologies, which is covered in Chapter 4. This may be seen as an example of technological coevolution, indicating that comparable combinations of boundary conditions and problems frequently lead to comparable solutions.

6.4 Thermoplastic Elastomer the Better Elastomer?

Many plastic medical devices combine several different materials to implement the desired functionalities. Thereby frequently hard and soft (elastic) materials are combined. Prominent example is a manual toothbrush, where the shaft features soft section for improved grip and use that is more convenient. Do not get confused, a manual toothbrush is classified as medical device (Class I) within many countries, including the US[2]. But many more medical devices for clinical application feature hard–soft combinations, such as respiratory masks, precision syringes, or any device very (re-)sealing is required, whereas two materials are applied for long time.

Natural rubber is a natural product harvested from the Pará rubber tree that is indigenous to South America. Native Indians have been using it as elastomeric material for a time long prior Europeans discovered this material. Anyhow, as natural rubber is thermoplastic in nature, it becomes rather rigid when cold, and very sticky and soft when warmed. In result, first products made from natural rubber, such as ponchos or rubber boots, totally failed in business. This was until Charles Goodyear discovered the process of vulcanization in 1839, that this material became successful and soon developed to a widely traded commodity and important material. It soon found application in chemical and pharmaceutical industry and subsequent application in medical devices. As cut from supply lines during World War II, German chemists developed a synthetic rubber as substitute material for tires. Basic element is **styrene–butadiene rubber** that since then consistently was evolved, creating a huge family of synthetic rubbers. The paramount medical application for rubber (natural as well as synthetic) beyond gloves is as plug in perforable ampoules (see Figure 2.6) or precision syringes. It does exhibit an excellent biocompatibility and features negligible interaction with close to any medicinal fluids, chemicals, and pharmaceuticals. Anyhow, as fine-dispersed particles within the body,

2. However, it is worth mentioning although classified as medical device by the FDA, a nonsterile toothbrush is exempt from most still not every single regulation for medical devices.

it shows a strong tendency to provoke fever. Further, a few number of global companies share the world market for medical natural rubber plugs, making it sometimes difficult to find appropriate pricing. Further, processing of an elastomeric duromer requires technical infrastructure that significantly differs from that for processing of thermoplasts. This did trigger the development of alternative materials that, while exhibiting comparable properties, allow easy processing. Prominent candidates are thermoplastic elastomers (TPEs), which will be presented further down this Chapter. It is worth mentioning that latex is not a synonym for natural rubber. Latex rather refers to a super group of natural elastomeric materials, whereas natural rubber (or caoutchouc) is the most prominent representative. Other sources for latex may be among others opium poppy, common dandelion, or rubber tree.

In comparison, **silicone** materials are always man-made. These are synthetic compounds made from repeating units of siloxane, a chemical compound with its characteristic the Si–O–Si linkage. They are rubber-like, very heat-resistant and inert to many aggressive chemicals. Striking is the large scale of available softness, ranging from jelly-like to almost rigid, their long-term stable and exquisite elasticity as well as considerate chemical inertness. They are available in many modifications such as oil, greace, rubber, or resin, and hence utilized in widespread applications, e.g., for sealing, lubrication, electrical insulation, or adhesion. A frequent application is thermal-resistant cooking utensils. Silicone oil does exhibit a very good biocompatibility, resistant to most disinfectants and well suited for repeated sterilization with hot steam, making it a very interesting material for medical devices. Standard applications are such as tubes, catheters, respiratory masks, anesthesia bags, and long-term implants. While small amounts of silicone oil within the body are harmless, greater amounts will provoke an inflammatory reaction called silicone-induced granuloma (siliconoma). This is why leaking of silicone oil-filled aesthetic implants will induce severe health conditions. Processing of silicone requires a process of curing that generates considerate amounts of heat. While this may be handled with moderate effort in extrusion, processing by injection molding, and then called **injection molding of liquid silicone rubber**, requires especially adapted equipment. In consequence, it is expensive compared to classical thermoplastic plastic processing. Anyhow, due to its superior material properties, many applications are not feasible with other materials than silicone. Thereby LSR enables to produce very complex geometries. Especially for devices that require high elasticity and that frequently are sterilized, no substitute materials are currently foreseeable. Prominent examples are respiratory masks and anesthetic bags.

As explained, major disadvantage of silicone and natural rubber is the comparable high prices due to elaborate technical infrastructure required for processing. An interesting alternative is TPEs, sometimes also called thermoplastic rubber. These are synthesized from a classical thermoplastic polymer and a synthetic elastomer, either by copolymerization or by physical mix. The major groups of TPEs available do on base styrene–butadiene copolymers (TPE-S), polyolefins (TPE-O), cross-linked elastomers basing on polyolefins (TPE-V), thermoplastic polyurethanes (TPE-U), or polyamides (TPE-A). But the precise formula of a TPE may be ways more confusing as the five groups mentioned frequently are combined during polymerization or subsequent compounding. In result, a wide range of those materials is available, and thus for many applications a candidate does exist that is suitable to replace rubber or silicone. Doing so comes along with some advantages. TPEs in close to any cases are cheaper and have a significantly longer shelf life than silicone. They may be processed with the identical equipment as classical thermoplastic and so additional costs for machinery or training of staff is not necessary compared to silicone. As no curing is necessary, processing may be performed in shorter time and differing from silicone hot runner or classical cold runner systems (short sprue) may be utilized, resulting in less material consumption. From a technical view, TPEs easily may be reprocessed due to their thermoplastic nature, this rarely is done for medical devices due to aspects of regulations and liability. Anyhow, utilization of TPEs involves some disadvantages as well. When very soft or jelly-like structures are required, suitable TPE materials often are not available. Due to their chemical and physical nature, a minimal content of rigid thermoplastic polymer is required. Further, TPEs become softer when heated, different from silicone that features identical flexibility over a wide range of temperatures. Most types face an alteration in material properties when sterilized with radiation, an aspect that may be problematic for sterile, low-price SUDs, but could be resolved by autosterile manufacturing (see Section 5.3). Currently no thermoplastic elastomer is available that withstand repeated sterilization with hot steam and resistance to aggressive chemicals and disinfectants may be an issue. Moreover, flexibility may change over product cycle and, compared to silicone, the material will rupture at lower deformation rates and does exhibit a tendency to creep when heavily loaded for a longer time. Therefore, TPE is not an adequate substitute for silicone in medical devices with challenging applications that combine reprocessing for reuse, long life cycle, and high deformation rates. A good example once more is an anesthetic bag. Anyhow, for many SUDs, silicone successfully was replaced by TPE. Currently the standard material for an atraumatic tip of a catheter for coronary intervention is TPE-A. Currently many manufacturers of syringes are about to replace the synthetic rubber plugs with ones basing on TPE. This will have significant impact on the world market and trigger the development of medical grade materials. This in turn will generate more trust in its application and lead to more medical devices where silicone is replaced, e.g., where (re-)sealing functionality is required.

6.5 Emerging Biopolymer Materials

The vast majority of polymers are based on crude oil and synthesized by inorganic chemical reactions. Triggered by peak oil, all polymer-related industries are seeking new sustainable sources for polymer. Promising approaches already found application in plastics based on organic precursors such as rapeseed oil or starch. Contrary to most oil-based ones, these usually are compostable and thus considered as less harmful to the environment. Comparable efforts pullulate in the world of medical devices, hence primarily driven by differing scopes. In fact, the very first compostable polymers have been developed for medical applications. Most biopolymers show material characteristics that are from great interest, as these enable innovative approaches for device design. You are presented three aspects that explain their importance for current and future prospective medical devices.

6.5.1 Biodegradable Polymers

Generally spoken, this class of plastics does comprise any polymer that will disintegrate in a biological system in reasonable timescale. This does include bioplastics that currently find increasing applications for products such as bags (Figure 6.5), disposable plates, or drinking cups, which easily can be composted after use. Within the world of medical devices, biodegradable polymer usually rather does refer to a plastic that will be dismantled inside the human body by means of metabolism within a period between several days and years. Put simply, an implant manufactured from these materials will completely disappear without further action. Thereby, a biodegradable exhibits two processes of degradation. In **bulk erosion**, degradation will commence equally within the entire body, so the ratio of volume to surface remains the same. The implant will remain about the same in size, but the internal structure will change significantly, altering to a jelly-like state. It may occur that this bubble like structure does rupture and spill its content at once. In **surface erosion**, degradation occurs on

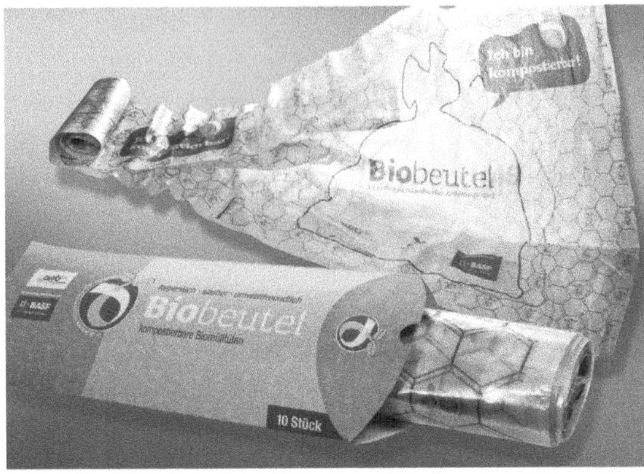

Figure 6.5 Biodegradable polymers already have widespread applications for compostable consumer products, such as bags (as displayed), disposable plates, or drinking cups. The increasing application as consumer products presumably will trigger more efforts for development, what in turn will lead to increased availability for medical applications. *Image courtesy of BASF.*

the surface mainly, and the implant disintegrates layer by layer, like an ice cube melting in the sun. Thereby, the aspect of volume to surface does change significantly. Both means of erosion are not exclusive, and many biodegradable polymers undergo a combination of both, yet one unusually clearly is dominating.

A well-established medical application is absorbent surgical suture materials that were introduced in the early 1960s. The advantages are obvious: while a conventional thread requires removal after healing, a biodegradable one does not require this after treatment, a striking advantage if you consider surgical interventions deep inside the body. Inspired by this idea many more materials and applications were developed and introduced. Currently there are five major groups of biodegradable plastic materials commercially available. However, by combining these by means of copolymerization or compounding, an enormous variety of materials may be obtained.

6.5.1.1 Polyglycolic Acid (PGA)

- Material for the first absorbable surgical suture (early 1960s)
- Wide application for absorbable suture
- Utilized for implants such as plates, pins, rods, and screws
- Shows bulk degradation in 30–90 days

6.5.1.2 Polylactic Acid (PLA)

- Well-processable by standard technologies for plastic processing
- Wide application for compostable consumer goods (e.g., plastic bags)
- Utilized for implants such as anchors, meshes, pins, rods, and screws
- Applied as dermal filling material in cosmetic surgery
- Shows Bulk degradation in 6–24 months
- Process of dismantling is beneficial for supporting structures
- Found hobby application as feed-material for 3D printers

6.5.1.3 Polycaprolactone (PCL)

- Degradation in 2–4 years
- Utilized for implants such as adhesion barriers, suture, or drug delivery
- Hobby application as feed-material for 3D printers
- The Melting point of 60 °C (140 F) makes it appealing for handicrafts, it is available as InstaMorph®, Plaast®, or ShapeLock™ (many more)

6.5.1.4 Polyanhydrides

- Very low hydrolytic stability
- Degradation rate may be adjusted in very wide range
- Shows surface degradation, thus material of choice for drug delivery

6.5.1.5 Polylactic-Co-Glycolic Acid (PLGA)

- Copolymer of PLA and PGA
- Hobby application as feed-material for 3D printers
- Due to the wide range of material properties utilized for implants such as grafts, sutures, surgical films, and nanoparticles

An implant basing on one of these biodegradable polymers subsequently will be replaced by body's own material, making implant removal after healing superfluous. Widespread applications are screws, plates, and fixing pins for osteosynthesis. This comes along with several advantages. The implant does bear the entire load direct after implantation. The patient regains mobility immediately and the body gets time to start bone healing. At one hand, while degrading subsequently, the **load is slowly deflected** to the skeletal system, what is known to further trigger the process of healing. This avoids the effect of stress shielding known from metal-based implants that feature close to equal rigidity over their lifetime what even may impede bone healing. On the other hand, an implant vanishing does not require any removal. Usually conventional plates and screws are explanted surgically, resulting in increased treatment expenses and the reoccurring risks accompanied with every operation. Additionally this will lead to more or better visible scars that are objectionable from an aesthetic aspect, especially when located at easy visible body parts. Biodegradable implants are the standard for the treatment of bone fractures within the face.

Recently biodegradable implants found widespread application as **material for stents**, especially those for coronary applications. Among the diseases of our affluent society in industrialized countries, coronary artery disease plays a dominant role. One of its most frequent causes is a constriction (stenosis), induced by deposits creating a plague, of one or several coronary arteries that are feeding the heart muscle (myocard). If untreated, this condition will eventually lead to stable or unstable angina, heart attack with subsequent death. Besides bypass operation, coronary heart disease may be treated by a therapy called percutaneous transluminal coronary angioplasty: via a peripheral access to the arterial system (e.g., groin), a catheter exhibiting a small balloon at its end is placed within the stenosis. The balloon is expanded, blasting the stenosis and reopening the coronary artery to its original diameter. To avoid elastic recovery of the artery, in most cases subsequently an implant known as stent is implanted, whereas currently most of them still are metal based. As first approach toward biodegradable polymers, some metal stents were coated with these plastics to implement a drug delivery functionality. Nevertheless, it is known that after a period of 6–12 months, the coronary artery has undergone a remodeling and the stent as support structure actually no longer would be required. Consequently, after a given time, metal stents represent a foreign body without actual benefit for the patient. An appropriate solution to this problem is stent basing on biodegradable polymers, designed in a way that these disappear when no longer needed. Moreover, these implants are ideal for the integration of drug delivery. Hence, the medical device market currently sees an impressive number of biodegradable stents brought to the market (see Figure 6.6).

Although established as medical device materials for several decades already, biodegradable polymers have seen an increasing application mainly in the recent years. With expanding applications, the price for

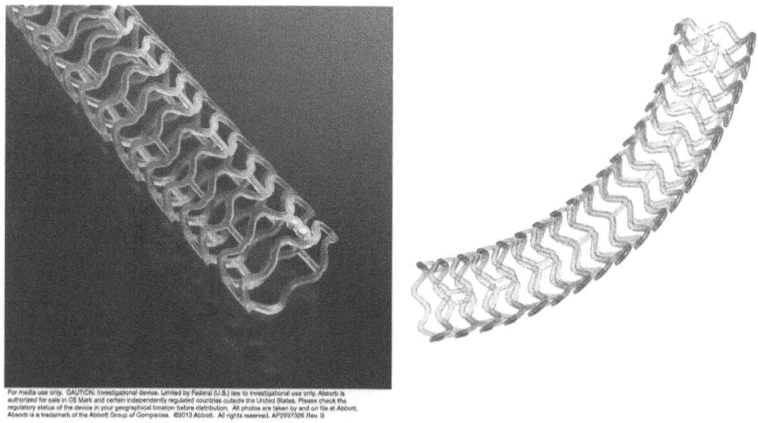

Figure 6.6 After a period of 6–12 months, coronary stents, utilized to support the artery after balloon dilatation, in most cases no longer are required due to remodeling of the vessel. Contrary to the established metal-based ones, stents produced from biodegradable polymers, like the ones on display, vanish after the desired period and no foreign body remains. As additional advantage, these easily may be combined with a drug delivery functionality, which is why the medical device market currently sees many of those systems being brought to market. *Left image courtesy of Abbott Vascular, right image curtesy of REVA Medical Inc.*

raw material is dropping, which in turn expands the range of commercial meaningful devices basing on them. Moreover, medical device engineers are becoming more aware of the enormous potential linked to the application of these plastics. Therefore, the world of medical devices will see a significant increase in applications of biodegradable polymers, not least to other features that frequently may be implemented in this class of materials.

6.5.2 Shape-Memory Polymers

Another interesting group of plastics are shape-memory polymers (SMPs). Just alike the better-known shape-memory alloys, these will "remember" their original shape when deformed, and **flip back** to the initial shape when exposed to an external stimulus (Figure 6.7). These stimuli may be an electric field, light, changes in pH-value, or, as most commonly, changes in temperature. Some SMPs even can retain three shapes, their initial (permanent) shape and two deformed morphologies. This effect offers several interesting options.

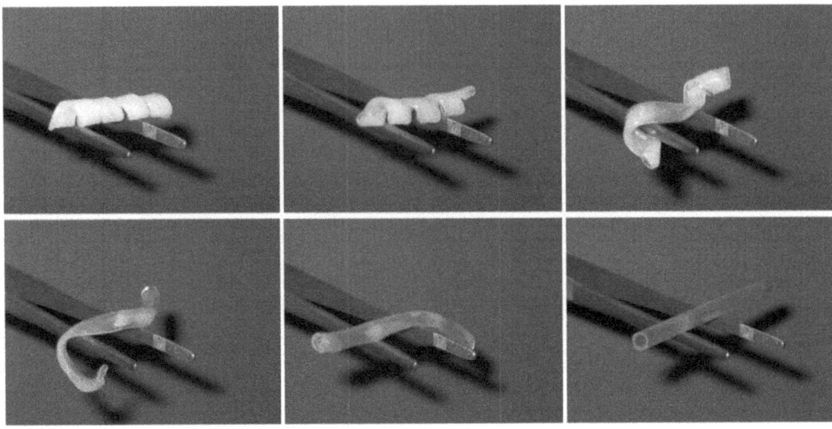

Figure 6.7 Shape-memory polymers (SMPs) offer wide ranges of applications for medical devices, e.g., for applying constant forces or as actuators. In display, there is a tube that was spirally winded, regaining its initial shape when exposed to the appropriate stimuli. This is just one example for the countless opportunities for device design, given by the application of SMPs. *Image courtesy of Springer, Marc Behl and Andreas Lendlein.*

The recovery triggered by the external stimuli does occur with considerable force. That way a **constant tension or compression** to surrounding tissue may be applied. To do so, the device is manufactured in the shape required to execute the desired influence. Prior application, it will be deformed in order to allow facilitated insertion. Using the appropriate stimuli, the SMP will retrieve its initial shape and constantly will perform the way desired. By applying a constant puissance, the body is forced to slowly alter its shape. A commonly known application is bracelets that alter the position of teeth over a period of several months, or coronary stents that strut the artery and prevent an elastic recoil. The alteration in shape also may be used for **clamping**. Feasible are form- and/or force-fitting fastenings. Applications for that are devices such as surgical staplers, remotely controlled switchable implants, or clamps to fix artificial heart valves. Using an appropriate sequence of different stimuli, an SMP may perform a periodically repeating movement that may be used as an **actuator**. Imaginable are valves that open and close automatically according to the surrounding conditions or tools for microsurgery. While shape-memory alloys already found widespread applications in medical devices, such as dental wires, cardiovascular stents, or orthopedic implants, the utilization of SMPs still is in its very beginnings.

6.5.3 Engineering with Biopolymers

Utilizing biodegradable polymers that additionally feature a shape-memory function, many novel designs for medical devices become imaginable. The following section shall give you some examples for such applications and so trigger your imagination. The important point for this is to think beyond classical boundary conditions.

A rather young, still emerging technology within bioengineering is **3D cell culture**. For biological analyses, like biological testing as covered by ISO 10993 (see Section 2.3.4), an encasing is required to simulate the conditions alike in the biological system (in vivo, Latin for *within the living*) as realistic as possible. For this, established techniques for cell culture currently predominantly utilize petri dishes or well plates, which by their nature only allow a two-dimensional cultivation (thus 2D cell culture). Anyhow, it is obvious that growing cells in three dimensions more accurately model the in vivo and presumably will lead to more accurate results. Two terms closely related to the approach of 3D cell culture is **scaffold**, as it describes a three-dimensional support structure intended to serve as "housing" for growing cells. Thereby, the application of scaffolds does range far beyond cell culture for biological in vitro analyses. In fact, scaffolds are an essential component for any attempt to artificially generate living structure for tissue or even entire organs, an approach commonly known as **tissue engineering**. This already is done successfully, e.g., for generating the cartilaginous structure of the human ear, that then is utilized for aesthetic reconstruction. Anyhow, the major objectives go ways further. For instance, replacing a damaged human heart valve is an established surgical procedure. As replacement may serve a plastic-based implant that features an appropriate life span while showing negative influence on the blood circulation, as the rate of hemolysis is rather high. As alternative, devitalized heart valves (only the cartilaginous structures remain) taken from cattle (bovine) or swine (porcine) may be utilized, which show a significant lower hemolysis rate, but exhibit a life span not really satisfactory. Thus, current research does focus on approaches to solve these problems by utilizing scaffolds made from biodegradable polymers. The following idea is partially, not yet fully, implemented: **creating a living replacement heart valve**, made from the body's own cells. In a first step, using a biodegradable polymer, a three-dimensional scaffold is created, featuring the shape and dimensions of the desired tissue structure (here: the heart valve). It is now colonized with appropriate cells, taken from the patient, and subsequently placed inside a bioreactor that performs the pulsatile movement of the bloodstream, simulating the in vivo condition as accurate as possible. The cells will start growth while the polymer scaffold starts to degenerate. After a given time, once obtains a heart valve, partially consisting of the initial scaffold, partially or even entirely of living tissue, as displayed in Figure 6.8. The heart valve now is implanted, whereas specific structure of the polymer scaffold, which features a shape-memory effect, could be used for anchoring the implant during surgery. Postsurgery, the implanted heart valve will be nourished by blood vessel growing into it, further promoting its biointegration, while the initial scaffold continues its dismantling until vanishing. The final result would be a newly created, body's own heart valve. Of course, it still will take years until this idea will come into reality. Still, research on these aspects fuels the knowledge upon the field of regenerative medicine. And within this discipline, biodegradable polymers play a vital role. With time, more elaborate techniques of tissue engineering will find techniques to artificially generate entire working organs, the ultimate solution to the problem of lacking transplants. Maybe one day, these techniques even find applications for the biotechnological production of food, an idea known as in vitro meat. Although this does sound (and most presumably is) very futuristic, it shows that it can be expected that in future the distinctions between the scientific fields of (micro)-biology, medicine, and medical engineering see a merger.

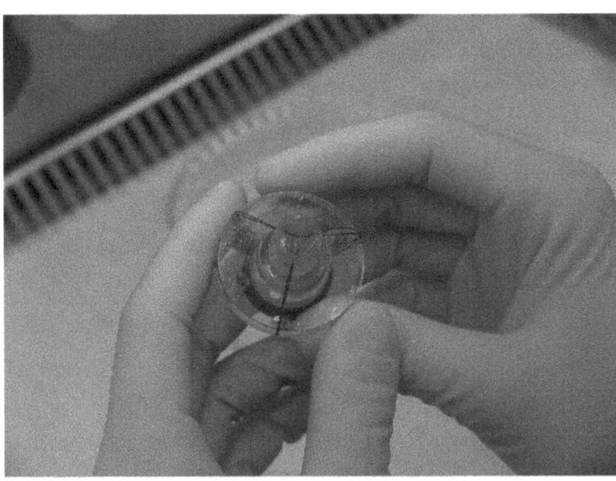

Figure 6.8 Artificial heart valve, created by tissue engineering. A scaffold, made from biodegradable polymers is colonized with living cells, and subsequently placed within a bioreactor, performing the pulsatile movement of the bloodstream, simulating the in vivo condition as accurate as possible. The cells start to grow, while the scaffold degenerates until vanishing, with only living tissue remaining. *Image taken from commonswiki, user: health-associated infections, published under Attribution-ShareAlike 3.0 Unported (CC BY-SA 3.0).*

Another interesting idea that might fuel your imagination is a micro device made from SMPs, which may serve as gripper or micro actuator. A star-shaped structure is made from a combination of soft hydrogels and a stiff biodegradable polymer that allows to perform a movement of folding it into itself, as displayed in Figure 6.9. The device could be used to perform challenging biopsies at complicated to access locations, or to perform interventional surgical procedures. The necessary navigation to perform these tasks could be implemented by adding magnetic nanoparticles into the system, allowing external magnetic fields to be used for moving the gripper to the position desired. Another imaginable application could be for targeted drug delivery (see Section 6.5.3). The device, encasing the pharmaceutical, is navigated at the appropriate location and then triggered to release its content. When selecting the appropriate hydrogel, this action can be triggered by light, acidity, or temperature variations, respectively. Although still subject to basic research, many applications for this approach are imaginable that appear realistic for implementation in a reasonable timescale.

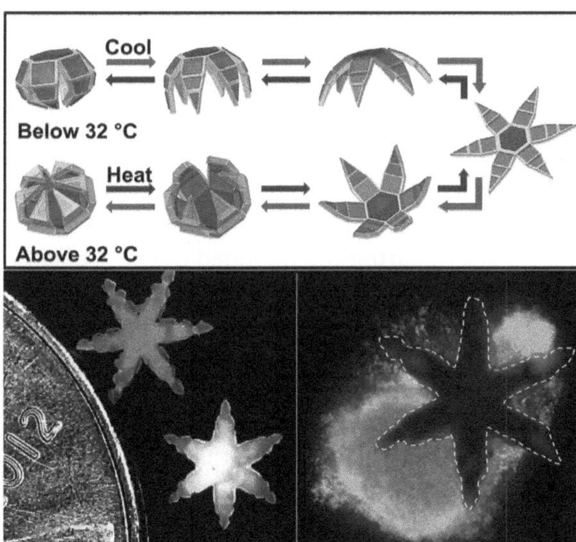

Figure 6.9 A star-shaped micro device is made from a combination of soft hydrogels and a stiff biodegradable polymer that allows to perform a movement of folding it into itself. By selecting the appropriate hydrogel, this action may be triggered by light, acidity, or temperature variations, respectively. Possible applications include, among others, biopsies at difficult to access locations, interventional surgical procedures, or targeted drug delivery. *Image courtesy of David Gracias, ChangKyu Yoon, and ACS Publications.*

Ideally, these examples showed you the enormous potential associated with the engineering of biopolymers. As indicated, many applications still are subject to research and development, may be expected to become a vital part of the polymer-based medical device world soon. This is not least to their enormous potential within the field of drug delivery technologies.

6.6 Drug Delivery Devices

Within the worlds of health care and medical engineering, you frequently will encounter the catchword **(targeted) drug delivery**. As frequently when dealing with subjects of comparatively young research, covered by many different scientific disciplines, such as pharmacology, chemistry, (bio)-chemistry, medicine, and medical engineering, there are many different understandings for this term. To come closer to a meaningful understanding of them, it is necessary to take a closer look to the way drugs usually are administered. Common techniques comprise either oral uptake (pills and capsules), dermal application (creams and ointments), or subdermal or intravenous injection. Common to all approaches is the fact that the pharmaceutical will be distributed over (almost[3]) the entire body and thus will affect the metabolism of all cells, even on those were this is not desired. This effect requires an increased dosage of the drug in order to achieve the desired level at the location where effect is desired. Moreover, any drug entering the human body via the digestive system will pass the liver, where considerate amounts will be transformed as part of the normal metabolism, no longer featuring the intended effect. This not only reduces the effective share of the initial administered amount, but also represents a considerate still unnecessary burden for this organ. Avoiding these and many more undesired side effects not mentioned, is the primary goal of targeted drug delivery, as it refers to approaches, formulations, technologies, and systems for transporting a pharmaceutical compound in the body as needed to safely achieve its desired therapeutic effect, while reducing undesired side effects as much as possible. Put simply, the deal of it is to bring the required amount of drug into the body only to the region, where the effect is required. And of course this aim may be reached by many

3. As the physiological metabolism of the human body is very complex, this restriction is necessary. For example, some chemicals are unable to pass the blood–brain barrier, a highly selective permeability barrier that separates the circulating blood from the brain. This is the reason why pharmaceuticals intended for showing effect in the brain must comply with specific biochemical requirements.

different approaches, including those utilizing mechanical-based solutions only. However, reflecting the subject of the book, we will focus on those involving biopolymers only.

Over the past decades, **biodegradable polymers** have proven to be a very **meaningful approach for targeted drug delivery**. As explained in Section 6.5.1, these types of polymers will disintegrate and eventually vanish when implanted into the human body, whereas the time and process of disintegration may be actively influenced by engineering. For instance, many medical devices are used as implant, serving as drug delivery system, intended to continuously administering a drug without any need for repeating intake of medicines. This offers diverse benefits. Drugs may be delivered continuously right at the desired location within the human body, bypassing the digestive system and the liver. This allows lower dosages, reducing undesired side effects, and ameliorates the effectiveness of substances that require constant drug level. Further convenience of the patient is increased as he is released from remembering when and how to intake drugs or any additional surgical intervention to remove the implant. Prominent example is small subcutaneous rod-shaped implants, a few millimeters in diameter and 5–10 mm in length, applied as a contraceptive. A polymer structure contains the hormones required to prevent an undesired pregnancy. The porter must not remember to take a contraceptive pill on daily basis, and thus may experience an improvement in quality of life. Nevertheless, it must be mentioned that these systems usually do not base on biodegradable polymers for simple reasons. Especially at the end of degradation, such an implant would be difficult to spot and/or remove, significantly complicating its application. Thus it is more reasonable to have it removed after its life span and, if desired, to have it replaced by a new one. However, all the opportunities of biodegradable polymers presented are combined in a drug called Ozurdex®, intended to treat a couple of diseases affecting the functionality of the eye (Figure 6.10). The system's core is a biodegradable implant about the size of a rice grain, containing the active pharmaceutical ingredient(s). Using a device resembling a ball pen, the implant is implanted into the eyeball. While being disintegrated over the following months, it does release the drug and thus continuously administers a constant drug level as close to the desired location as possible. And this does combine several advantages. The constant drug level, compared to the approach of taking eye drops several times a day, does lead to improved treatment. Further, as the diffusion of the pharmaceutical stretches over a shorter distance, as the drug is administered inside instead of outside the eyeball, a reduced dosage may be applied that still shows more effect. And finally, compliance of and convenience for the patient

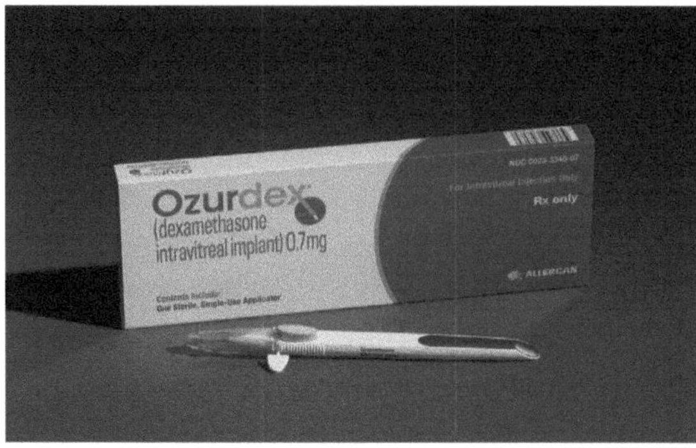

Figure 6.10 Image of the Ozurdex® drug delivery system, consisting of a biodegradable implant that contains the drug and a single use device as applicator. After injection into the eyeball, the implant will dissolve within a defined period and so administer the medicine at constant drug level directly in the target area. *Image courtesy of Allergan.*

are improved, as the cumbersome routine of taking the drug (e.g., the eye drops) repetitive and not forgetting to do so.

You probably will see the enormous potential for drug delivery systems when utilizing biodegradable polymers. And so many more of those medical devices may be expected to come. This not least to the fact that these may significantly improve the convenience for the patient, an aspect definitely the mere therapeutic aims, still gaining more and more importance (see Chapter 7). Anyhow, using biodegradable polymers for drug delivery devices usually necessarily requires to combine a conventional medical device with a pharmaceutical, an approach that may lead to significant regulatory issues, as these are explained in Section 2.7.2.

6.7 Health-Related Wearables

As early as the dawn of mankind, humans started to fabricate and utilize tools to ease the daily work, which is why these soon became an integral part of our life. Soon, many tools, such as weapons or religious symbols emerged to a status symbol, were carried around for representative purposes beyond mere utilization. Human and tools slowly merged into one unity, and nowadays some tools are linked that tight to a specific profession, that the device alone may be used to represent the occupation. Just think about a stethoscope, probably one of the most frequently used symbol to represent a medical professional. In parallel, authors of science fiction started to fantasize about tools being integrated into the human body, either to ease disabilities and injuries or to even expand the abilities of the human being wearing those. And as soon as electronics and computers became part of our daily life, integrating those into the human body became object of desire for many. The merger of organic and biomechatronic parts is called **cyborg** and it is subject of many activities in current research. Among those how major impact had on the evolution of this discipline probably is **Steven Mann**, a researcher and inventor known for his work on wearable computing, probably has had a major impact on the evolution of this discipline. Since the 1980s he has been evolving the idea of fusing a human being and a wearable computer, as illustrated in Figure 6.11, and has demonstrated the resulting opportunities for the evolution of mankind.

You might consider this rather as science fiction or hogwash of a freaky scientist. But in fact, wearable computers are close to market. Just think about the Google Glass. Although this item is subject to vivid discussions upon ethical aspects and a broad commercial accessibility still is pending, it clearly shows that wearable computers or cyborg systems are close to get part of our daily life. Self-speaking that the opportunities of wearable computers are from greater interest for modern medicine as these represent the first meaningful approach to cure diseases and disabilities that formerly were considered as incurable. Many people who suffer from congenital deafness are treated with a cochlea implant, an implantable computer giving them ability for acoustical perception. Depending on the

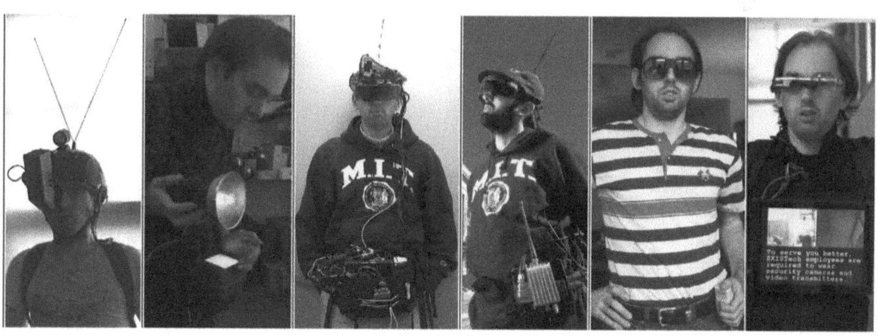

Figure 6.11 Steve Mann, a researcher known for his work on wearable computing, is pushing the idea of fusing a human being and electronics in order to form a cyborg since the 1980s. Although this might sound as science fiction, these developments already have impact and applications in our daily life in general, and the world of medical devices in particular. *Image taken from commonswiki, user: glogger, published under Attribution-ShareAlike 3.0 Unported (CC BY-SA 3.0).*

definition, you might call these people cyborgs, just alike those wearing an implanted pacemaker. Current research within ophthalmology follows the approach to restore vision for the blind by an implantable computer for optical processing. In parallel, current developments focus on curing or easing paraplegia. Another very advanced approach is an exoskeleton, a wearable machine, that is put on like a suit. This allows the porter to walk and move almost like a healthy person. These systems, as depicted in Figure 6.12, currently see wide application in orthopedic rehabilitation, but may be expected to become a meaningful approach to help people suffering from paraplegia.

All well and good, you might think now. But where is the relevance for medical plastic engineering? In fact, the introduction is intended to give you a feeling upon how much influence biomechatronics already has on medical engineering—and presumably will have even more in the future. Due to the general evolvement of microelectronics, computer and mechatronic systems see increasing capabilities while their prices keep decreasing (see Sections 5.5. and 5.6.2). Just think about the smartphones that basically are computers that feature a processing power you only could dream about in the end of the millennium—and that all to the size of a pocket. The unprecedented commercial success of smartphones allowed

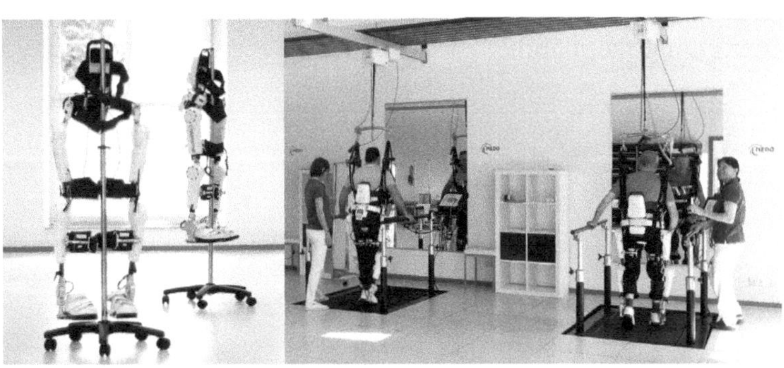

Figure 6.12 The robotic system HAL I is intended for the rehabilitation of people suffering from disorders in walking, e.g., induced by paraplegia or stroke. Its exoskeleton is operated by nerve impulses that are monitored by sensors placed on the patient's skin, and so significantly may contribute to restoring the ability to walk, as far as possible. This is an impressive example demonstrating how far the fusion of human being and mechatronics has come so far. The HAL system displayed is not intended to restore the ability to walk as an exoskeleton but rather is used as medical device for the purpose of rehabilitation only. *Image courtesy of Cyberdyne Care Robotics GmbH.*

to develope very small still powerful micro computer platforms that now find application in many other aspects of mechatronics (see Section 6.3, detection of diseases in third world countries). Moreover, any kind of microelectronic systems benefit from the impressive market demand for more and more powerful smartphones, which is why microelectronic elements are getting smaller, more robust, and cheaper in price. The logic consequences are single-use consumer electronic products, like it already is expressed as disposable cell phones. And further, single-use medical devices may be equipped with integrated mechatronic systems (see Section 5.6.2, sensor integration) that are of remarkable complexity.

All these technological developments triggered a new market segment, called **health-related wearables** (Figure 6.13). Its products comprise manifold products of consumer products that somehow are connected to the body in order to measure, track, analyze, and store vital parameters, such as pulse, blood pressure, body temperature, any kind of movement, and many more. You probably already have seen or even pose a bracelet or wrist watch, utilized as fitness tracker. Most recently, health-related wearables also are available as SUDs, skin patches that are ported for a designated time, and the disposed, just alike a single-use medical device. Beyond maybe serving a status symbol, the primary scope of these devices in fact is to monitor the personal lifestyle. Currently it is *en vogue* for many people to live a **lifestyle of health and sustainability** (LOHAS) and thus the personal health consequently is integrated into the all-embracing network of mobile communication and data storage. Just think about the fast-growing number of fitness trackers that are connected to the smartphone, used to optimize the personal fitness goals, as these might be used to reduce weight, or just to maintain a healthy status. And many systems allow to instantly share any fitness success via social networks. Sure, any approach to increase ones personal fitness is to be welcomed, and doing sports in at reasonable extent doubtless is the most appropriate way to maintain one's health, making it the ultimate virtual medical device. This does sound funny to you? Take a closer look to the definition of medical devices, as given in Section 1.1 (What is a medical device?), as this does comprise any device to detect, prevent, monitor, treat, or alleviate diseases, injuries, or disabilities. Anyhow, this development exhibits some aspects that should not be embraced without questioning.

It is obvious that data derived from a health-related wearable have impact on our behavior. If not, why should someone be using one? And it is unquestionable that the data generated may have significant benefit for our lifestyle. Those systems may indicate that you are not showing sufficient activity, or that your training did help to improve your endurance. In case of sudden

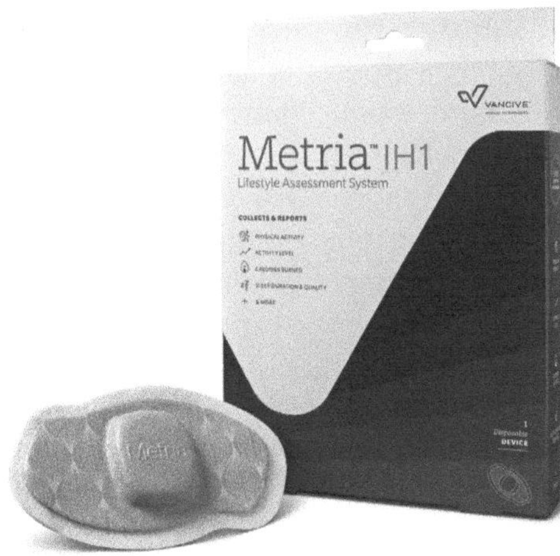

Figure 6.13 The Metria™ IH1 is a single-use fitness tracker, representing the latest development in health-related wearables. The patch is applied to the skin and monitors vital parameters, such as pulse, temperature, or movement for a designated period. After this, it is removed and disposed, just alike a single-use medical device. The system displayed is not a medical device and is not to be marketed as one. *Image courtesy of Vancive Medical Technologies™, an Avery Dennison business.*

sickness, the long-term measurement of body temperature or breathing frequency over day and night may significantly help a treating medic to find the appropriate therapy. But you see, exactly all this does place a **health-related wearable very close to a medical device**. If a fitness tracker does analyze your vital parameters and subsequently gives behavioral advices, it may be considered a device influencing your health. And this may be seen for any of those products of our postmodern times, such as fitness or health-related apps. Depending on how far the health recommendations of those health-related wearable devices and apps go, these easily may see a transition into the market of medical devices, making a subject to all the related rules and regulations as the most relevant ones are presented in Chapter 2. It is not surprising that the FDA recently addressed these developments by issuing a relevant draft guideline in February 2015. Consequently, some health-related wearables as well as related software and apps are developed and marketed as medical devices, such as the smartphone-based medical kit displayed in Figure 6.14. The transition between a health-related wearable, clearly an unregulated consumer product, and medical device, unquestionable subject to many rules and regulations, sometimes is subtle. You should remember this if getting involved in one type of them occupationally.

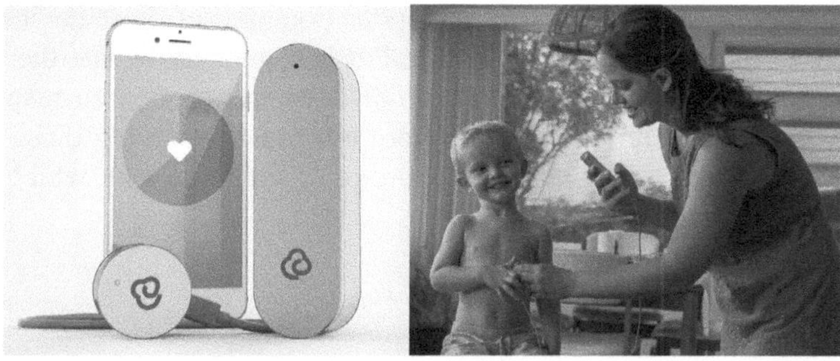

Figure 6.14 CliniCloud is a smartphone-based medical kit intended for home application. It allows you to closely monitor every fever, chill, cough, wheeze, or cold, and even enables to get a medical consultation in the comfort of your own home. It does comprise guided checkup, review, analysis, and records of the health status. This shows that the transition from health-related wearable to medical device (the CliniCloud system adheres to the calibration standards set forth by CE and FDA for Class II medical devices) is very smooth and the differences sometimes are subtle. *Image courtesy of CliniCloud.*

Another aspect concerning health-related wearables that should be considered is the amount of very personal data that is created and stored, making private affairs prone to data abuse. Many of those systems exhibit the convenient function of automatically uploading the generated data into the cloud. This allows remote access and does release the user of caring about data-backup. Nevertheless, you probably are aware that anything uploaded to the Internet presumably will be accessible for ever, even for those you maybe not want to gain insight into information that is private. Moreover, some health insurance companies already offer special health plans with reduced costs, when utilizing health-related wearables and sharing the related information upon your health. At first sight, the idea does sound fair. Exhibiting a healthy lifestyle that does lead to a reduced probability of getting sick is rewarded. But when taking a second look: do you want your insurance company monitoring your lifestyle, and disciplining any behavior not compliant to a healthy lifestyle?

You might get the impression that we, the people, are rather critical about these developments. And in fact this partially is true. We are critical about any health aware individual becoming a glass human being. And we see the risk that some health-related wearables and apps might be indeed health-related, but pointing a negative direction. Meantime, we acknowledge and appreciate the enormous potential of these devices and products to increase the public health. Further, we believe that the future will see a merger of many aspects of our daily living, as their respective boundaries will become more and more blurred. But giving those statements rather is an aspect of looking through the crystal ball, which leads us to the next chapter.

7 Looking through the Crystal Ball

OUTLINE

As we have started to work on this book project, our first intention was simply to introduce emerging technologies in medical plastic engineering by having a deep look into the existing technologies and upcoming trends. As the project advanced, it has become more and more clear to introduce a bigger picture about medical devices, product development, plastics, and of course, the manufacturing processes. And of course, how will future medical devices look like, and what will their respective markets be? It is our self-conception to interpret the term technologies more widely, because in our opinion it is no longer possible to draw a clear picture of upcoming technological trends without having a look into all aspects of the medical product life cycle, beginning with the development, regulatory affairs, manufacturing and ending with interaction with the end-consumer, the medical professionals and patients around the world. As it is consequently done throughout every single chapter, also this chapter, dedicated a look through the crystal ball, is beginning by having an overall impression of the current situation.

7.1 Contemporary Medical Device Life Cycle

Our definition of a medical device life cycle is as next: it begins with an idea for a new product, followed by development, testing and evaluation, manufacturing, and finally by its application. An overview scenario is shown for better understanding in Figure 7.1. Typically, each step works for itself. At certain points of the life cycle, predefined interactions between steps like development and manufacturing are taking place. Each department within a business unit works for itself, some to a bigger and

Emerging Trends in Medical Plastic Engineering and Manufacturing
http://dx.doi.org/10.1016/B978-0-323-37023-3.00007-5

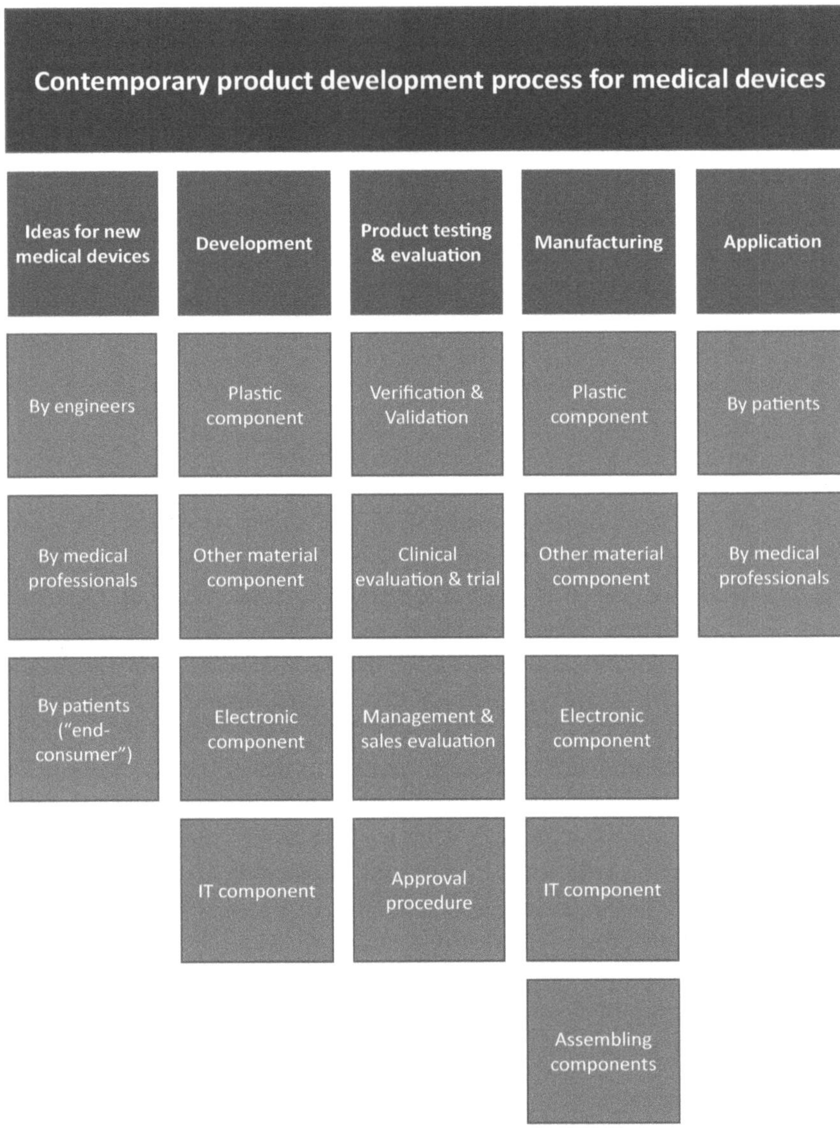

Figure 7.1 Contemporary product development process for medical devices: The current situation is characterized by many interfaces, which can cause a lack in flow of information (e.g., ideas, improvements, errors) and may offer huge potential for future improvements. Especially, the knowledge derived during application by "end-consumer" is currently tough to introduce to development, testing, or even production processes. Exemplarily spoken: sometimes a simple change in a surface condition, which occurs during production, may lead to an easier handling for medical professionals. Especially for simple products, there is often no accurate flow of information possible.

some to a smaller extent, surely with some interaction, when needed. The bigger the interface between major or even little steps, the more interesting and difficult is the information transfer. Think about a medical device, which is in application regularly within surgery procedures, like a stapler. The existing stapler may have some glitches due to some design issues, but it works actually to a certain extent quite well. Due to the fact that most medical professionals seldom find time for or maybe just are not really interested in the design of medical devices, they do just accept the minor difficulties without trying getting in touch with the medical device manufacturer. There might be a benefit of having less trouble with the device, but overall there is not big need for improvement. On the other hand, the R & D departments are constantly looking for new ideas. However, the actually best source for ideas, the end-user, cannot participate usually due to the existing boundaries. Only few companies and also medical professionals try to overcome these hurdles by contacting each other directly. This might not be an appropriate way for the vast majority of medical devices, simply due to the fact of huge amount of applicants and medical device companies. Who would be able to handle all the interactions? The same problems can be seen in most companies as well. Most R & D departments may work smoothly, if they are located at one point, but for bigger companies, there might be a location for the design unit, another for the packaging unit, a manufacturing unit elsewhere, and so on.

And don't forget about the usually biggest hurdle in companies: information transfer between the product design and actual product manufacturing. There is usually an improvable information policy. Within the manufacturing processes, there is a huge potential for medical device improvements hidden: broken down to the fact "flow of information." This brings us to the future integrated product development processes.

7.2 Future Integrated Product Development Processes

It is easily written about a fully integrated product development process. Imagine a system with the idealistic idea of a perfect flow of information as described in Figure 7.2. Surely, there are some critical issues like secret policy or marketing questions, but at least a perfect flow of information from manufacturing, medical professionals, and even patients to the development parties may have enormous potential for future medical devices. We are thinking about the aspect of crowdsourced innovation to bring all necessary information together plus having the right tools to evaluate the deriving

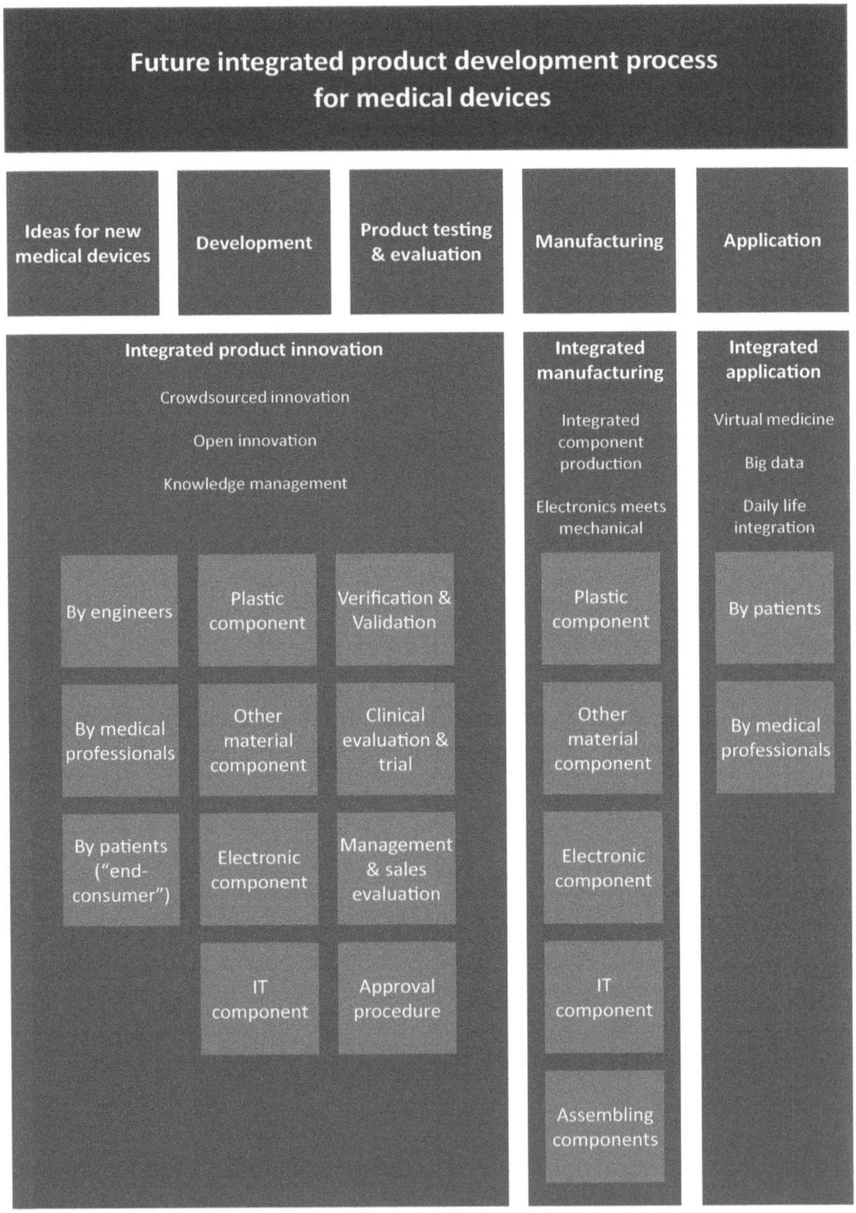

Figure 7.2 A scenario for future medical device development: little by little the major steps of a product life cycle will become more and more integrated by increasing the flow of information and reducing existing hurdles between. The flow of information is triggered by applicable interfaces like crowd-sourced information, a part of future knowledge management approaches. This will also affect the manufacturing of new devices: technologies from various engineering directions will interact more and more, as it is already seeable in some emerging technologies as described in Chapters 5 and 6.

ideas. Why not use the experiences of patients, medical professionals, and so on to evaluate actual ideas for new medical devices? First experiences with crowdsourced innovation have been realized within different fields like service sectors, fast food restaurant, end-consumer electronics, or agriculture. You may wonder, why it is worth having a look into the field of agriculture. Employees in agriculture are usually highly committed to their work environment and they are interested in improving the technological possibilities regularly. Therefore, first crowdsourcing innovation projects have been realized successfully within. Medical professionals can be considered of having a similar commitment to their jobs. It would be a perfect source of know-how, innovation, and new ideas for future medical devices. This combined with the new technological integrated possibilities, whose boundaries are not really discovered, yet. The combination of electronics, information technology, and plastic will influence future medical devices magnificently. But, how does this fit to our demand for classic engineering disciplines for future medical device employees, which we have proposed within the previous chapters. It does fit perfectly. The overall available knowledge is growing constantly in a progressive manner that nobody can ensure of having all necessary knowledge of all technical, medical, or biological fields. Future employees should focus on their specific field, but have to be able to interact with other disciplines, which is currently often a major hurdle. Technological approaches will help to cover these hurdles. The same principles used for getting in touch with end-consumers like Internet-based crowdsourcing platforms may be used to improve the flow of information between different disciplines, which are working on plastic medical devices. This brings us to the mystic expression of Internet of the things and industry 4.0.

These aspects are definitely interesting for the manufacturing processes. But, the really amazing opportunities are achievable by integrating the perfect flow of information by using these approaches within the product development process and the interface of patients and medical professionals.

7.3 The Perfect Future Medical Device

What does perfect mean in this context? Uncountable different definitions may seem reasonable. We have chosen this approach: gathering as many information by using sensors, data collecting, or patient interaction as possible, help to see the right coincidences, all with the major aim to reveal possible illnesses as soon as possible and evaluate applied treatments the best way possible. Wouldn't it be a great benefit of having, for example, plastic hip socket implants, which can monitor the current state of mechanical load, abrasion, or the "health" of the surrounding tissue by measuring inflammation parameters (some sound simple like pH levels)? Besides monitoring sensors, the plastic hip socket has some sort of wireless data transfer implemented. This could help to improve future device designs on the one hand, but also would help the actual patient by detecting extraordinary circumstances before it affects the whole body and probably quite early in comparison. The question is now, how to ensure patients' data are collected adequately, the information is provided to the necessary extend (e.g., R & D departments and medical professionals) without hurting privacy concerns. The perfect plastic medical device will have no success if there is no medical professional or patient, who is willing to work with it. But, the possibilities of the Internet of things approaches are enormous and have to be taken into account by future plastic medical device engineers.

7.4 Future Medical Devices as Part of Smart Living

We expect further that future medical devices will see applications going ways beyond their objective of healing. They rather will become a part of the integrated, intercommunicating network of things and information embracing our daily life, and they will be **integrated into our smart living**. We'll explain the details and why we state this. Initial approaches to this development already can be seen. Taking the example of the drug delivery device, presented in Figure 6.10, you see a medical device featuring a technology that significantly does increase the convenience of the patient. First of all, an increased compliance with the patient will increase the outcome of any therapy. Nevertheless, in parts, the comfort does go further than the initial intention of healing would require. The decision to select a specific medical device, regardless weather done by the patient or a medical professional, is triggered by aspects beyond their sheer biomedical effect. For market success of a medical device, it will get more and more important to mediate a specific lifestyle beyond the mere promise to heal a disease. For centuries, a patient was tolerating a lot of pain and willing to accept even horrible treatments. Think about how dentistry was alike just a century ago. Today, a patient is well informed by many media, especially the Internet, and frequently has a profound understanding about how an appropriate treatment for his condition should look alike. This change of mind in our society is reflected by the movement to replace the noun *compliance* (is the patient doing what I said him to do) by *adherence* (how effective did we, the patient and I, follow the agreed plan of treatment). This shows that by many people, an occurring sickness or disease, as well as its treatment, no longer is considered as an occurring event, outside the normal life but rather as a part of their life. The once present understanding of two possibilities, binary conditions *healthy or sick*, whereas one does exclude the other, is getting replaced by the idea that the general being rather is a continuous ongoing. Just alike the catchword work–life balance that now is being replaced by life balance. This evolution is very helpful to dismantle barriers and fears of contact to medical devices and their applications. The consequence is that more and more medical treatments and surgical interventions are performed without any real health-related reason. A good example for this beyond aesthetic and plastic surgery is the laser-based treatment of defective vision. These medical procedures are advertised currently heavily as a lifestyle accessory. In parallel, a fast-growing number of people are getting more and more aware of their personal being and care about their lifestyle. Some sociologists claim that special nutritional habits and self-imposed fitness programs may be seen as a modern substitute for religion. This probably is not least to our general increasing prosperity, as we are able to generate more wealth in less time. Hence, the time required to assure the daily living is shortened, giving room to focus on one's personal health status. The rapid-growing number of health-related wearables and fitness apps is reflecting these developments. If appreciated or not, these devices and products will become part of the medical device world too, even if many of these manufacturers try to avoid this currently due to the regulatory burden involved. Beyond the critics we stated about health-related wearables, we actually are thrilled about the possibilities opening up. It is beyond any doubt that as more data upon a patient are available, the easier it is to develop a holistic therapy concept. It is easy to predict that medical devices will become part of the big data.

7.5 Grand Unified Well-Being[1]

We already introduced the concept of life sciences (see Chapter 1) and showed that these already are subject to a rapid merger. When dealing with combination products, even competent authorities struggle to distinguish between medical device and pharmaceutical. If thinking about the emerging technologies coming along with bio and tissue engineering, the boundaries between all sciences involved in the art of healing will get more and more blurred. When taking a short look into the scientific field of physics, you see comparable results: researchers try to combine three out of four existing fundamental interactions with into a model called Grand Unified Theory. We expect parallel developments for the world of medical devices, as many different aspects of life are integrated into one big model, focusing on a holistic approach to maintain and restore health. Medical devices are

1. Term coined by Dr Marc Hoffstetter

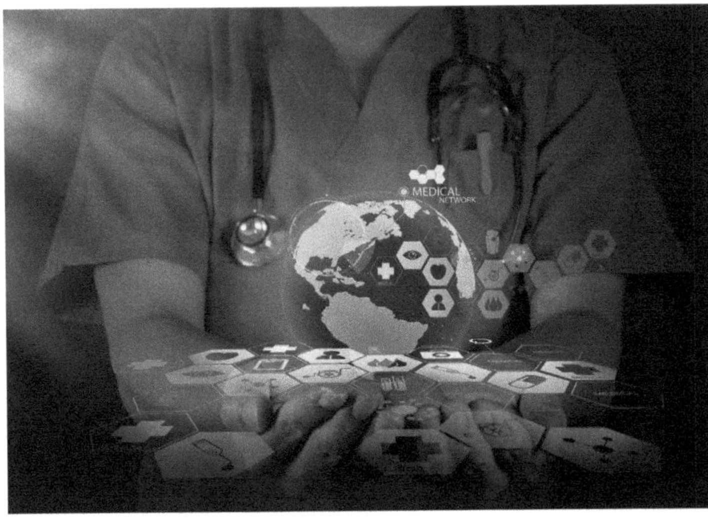

Figure 7.3 The future will see a further merging of all life sciences, further blurring their boundaries. Moreover, many more aspects of our daily living are pushing into the health-related sciences, and nowadays medical devices are used as consumer products for convenience, food is considered as a pharmaceutical, and consumer electronics are used to maintain and restore health. Influenced by less-natural science-based aspects, like those focusing on the general well-being, this will expand the life sciences toward a broader understanding, creating a model we call Grand Unified Well-being. Whatever there may be expected to come due to the increasingly rapid technological development, you should actively participate. Thus, stay interested, stay tuned, and stay enthused! *Image courtesy of Dr Bertalan Meskó, published under Attribution-ShareAlike 2.5 Generic (CC BY-SA 2.5).*

used as consumer products for convenience, food is considered as a pharmaceutical and consumer electronics are used to maintain and restore the health. Thereby, many less-scientific aspects are pushing in that focus rather on one's personal well-being. It is doubtless that these have a positive effect on our health as well. So, the life sciences presumably will be expanded to a bigger model dealing with our health, a model we want to call **Grand Unified Well-being**. It is obvious that we are unable to predict the future. Nevertheless, it is equally obvious that the increasingly rapid technological development will lead to products and (medical) devices, we are unable to imagine yet. Moreover, alike any passionate engineer, we are excited about what there is to come and want to contribute actively to these developments. If we manage to enthuse you about medical engineering and its emerging technologies, you will participate presumably in this technological evolution. As news anchors would finish: stay interested, stay tuned, and stay enthused (Figure 7.3).

Glossary

AAL Ambient Assisted Living

ABR Antibiotic resistance

AIDC Automatic identification and data capture

AKF Arburg plastic freeforming

AMR Antimicrobial resistance

BRICS Brazil, Russia, India, China, and South Africa

CAD Computer-aided design

CAE Computer-aided engineering

CAI Computer-aided innovation

CBER Center for Biologics Evaluation and Research

CDER Center for Drug Evaluation and Research

CDRH Center for Devices and Radiological Health

CFDA China Food and Drug Administration

CNC Computer numerical control

CNT Carbon nanotube

D-value Decimal reduction time value

DLP Digital light processing

ERP Enterprise recourse planning

ETO Ethylene oxide

EUDAMED European Database on Medical Devices

FDA Food and Drug Administration

FDM Fused deposition modeling

GDP Gross domestic product

GLP Good laboratory practice

GS1 Global Standards One

GUDID Global Unique Device Identification Database

HA Hydroxylapatite

HAI Health-Associated Infection

HIBCC Health Industry Business Communications Council

HRI Human readable interpretation

ICCBBA International Council for Commonality in Blood Banking Automation

ISO International Organization for Standardization

IT Information technology

LED Light-emitting diode

LOC Lab-on-a-chip

MAF Master file for devices (technical file/design dossier for FDA approval processes)

MAUDE Manufacturer and User Facility Device Experience

MDD Medical Device Directive, common name for 93/42/EWG

MDR Medical Device Regulation

MJM Multijet modeling

μTAS Micro total analysis system

OPC Office for Combination Products

PDM Product data management

PEEK Polyetheretherketone

PMOA Primary mode of action

QMS Quality management system

RODAC Replicate Organism Detection and Counting

ROS Reactive oxygen species

SCENHIR Scientific Committee on Emerging and Newly Identified Health Risks

SEM Scanning electron microscope

SLS Selective laser sintering

STL Stereolithography (language)

SWOT Strengths, weakness, opportunities, and threats

TC Technical Committee (of ISO)

TIPS see TRIZ for explanation

TRIZ A Russian acronym for "Teoria reschenija isobretatjelskich sadatsch," which is regularly translated to "Theory of Inventive Problem Solving" (TIPS)

UMDNS Universal Medical Device Nomenclature System

UV Ultraviolet radiation

Index

Note: 'Page numbers followed by "f" indicate figures and "t" indicate tables.'

R

S

T

FSC
www.fsc.org
MIX
Papier | Fördert
gute Waldnutzung
FSC® C083411

Kolibri 360 GmbH
Ferdinand-Jühlke-Straße 7
99095 Erfurt, Deutschland
produktsicherheit@kolibri360.de